The NEW DIABETIC COOKBOOK

More than 200 Delicious Recipes for a Low-Fat, Low-Sugar, Low-Cholesterol, Low-Salt, High-Fiber Diet

FIFTH EDITION

MABEL CAVAIANI

McGraw·Hill

New York   Chicago   San Francisco   Lisbon   London   Madrid   Mexico City
Milan   New Delhi   San Juan   Seoul   Singapore   Sydney   Toronto

The McGraw·Hill Companies

Library of Congress Cataloging-in-Publication Data

Cavaiani, Mabel.
The new diabetic cookbook : more than 200 delicious recipes for a low-fat, low-sugar, low-cholesterol, low-salt, high-fiber diet / Mabel Cavaiani ; foreword by Joseph Turner Crockett. — 5th ed.
    p.   cm.
Includes index.
    ISBN 0-07-139135-5
    1. Diabetes—Diet therapy—Recipes.   I. Title.

RC662.C38   2002
641.5'6314—dc21   2001053689

9 10 11 12 13 14 15 16 17 18 19 20   FGR/FGR   0 9 8 7

ISBN 0-07-139135-5

Cover design by Monica Baziuk
Cover photograph copyright © Foodpix/Brian Hagiwara
Featured on the cover: Italian Chicken over Linguine, page 173.

McGraw-Hill books are available at special quantity discounts to use as premiums and sales promotions, or for use in corporate training programs. For more information, please write to the Director of Special Sales, Professional Publishing, McGraw-Hill, Two Penn Plaza, New York, NY 10121-2298. Or contact your local bookstore.

This book is printed on acid-free paper.

Contents

Foreword

There are estimated to be approximately 16 million persons in America with diabetes—and about 8 million of these people are unaware of having the disease.

The most usual form of diabetes is diabetes mellitus, which has both metabolic and vascular components that are interrelated. The metabolic component is related to a deficiency of insulin activity and is associated with hyperglycemia and altered fat and protein metabolism. Vascular components consist of a speed-up of fatty deposits in the blood vessels and changes in the kidney and eye blood vessels. Treatment of diabetics aims to keep the blood sugar as close to normal as possible. This requires maintaining a balance between diet, blood glucose levels, and exercise.

Most people are aware of the importance of diet in the treatment of diabetes. In fact it is possible to completely control the milder forms of diabetes with diet alone without added insulin. The usual diet for persons with diabetes is a balance of carbohydrates, fats, and proteins specifically computed for each individual. It is extremely important that an individual adhere closely to the given diet in addition to eating at regular intervals. It is also important that the individual exercise and maintain a normal weight for his or her sex, type, and build.

There has been much research done on the components of diabetic diets. These researchers recommend that the old diabetic diets be changed to include more carbohydrates of the polysaccharides type and less fat of the saturated type. The American

Diabetes Association also suggests that high-fiber, unrefined carbohydrates be substituted for highly refined carbohydrates with low fiber content. The addition of dietary fiber may reduce blood sugar levels after meals. The British Diabetes Association basically agrees and also discourages high salt intake to help control cardiovascular complications.

Recommendations on diet alone will be useless if the person does not comply. The diets must be acceptable to individuals in terms of both palatability and the availability of the foods. Diets should interfere as little as possible with the dietary habits of the individual.

This new book by Mabel Cavaiani is a compilation of recipes for use by persons with diabetes. She has taken many commonly known recipes and adapted them to comply with the latest recommendations of the American Diabetes Association and the American Dietetic Association. Her recipes replace much of the monosaccharides and disaccharides with polysaccharides, increase the amount of dietary fiber, decrease the amount of salt, and replace the cholesterol and saturated fats with unsaturated fats. In the process she has brought much more interesting variety into the diet for persons with diabetes. She has diabetes herself, is a member of the American Diabetes Association, and a retired member of the American Dietetic Association who recognizes the need for a book such as this. We both hope you will enjoy this book and use it to add interest and variety to your own unique diet.

—Joseph Turner Crockett, M.D., L.F.A.P.A.
San Diego, California

Introduction to the Fifth Edition

This fifth edition of *The New Diabetic Cookbook* includes the recently published *American Heart Association 2000 Dietary Guidelines, Major Changes and Revisions*. These simplified guidelines focus on an overall dietary pattern based on foods, rather than nutrient components.

Today, many doctors, dietitians, and nutritionists are advocating counting your carbohydrate intake instead of using the exchange lists. Therefore, included in this edition is a new chapter on carbohydrate counting so that you can have more flexibility in the way you manage your food choices and blood glucose levels.

In addition, there are changes to the nutrient information tables in Chapter 3 that will make it easier to calculate your own recipes and a new chapter that will help you make your own dry mixes.

The American Diabetes Association, Inc. provides the following guidelines regarding sugar: recipes containing more than 1 teaspoon but less than 1 tablespoon (5–15 gm) of caloric sweetener per serving are for occasional use only; try to limit the number of servings of these foods to one a day. Recipes containing more than 1 tablespoon (15 gm) of caloric sweetener per serving are generally not recommended for people with diabetes.

None of these recipes contain one or more tablespoons of sugar, but I thought it might be helpful to list the amount of sugar per serving along with other nutritive values whenever sugar is an ingredient in a recipe. Honey, corn syrup, and molasses are considered the equivalent of sugar (sucrose). No fructose, maltose, lactose, dextrose, or fruit juice concentrates are used in the recipes, but they should also be considered the equivalent of sugar if you use them or see them listed as an ingredient.

A great deal of study on the advantages of fiber in the diabetic and low-cholesterol diets has shown that we should take the use of an increased amount of fiber very seriously. Fiber-rich recipes are used as often as possible, and you should take advantage of them to increase the fiber in your diet. Remember that fiber needs liquid to expand, and the indiscriminate addition of fiber without enough water can cause complications.

Please keep in mind that this is a cookbook, not a diet manual. Many books that are written to help people on a special diet are filled with "you can't do this" or "you must do that." No matter what your special diet may be, there are many familiar foods that you can and should have in your diet. Unless a diet includes familiar foods, it will not be followed, and it is better to talk about the foods you are allowed rather than the ones that are no longer allowed on your diet.

When I first developed diabetes I felt as though the world had dropped out from under me. I remember telling my mother, "I'm such a good cook—and now I can't ever cook anything good again." That was a ridiculous statement, but it expressed my feelings at the time. It was a shock to me to discover that I had diabetes. We had always worried that my husband Chuck might develop diabetes because his mother, brother, sister, and nephew were all diagnosed with diabetes at different times—but we had never worried about me being diagnosed because no one in my family had diabetes.

I am a dietitian and should have recognized the symptoms, but I didn't. I only knew I felt terrible and didn't seem to get any better. I consulted Dr. Susan Urbatsch, my family doctor, who ordered a blood profile, and when the results were returned it was evident that I had diabetes. Of course, she investigated further but there wasn't much doubt about it after that first test.

I don't know if coping with diabetes is easier or harder for a diabetic who is also a dietitian. In one way it is easier because you don't need any diet counseling, you don't have questions regarding the suitability of different foods for your diet, and you don't have much trouble deciding if you can or can't have a certain food. However, I think it may actually be more difficult to be a dietitian because you are seldom free to relax and forget about your diet—you know what will happen to you if you do. I've seen too many people in the hospital or nursing home who were minus a foot or a leg or blind because they didn't think it made any difference whether they followed their diet and exercised regularly. It is so easy to say that you will put it off until tomorrow—but for a person with diabetes that tomorrow is right now and you'd better get with it or you will pay dearly for it later.

The low-cholesterol part of my diet didn't bother me because I had been keeping a low-cholesterol kitchen for many years. The doctor put my husband Chuck on a low-cholesterol diet when we were first married, and because I liked the diet and thought the food was good, I had always followed it right along with him. Dr. Urbatsch didn't tell me that I had a high cholesterol count or put me on a low-cholesterol diet, but the fact that 75 percent of all persons with diabetes die of atherosclerosis or related diseases convinced me that I should follow a low-cholesterol diet even more carefully when I knew I had diabetes.

All of the recipes in this book are suitable for persons with diabetes on a low-cholesterol diet. I might even suggest that if you are on a low-cholesterol diet and want to lose weight (even if you don't have diabetes), you might find it useful to use these recipes to help take off those extra pounds. Fiber is included in many of these recipes because research has shown that fiber helps keep blood sugar lower for a diabetic and helps bring down the cholesterol count. Low-sodium variations are given for recipes whenever it is possible—I have found that so many people who need the low-cholesterol diabetic diet also have some restrictions on their acceptable sodium intake.

Our local diabetes association branch has been a big help to me. The support of others who have similar health concerns seems to be particularly helpful, and this association is very active in providing information that is most useful to diabetics.

You should contact your own local association for additional information and support.

I hope you will find these recipes beneficial. I have tried to use foods that are nationally available and foods that most people stock regularly because I dislike cookbooks that use recipes with unusual and hard-to-find ingredients. These are recipes that my family and I use regularly, and I hope they will become standards in your home also.

I would like to thank the following persons for their encouragement and professional help in developing and writing this book. Without their support I could never have written it.

Dr. Susan Urbatsch, Mary Agnes Jones, R.D., Muriel Urbashich, R.D., Nancy Johnson, R.D., Dorothy Berzy, R.D., Mabel Frances Gunsallus, R.D., M.S., Edith Robinson, R.D., M.S., Eva Burrack, F.S.S., Mary Klicka, R.D., M.S., Frances Lee, R.D., M.S., Patti Dillon, M.S., Julie M. Cull, R.D., Mindy Greufe, R.D., "Chef Dave" Hutchins, Frances Nielsen, Vera and Aulden Wilson, Hazel and Ed Gernand, Patricia Ziegenhorn-Erbach, M.S., R.D., CNSD, L.D., Anne Kriener Blocker, R.D., L.D., and finally my husband, Charles Cavaiani, and my sister, Shirley Sniffin. Their patience and support while I was writing this book helped make it all possible.

I would also like to thank the following organizations for background information and resource material used in this book.

The American Diabetes Association, Inc.
The American Dietetic Association
The American Heart Association
Iowa State University Extension Service
U.S. Department of Agriculture
U.S. Food and Drug Administration
HCF Nutrition Research Foundation, Inc.
Hill Nutrition Associates, Inc.

—Mabel Cavaiani
West Union, Iowa

1

Diabetes

Diabetes is a very common disease, and there seem to be more people diagnosed as diabetics every day. According to the American Diabetes Association, there are 16 million people with diabetes in the United States, half of whom don't know they have diabetes. Each day, 1,800 new cases of diabetes are diagnosed, and 665,000 new cases are diagnosed in the average year. It has become the seventh leading cause of death among Americans.

Diabetes is not something that happens to other people. One out of 17 people in the United States has some form of diabetes, and one out of four families is affected in some way by it. Although there is no cure for diabetes at this time, a great deal of research is being done, and it is hoped that sometime in the near future diabetes can be prevented or cured.

There are several different types of diabetes:

1. *Type 1*, insulin-dependent diabetes, is generally found in children and young adults. Patients with Type 1 diabetes must take insulin because their bodies produce little or no insulin, which is needed for utilization of glucose in the body.

2. *Type 2*, non-insulin-dependent diabetes, usually occurs in overweight adults 40 years or older; however, it is being diagnosed in overweight children as well. It can generally be controlled by exercise, weight loss, diet, and sometimes oral medication. In this type of diabetes, some insulin is produced, but it isn't used effectively. It can often be prevented or controlled if the person maintains a normal weight and performs regular exercise.

3. *Gestational diabetes* occurs in some pregnant women and can sometimes be controlled by diet; occasionally, insulin is necessary. Most of these women return to normal after their babies are born, but they need to watch their weight and get regular exercise because they are at a greater risk for developing diabetes as they get older.

4. *Impaired glucose tolerance* is diagnosed when a patient's blood sugar levels are between normal and diabetic. This condition is generally treated with diet and weight loss to prevent the development of diabetes later in life.

5. *Secondary diabetes* can be caused by drugs or chemicals as well as pancreatic or endocrine disease.

The warning signs of diabetes are:

Type 1
Frequent urination
Abnormal thirst
Unusual hunger
Weight loss
Irritability
Weakness or fatigue
Nausea and vomiting

Type 2
Excess weight
Drowsiness
Blurred vision
Tingling and numbness in hands and feet
Skin infections
Slow healing of cuts, especially on the feet
Itching, particularly in the vaginal area

When your doctor tells you that you have diabetes, the doctor will probably discuss your diet with you or send you to a registered dietitian, nutritionist, or a certified diabetes educator who can discuss your diet with you. Don't let your doctor send you off with just a sheet of paper with instructions to follow that diet. You need more than that. Each patient's diet should be developed and individualized especially for him or her, considering his or her age, weight, physical condition, lifestyle, and eating habits. A diabetic diet can be challenging to follow at first, and you need all the help you can get . . . and remember, once you develop your meal plan, you must follow it. You can make some modifications after you are familiar with the diet, but it is important to follow it faithfully at first.

Many doctors don't have the time to spend with you discussing your diet, but they can and should recommend someone who can answer your questions and concerns. Your local medical clinic or hospital may have a diabetes support group, or it can recommend someone to help you.

Once you find a knowledgeable person, be perfectly frank with him or her and discuss your lifestyle, likes and dislikes, budgetary problems, and whether you are willing to cook special foods or if you want very simple foods. Tell them if you take a bagged lunch to work or if you depend on restaurants at noon. Help them help you plan a diet that fits your lifestyle, budget, and capabilities.

Diabetes can be overwhelming at first. It can make you feel as though you are alone in the world. Trying to cope with a new diet, medication or insulin shots, establishing an exercise program, and losing weight can be overwhelming. Life may be pretty grim around your house for a while, but you'll learn to cope with it before long and discover there is life after diabetes.

Now that I have had diabetes for 14 years and have learned to live with it, I always tell new diabetics that one of the biggest helps, next to a supportive family, is a group of people who also have diabetes and know what you are experiencing. The best way to find this supportive group is to join your local chapter of the American Diabetes Association. If you don't have a local association, you may be able to find one in a neighboring community. If you aren't able to find a local group, write to: The American Diabetes Association, National Service Center, 1660 Duke Street, Alexandria, VA 22314, or visit their website at www.diabetes.org.

They can give you the address of your state association, which can help you find the nearest local chapter. After you find the nearest chapter, attend the meetings. You will meet other diabetics and discover you aren't alone; there are others out there who care and are trying to help each other. Don't feel bewildered—search for information and use it to make your life happier, healthier, and more comfortable.

2

Food Exchanges

Developing a meal plan is one way to manage your diabetes. Exchange lists are the backbone for one type of diabetic meal planning. The number and kind of exchanges you can have for each meal will be determined by your doctor and/or dietitian, depending upon your age, sex, amount of activity, and your personal eating style. Each exchange has an established nutritional value. The total of your exchanges during the day is the total amount of carbohydrate, protein, and fat that your body needs to feel its best. Each of the items in an exchange list has approximately the same nutritional value.

The following exchange lists (copyright © 1995 American Diabetes Association, Inc., American Dietetic Association) have been reprinted with permission. The exchange lists are the basis of a meal planning system designed by a committee of the American Diabetes Association and the American Dietetic Association. While designed primarily for people with diabetes and others who must follow special diets, the exchange lists are based on principles of good nutrition that apply to everyone. There are seven basic exchanges with variations in some of the lists. They are starches, fruit, milk, other carbohydrates, vegetables, meats, and fats.

Foods are listed with their serving sizes, which are usually measured after cooking. When you begin, you should measure the size of each serving. This may help you learn to "eyeball" correct serving sizes.

The following chart shows the amount of nutrients in one serving from each list.

Food exchanges	Carbohydrate (grams)	Protein (grams)	Fat (grams)	Calories
Carbohydrate Group				
Starch/bread	15	3	1 or less	80
Fruit	15	–	–	60
Milk				
Skim	12	8	0–3	90
Low-fat	12	8	5	120
Whole	12	8	8	150
Other				
Carbohydrates	15	varies	varies	varies
Vegetables	5	2	–	25
Meat and Meat Substitute Group				
Very lean	–	7	0–1	35
Lean	–	7	3	55
Medium-fat	–	7	5	75
High-fat	–	7	8	100
Fat Group	–	–	5	45

The new exchange lists emphasize that healthy eating is the first step in taking care of your diabetes. You can make a difference in your blood glucose control through your food choices. You do not need special foods. In fact, the foods that are good for you are good for everyone.

If you have diabetes, it is important to eat about the same amount of food at the same time each day. Regardless of what your blood glucose level is, try not to skip meals or snacks. This may lead to large swings in blood glucose levels.

To keep your blood glucose levels near normal, you need to balance the food you eat with the insulin your body makes or gets by injection and with your physical activities. Blood glucose monitoring gives you information to help you with this balancing act. Near-normal blood glucose levels help you feel better and they may reduce or prevent complications from diabetes.

The number of calories you need depends on your size, age, and activity level. Children and adolescents must eat enough calories so they grow and develop normally. Don't limit their calories to try to control blood glucose levels. Instead, adjust their insulin to cover the calories they need.

Of course, everyone needs to eat nutritious foods. Our good health depends on eating a variety of foods that contain the right amount of carbohydrate, protein, fat, vitamins, minerals, fiber, and water.

Carbohydrate, protein, and fat are found in the food you eat. They supply your body with energy, or calories. Your body needs insulin to use this energy. Insulin is made in the pancreas. If you have diabetes, either your pancreas is no longer making insulin or your body can't use the insulin it is making. In either case, your blood glucose levels are not normal.

Carbohydrate: Starch and sugar in foods are carbohydrates. Starch is in breads, pasta, cereals, potatoes, peas, beans, and lentils. Naturally present sugars are in fruits, milk, and vegetables. Added sugars are in desserts, candy, jams, and syrups. All these carbohydrates provide 4 calories per gram and can affect your blood glucose levels.

When you eat carbohydrates, they turn into glucose and travel in your bloodstream. Insulin helps the glucose enter the cells, where it can be used for energy or stored. Eating the same amounts of carbohydrate daily at meals and snacks can help you control your blood glucose levels.

Protein: Protein is in meats, poultry, fish, milk and other dairy products, eggs, dried beans, and peas. Starches and vegetables also have small amounts of protein.

The body uses protein for growth, maintenance, and energy. Protein has 4 calories of energy per gram. Again, your body needs insulin to use the protein you eat.

Fat: Fat is in margarine, butter, oils, salad dressings, nuts, seeds, milk, cheese, meat, fish, poultry, snack foods, ice cream, and desserts.

There are different types of fat. Monounsaturated fats are found in canola oil, olive oil, nuts, and avocados. The polyunsaturated fats found in corn oil, soybean oil, or sunflower oil are also good choices. (See Chapter 6 for saturated fats.)

After you eat fat, it travels in your bloodstream. You need insulin to store fat in the cells of your body. Fats are used for energy. In fact, fats have 9 calories per gram, more than two times the calories you get from carbohydrates and protein.

Vitamins and minerals: Most foods in this book are good sources of vitamins and minerals. If you eat a variety of these foods, you probably do not need a vitamin or mineral supplement.

Salt or sodium: High blood pressure may be made worse by eating too much sodium (salt and salty foods). Try to use less salt in cooking and at the table. In the exchange lists, foods which are high in sodium (400 milligrams or more sodium per exchange) have an asterisk by them.

Alcohol: You may have an alcoholic drink occasionally. If you take insulin or a diabetic medication, be sure to eat food with your drink. Ask your dietitian about a safe amount of alcohol for you and how to work it into your meal plan.

What to eat and when: You and your dietitian will work out a meal plan to get the right balance between your food, medication, and exercise/activity. The list of food choices (exchange lists) in this book can help you make interesting and healthy food choices. Exchange lists and a meal plan help you know what to eat, how much to eat, and when to eat.

Exchange lists: These foods are listed together because they are alike. Each serving of food has about the same amount of carbohydrate, protein, fat, and calories as the other foods on that list. That is why any food on the list can be "exchanged" or traded for any other food on the same list. For example, you can trade the slice of bread you might eat for breakfast for ½ cup of cooked cereal. Each of these foods equals one starch choice.

Exchange information is based on foods found in grocery stores. However, food companies often change ingredients in their products. That is why you need to check the Nutrition Facts panel of the food label.

See your dietitian regularly when you are first learning how to use your meal plan and exchange lists. Your meal plan can be adjusted to fit changes in your lifestyle, such as work, school, vacation, or travel. Regular nutrition counseling can help you make positive changes in your eating habits.

Starch list: Cereals, grains, pasta, bread, crackers, snacks, starchy vegetables, and cooked dried beans, peas, and lentils are starches. In general one starch is: ½ cup cereal, grain, pasta, or starchy vegetable; 1 ounce of bread products such as one slice of bread; or ¾ ounce to 1 ounce of most snack foods. (Some snack foods may also have added fat.)

Bread exchanges with 15 grams carbohydrate, 3 grams protein, 0–1 grams fat, and 80 calories include the following items:

Bagel, ½ (1 ounce)
Reduced calorie bread, 2 slices (1½ ounces)
Bread, white, whole wheat, pumpernickel, rye, 1 slice
    (1 ounce)
Bread sticks, crisp, 4 inches long × ½ inch, 2 (⅔ ounce)
English muffin, ½
Hot dog or hamburger bun, ½ (1 ounce)
Pita, ½, 6 inches across
Roll, plain, small, 1 (1 ounce)
Raisin bread, unfrosted, 1 slice (1 ounce)
Tortilla, corn, 6 inches across, 1
Tortilla, flour, 7–8 inches across, 1
Waffle, 4½ inches square, 1

Cereals and grain exchanges with 15 grams carbohydrate, 3 grams protein, 0–1 grams fat, and 80 calories include the following items:

Bran cereals, ½ cup
Bulgur, cooked, ½ cup
Cereals, uncooked, ½ cup
Cereals, unsweetened, ready to eat, ¾ cup
Cornmeal, dry, 3 tablespoons
Couscous, dry, ⅓ cup
Flour, dry, 3 tablespoons
Granola, low-fat, ¼ cup

Grapenuts, 1/4 cup
Grits, cooked, 1/2 cup
Kasha, cooked, 1/2 cup
Millet, cooked, 1/4 cup
Muesli, 1/4 cup
Oats, cooked, 1/2 cup
Pasta, cooked, 1/2 cup
Puffed cereal, 1 1/2 cups
Rice milk, 1/2 cup
Rice, white or brown, cooked, 1/3 cup
Shredded wheat, 1/2 cup
Sugar-frosted cereal, 1/2 cup
Wheat germ, 3 tablespoons

Starchy vegetable exchanges with 15 grams carbohydrate, 3 grams protein, 0–1 grams fat, and 80 calories include the following items:

Baked beans, 1/3 cup
Corn, 1/2 cup
Corn on the cob, medium, 1 (5 ounces)
Mixed vegetables with corn, peas, or pasta, 1 cup
Peas, green, 1/2 cup
Plantain, 1/2 cup
Potato, baked or boiled, 1 small (3 ounces)
Potato, mashed, 1/2 cup
Squash, winter (acorn, butternut), 1 cup
Yam, sweet potato, plain, 1/2 cup

Crackers and snack exchanges with 15 grams carbohydrate, 3 grams protein, 0–1 grams fat, and 80 calories include the following items:

Animal crackers, 8
Graham crackers, 2 1/2 inches square, 3
Matzoh, 3/4 ounce
Melba toast, 4 slices

Oyster crackers, 24
Popcorn (popped, no fat added, or low-fat microwave),
3 cups
Pretzels, ¾ ounce
Rice cakes, 4 inches across, 2
Saltine type crackers, 6
Snack chips, fat-free (tortilla, potato), 15–20 (¾ ounce)
Whole wheat crackers, no fat added, 2–5 (¾ ounce)

Dried beans, peas, and lentils (cooked) which count as
one starch exchange plus one very lean meat exchange include
the following items:

Beans and peas (garbanzo, pinto, kidney, white, split,
black-eyed), ½ cup
Lima beans, ⅔ cup
Lentils, ½ cup
Miso, 3 tablespoons

Starchy foods prepared with fat which count as one starch
exchange plus one fat exchange include the following items:

Biscuit, 2½ inches across, 1
Chow mein noodles, ½ cup
Cornbread, 2-inch cube, 1 (2 ounces)
Crackers, round, butter type, 6
Croutons, 1 cup
French-fried potatoes, 16–25 (3 ounces)
Granola, ¼ cup
Muffin, small, 1 (1½ ounces)
Pancakes, 4 inches across, 2
Popcorn, microwave, popped, 3 cups
Sandwich crackers, cheese or peanut butter filling, 3
Stuffing, bread (prepared), ⅓ cup
Taco shell, 6 inches across, 2
Waffle, 4½ inches square, 1
Whole wheat crackers, fat added, 4–6 (1 ounce)

Fruit list with 15 grams carbohydrate and 60 calories includes fresh and canned fruits and fruit juices, all prepared without added sugar. Food labels for fruits may contain the words "no sugar added" or "unsweetened." This means that no sucrose (table sugar) has been added. Generally, fruit canned in light syrup has the same amount of carbohydrate per serving as the "no sugar added" or the juice pack. All canned fruits on the fruit list are based on one of these three types of pack. Portion sizes for canned fruits are for the fruit and a small amount of juice. Count ½ cup cranberries or rhubarb sweetened with sugar substitute as free foods.

Fruit exchanges with 15 grams carbohydrate and 60 calories include the following items:

Apple, unpeeled, small, 1 (4 ounces)
Applesauce, unsweetened, ½ cup
Apples, dried, 4 rings
Apricots, fresh, 4 whole (5½ ounces)
Apricots, dried, 8 halves
Apricots, canned, ½ cup
Banana, small, 1 (4 ounces)
Blackberries, ¾ cup
Blueberries, ¾ cup
Cantaloupe, small, ⅓ melon (11 ounces) or 1 cup cubes
Cherries, sweet, fresh, 12 (3 ounces)
Cherries, sweet, canned, ½ cup
Dates, 3
Figs, fresh, 1½ large or 2 medium (3½ ounces)
Figs, dried, 1½
Fruit cocktail, ½ cup
Grapefruit, large, ½ (11 ounces)
Grapefruit sections, canned, ¾ cup
Grapes, small, 17 (3 ounces)
Honeydew melon, 1 slice (10 ounces) or 1 cup cubes
Kiwi, 1 (3½ ounces)
Mandarin oranges, canned, ¾ cup
Mango, small, ½ fruit (5½ ounces) or ½ cup

Nectarine, small, 1 (5 ounces)
Orange, small, 1 (6½ ounces)
Papaya, ½ fruit (8 ounces) or 1 cup cubes
Peach, medium, fresh, 1 (6 ounces)
Peaches, canned, ½ cup
Pear, large, fresh, ½ (4 ounces)
Pears, canned, ½ cup
Pineapple, fresh, ¾ cup
Pineapple, canned, ½ cup
Plums, small, 2 (5 ounces)
Plums, canned, ½ cup
Prunes, dried, 3
Raisins, 2 tablespoons
Raspberries, 1 cup
Strawberries, 1¼ cups whole berries
Tangerines, small, 2
Watermelon, 1 slice (13½ ounces) or 1¼ cups cubes

Fruit juices

Apple juice/cider, ½ cup
Cranberry juice cocktail, ⅓ cup
Cranberry juice cocktail, reduced calorie, 1 cup
Fruit juice blends, 100 percent juice, ⅓ cup
Grape juice, ⅓ cup
Grapefruit juice, ½ cup
Orange juice, ½ cup
Pineapple juice, ½ cup
Prune juice, ⅓ cup

Milk list includes different types of milk and milk products. Cheeses are on the meat list and cream and other dairy fats are on the fat list. Based on the amount of fat they contain, milks are divided into skim/very low-fat milk, low-fat milk, and whole milk. Chocolate milk, frozen yogurt, and ice cream are on the other carbohydrates list. Nondairy creamers are on the free foods list. Rice milk is on the starch list and soy milk is on the medium-fat meat list. Milk and yogurt are good sources of calcium and protein. Check the food label. The higher the fat content of milk and yogurt, the greater the amount of saturated fat and cholesterol. Choose lower-fat varieties. For those who are lactose intolerant, look for lactose-free varieties of milk. One cup equals 8 fluid ounces or ½ pint.

Skim and very low-fat milk exchanges with 12 grams carbohydrate, 8 grams protein, and 0–3 grams fat per serving include the following items:

Skim milk, 1 cup
½ percent milk, 1 cup
1 percent milk, 1 cup
Nonfat or low-fat buttermilk, 1 cup
Evaporated skim milk, ½ cup
Nonfat dry milk, ⅓ cup dry
Plain nonfat yogurt, ¾ cup
Nonfat or low-fat fruit flavored yogurt sweetened with
    aspartame or with a nonnutritive sweetener, 1 cup

Low-fat milk exchanges with 12 grams carbohydrate, 8 grams protein, and 5 grams fat include the following items:

2 percent milk, 1 cup
Plain low-fat yogurt, ¾ cup
Sweet acidophilus milk, 1 cup

Whole milk exchanges with 12 grams carbohydrate, 8 grams protein, and 8 grams fat include the following items:

Whole milk, 1 cup
Evaporated whole milk, ½ cup
Goat's milk, 1 cup
Kefir, 1 cup

Other carbohydrates list with 15 grams carbohydrate or one starch, or one fruit, or one milk. Items on this list can be substituted for a starch, fruit, or milk choice in your meal plan. Some choices will also count as one fat exchange. They can be substituted in the meal plan even though they contain added sugars or fat. However, they do not contain as many important vitamins and minerals as the choices on the starch, fruit, or milk list. When you plan to use these foods in your meal plan, be sure to include foods from all of the lists to eat a balanced meal. Always check the nutritive information on the food label. It will be your most accurate source of information. Because many of these foods are concentrated sources of carbohydrate and fat, the portion sizes are often very small. Look for salad dressings in smaller amounts on the free foods list. Many fat-free or reduced-fat products made with fat replacers contain carbohydrate. When eaten in large amounts, they may need to be counted. Talk with your dietitian to determine how to count these in your meal plan.

Other carbohydrates that count as one exchange with 15 grams of carbohydrate or one starch or one fruit or one milk include the following items:

Angel food cake, unfrosted, 1/12 cake, 2 carbohydrates
Brownie, small, unfrosted, 2-inch square, 1 carbohydrate, 1
  fat
Cake, unfrosted, 2-inch square, 1 carbohydrate, 1 fat
Cake, frosted, 2-inch square, 2 carbohydrates, 1 fat
Cookie, fat-free, 2 small, 1 carbohydrate
Cookie or sandwich cookie with creme filling, 2 small,
  1 carbohydrate, 1 fat
Cupcake, frosted, 1 small, 2 carbohydrates, 1 fat
Cranberry sauce, jellied, 1/4 cup, 2 carbohydrates
Doughnut, plain, cake, 1 medium (1 1/2 ounces),
  1 1/2 carbohydrates, 2 fat
Doughnut, glazed, 3 3/4 inches across (2 ounces),
  2 carbohydrates, 2 fats
Fruit juice bars, frozen, 100 percent juice, 1 bar (3 ounces),
  1 carbohydrate
Fruit snacks, chewy (puréed fruit concentrate), 1 roll
  (3/4 ounce), 1 carbohydrate
Fruit spread, 100 percent fruit, 1 tablespoon,
  1 carbohydrate

Gelatin, regular, ½ cup, 1 carbohydrate
Gingersnaps, 3, 1 carbohydrate
Granola bar, 1 bar, 1 carbohydrate, 1 fat
Granola bar, fat-free, 1 bar, 2 carbohydrates
Hummus, ⅓ cup, 1 carbohydrate, 1 fat
Ice cream, ½ cup, 1 carbohydrate, 2 fats
Ice cream, light, ½ cup, 1 carbohydrate, 1 fat
Ice cream, fat-free, no sugar added, ½ cup, 1 carbohydrate
Jam or jelly, regular, 1 tablespoon, 1 carbohydrate
Milk, chocolate, whole, 1 cup, 2 carbohydrates, 1 fat
Pie, fruit, 2 crusts, ⅙ pie, 3 carbohydrates, 2 fats
Pie, pumpkin or custard, ⅛ pie, 1 carbohydrate, 2 fats
Potato chips, 12 to 18 (1 ounce), 1 carbohydrate, 2 fats
Pudding, regular, made with low-fat milk, ½ cup,
    2 carbohydrates
Pudding, sugar-free, made with low-fat milk, ½ cup,
    1 carbohydrate
Salad dressing, fat-free, ¼ cup, 1 carbohydrate
Sherbet, sorbet, ½ cup, 2 carbohydrates
Spaghetti or pasta sauce, canned, ½ cup, 1 carbohydrate, 1
    fat
Sweet roll or Danish, 1 (2½ ounces), 2½ carbohydrates,
    2 fats
Syrup, light, 2 tablespoons, 1 carbohydrate
Syrup, regular, 1 tablespoon, 1 carbohydrate
Syrup, regular, ¼ cup, 4 carbohydrates
Tortilla chips, 6–12 (1 ounce), 1 carbohydrate, 2 fats
Yogurt, frozen, low-fat, fat-free, ⅓ cup, 1 carbohydrate,
    0–1 fat
Yogurt, frozen, fat-free, no sugar added, ½ cup,
    1 carbohydrate
Yogurt, low-fat, with fruit, 1 cup, 3 carbohydrates, 0–1 fat
Vanilla wafers, 5, 1 carbohydrate, 1 fat

Vegetable list includes vegetables with small amounts of carbohydrate and calories. You should try to eat at least two or
three vegetable choices each day. In general, one vegetable

exchange is ½ cup cooked vegetables or vegetable juice or 1 cup raw vegetables. If you eat one or two vegetable choices at a meal, you do not have to count the calories or carbohydrates because they contain small amounts of these nutrients. Fresh and frozen vegetables contain less salt than canned vegetables. Drain and rinse canned vegetables if you want to reduce the salt. Choose more dark green and dark yellow vegetables, such as spinach, broccoli, romaine, carrots, chilies, and peppers. Brussels sprouts, cauliflower, greens, peppers, spinach, and tomatoes are good sources of vitamin C. If you eat more than 4 cups of raw vegetables or 2 cups of cooked vegetables at one meal, count them as one carbohydrate choice. Starchy vegetables such as corn, peas, winter squash, and potatoes that contain larger amounts of calories and carbohydrates are on the starch list.

Vegetable exchange: one exchange, which is 1 cup raw vegetables or ½ cup cooked vegetables with 5 grams carbohydrate, 2 grams protein, 0 grams fat, and 25 calories, includes the following items:

Artichoke or artichoke hearts
Asparagus
Beans (green, wax, or Italian)
Bean sprouts
Beets
Broccoli
Brussels sprouts
Cabbage
Carrots
Cauliflower
Celery
Cucumber
Eggplant
Green onions or scallions
Greens (collards, kale, mustard, turnip)
Kohlrabi
Leeks

Mixed vegetables (without corn, peas, or pasta)
Mushrooms
Okra
Onions
Pea pods
Peppers (all varieties)
Radishes
Salad greens (endive, escarole, lettuce, romaine, spinach)
Sauerkraut*
Spinach
Summer squash
Tomato
Tomatoes, canned
Tomato sauce*
Tomato/vegetable juice*
Turnips
Water chestnuts
Watercress
Zucchini

Meat and meat substitutes list contains both protein and fat. In general, one meat exchange is: 1 ounce meat, fish, poultry, or cheese or ½ cup cooked dried beans. Based on the amount of fat they contain, meats are divided into very lean, lean, medium-fat, and high-fat. This is done so you can see which ones contain the least amount of fat. One ounce (one exchange) of each of these includes:

Very lean with 0 grams carbohydrate, 7 grams protein, 0–1 grams fat, and 35 calories.

Lean with 0 grams carbohydrate, 7 grams protein, 3 grams fat, and 55 calories.

Medium-fat with 0 grams carbohydrate, 7 grams protein, 5 grams fat, and 75 calories.

High-fat with 0 grams carbohydrate, 7 grams protein, 8 grams fat, and 100 calories.

* = 400 mg or more sodium per exchange

- Choose very lean and lean meat choices whenever possible. Items from the high-fat group are high in saturated fat, cholesterol, and calories and can raise blood cholesterol levels. Meats do not have any fiber but dried beans, peas, and lentils are good sources of fiber. Some processed meats, seafood, and soy products may contain carbohydrate when consumed in large quantities. Check the Nutrition Facts on the label to see if the amount is close to 15 grams. If so, count it as a carbohydrate choice as well as a meat choice.
- Weigh meat after cooking and removing bones and fat. Four ounces of raw meat is equal to 3 ounces of cooked meat. Some examples of meat portions are:

  1 ounce cheese = 1 meat choice and is about the size of a 1-inch cube.

  2 ounces meat = 2 meat choices, such as 1 small chicken leg or thigh or ½ cup cottage cheese or tuna.

  3 ounces meat = 3 meat choices and is about the size of a deck of cards, such as 1 medium pork chop, 1 small hamburger, ½ of a whole chicken breast, or 1 unbreaded fish fillet.

- Limit your choices from the high-fat group to three times per week or less.

- Most grocery stores stock Select and Choice grades of meat. Select grades of meat are the leanest meats. Choice grades contain a moderate amount of fat, and Prime cuts of meat have the highest amount of fat. Restaurants usually serve Prime cuts of meat.

- "Hamburger" may contain added seasoning and fat, but ground beef does not.

- Read labels to find products that are low in fat and cholesterol (5 grams or less of fat per serving).

- Dried beans, peas, and lentils are also found on the starch list.

- Peanut butter, in smaller amounts, is also found on the fats list.
- Bacon, in smaller amounts, is also found on the fats list.

Meal planning tips: Bake, roast, broil, poach, steam, or boil these foods rather than frying. Place meat on a rack so the fat will drain off during cooking. Use a nonstick spray and a nonstick pan to brown or fry foods. Trim off visible fat before and after cooking. If you add flour, bread crumbs, coating mixes, fat, or marinades when cooking, ask your dietitian how to count it in your meal plan.

Very lean meat and substitutes exchanges with 0 grams carbohydrate, 7 grams protein, 0–1 grams fat, and 35 calories include the following items:

Poultry: chicken or turkey (white meat, no skin), Cornish
   hen (no skin), 1 ounce
Fish: fresh or frozen cod, flounder, haddock, halibut, trout,
   tuna (fresh or canned in water), 1 ounce
Shellfish: clams, crab, lobster, scallops, shrimp, imitation
   shellfish, 1 ounce
Game: duck or pheasant (no skin), venison, buffalo,
   ostrich, 1 ounce
Cheese with 1 gram or less fat per ounce: nonfat or low-fat
   cottage cheese, fat-free cheese, 1 ounce
Other: processed sandwich meats with 1 gram or less fat
   per ounce, such as deli thin, shaved meats, chipped
   beef*, turkey ham, 1 ounce
Egg whites, 2
Egg substitute, plain, ¼ cup
Hot dogs with 1 gram or less fat per ounce*, 1 ounce
Kidney (high in cholesterol), 1 ounce
Sausage with 1 gram or less fat per ounce, 1 ounce

* = 400 mg or more sodium per exchange

Count as one very lean meat and one starch exchange: dried beans, peas, lentils (cooked), ½ cup.

Lean meat and substitutes exchanges with 0 grams carbohydrate, 7 grams protein, 3 grams fat, and 55 calories include the following items:

Beef: USDA Select or Choice grades of lean beef trimmed of fat, such as round, sirloin, and flank steak, tenderloin, roast (rib, chuck, rump), steak (porterhouse, cubed), ground round, 1 ounce

Pork: lean pork, such as fresh ham; canned, cured, or boiled ham; Canadian bacon*; tenderloin; center cut chop, 1 ounce

Lamb: roast, chop, leg, 1 ounce

Veal: lean chop, roast, 1 ounce

Poultry: chicken or turkey (dark meat, no skin), chicken (white meat with skin), domestic duck or goose (well drained of fat, no skin), 1 ounce

Fish:
  Herring (uncreamed or smoked), 1 ounce
  Oysters, 6 medium
  Salmon (fresh or canned), catfish, 1 ounce
  Sardines (canned), 2 medium
  Tuna (canned in oil, drained), 1 ounce

Game: goose (no skin), rabbit, 1 ounce

Cheese:
  4.5 percent fat cottage cheese, ¼ cup
  Parmesan, grated, 2 tablespoons
  Cheese with 3 grams or less fat per ounce, 1 ounce

Other:
  Hot dogs with 3 grams or less fat per ounce*, 1½ ounces
  Processed sandwich meat with 3 grams or less fat per ounce, such as turkey pastrami or kielbasa, 1 ounce
  Liver, heart (high in cholesterol), 1 ounce

* = 400 mg or more sodium per exchange

Medium-fat meat and substitutes exchanges with 0 grams carbohydrate, 7 grams protein, 5 grams fat, and 75 calories include the following items:

Beef: most beef products fall into this category (ground
    beef, meat loaf, corned beef, short ribs, Prime grades of
    meat trimmed of fat, such as prime rib), 1 ounce
Pork: top loin, chop, Boston butt, cutlet, 1 ounce
Lamb: rib roast, ground, 1 ounce
Veal: cutlet (ground or cubed, unbreaded), 1 ounce
Poultry: chicken, dark meat (with skin), ground turkey or
    ground chicken, fried chicken (with skin), 1 ounce
Fish: any fried fish product, 1 ounce
Cheese with 5 grams or less fat per ounce:
    Feta or mozzarella, 1 ounce
    Ricotta, ¼ cup (2 ounces)
Other:
    Egg (high in cholesterol, limit to 3 per week), 1
    Sausage with 5 grams or less fat per ounce, 1 ounce
    Soy milk, 1 cup
    Tempeh, ¼ cup
    Tofu, 4 ounces or ½ cup

High-fat meat and substitutes exchanges with 0 grams carbohydrate, 7 grams protein, 8 grams fat, and 100 calories include the following items:

Pork: spareribs, ground pork, pork sausage, 1 ounce
Cheese: all regular cheeses such as American*, cheddar,
    Monterey Jack, Swiss, 1 ounce
Other:
    Processed sandwich meats with 8 grams or less fat per
        ounce such as bologna, pimiento loaf, salami, 1 ounce
    Sausage, such as bratwurst, Italian, knockwurst, Polish,
        smoked, 1 ounce
    Hot dog (turkey or chicken)*, 1 (10 per pound)
    Bacon, 3 slices (20 slices per pound)

* = 400 mg or more sodium per exchange

Count as one high-fat meat plus one fat exchange:
Hot dog (beef, pork, or combination)*, 1 (10 per pound)
Peanut butter (contains unsaturated fat), 2 tablespoons

Fat list fats are divided into three groups based on the main type of fat they contain: monounsaturated, polyunsaturated, and saturated. Small amounts of monounsaturated and polyunsaturated fats in the foods we eat are linked with good health benefits. Saturated fats are linked with heart disease and cancer. In general, one fat exchange is: 1 teaspoon of regular margarine or vegetable oil or 1 tablespoon of regular salad dressing. All fats are high in calories. Limit serving sizes for good nutrition and health. If blood pressure is a concern, choose fats in the unsalted form to help lower sodium intake, such as unsalted peanuts. Check the Nutrition Facts on food labels for serving sizes. One fat exchange is based on a serving size containing 5 grams of fat. When selecting regular margarines, choose those with liquid vegetable oil as the first ingredient. Soft margarines are not as saturated as stick margarines. Soft margarines are healthier choices. Avoid those listing hydrogenated or partially hydrogenated fat as the first ingredient. When selecting low-fat margarines, look for liquid vegetable oil as the second ingredient. Water is usually the first ingredient. When used in smaller amounts, bacon and peanut butter are counted as fat choices. When used in larger amounts, they are counted as high-fat meat choices. See the free foods list for nondairy coffee creamers, whipped topping, and fat-free products, such as margarines, salad dressings, mayonnaise, sour cream, cream cheese, and nonstick cooking spray.

Monounsaturated fat exchanges with 5 grams fat and 45 calories include the following items:

Avocado, medium, ⅛ (1 ounce)
Oil (canola, olive, peanut), 1 teaspoon
Olives: ripe (black), 8 large green
    (stuffed)*, 10 large

---

* = 400 mg or more sodium per exchange

Nuts
    almonds, cashews, 6 nuts
    mixed (50 percent peanuts), 6 nuts
    peanuts, 10 nuts
    pecans, 4 halves
Peanut butter, smooth or crunchy, 2 teaspoons
Sesame seeds, 1 tablespoon
Tahini paste, 2 teaspoons

Polyunsaturated fat exchanges with 5 grams fat and 45 calories include the following items:

Margarine, stick, tub, or squeeze, 1 teaspoon
    lower fat (30 percent to 50 percent vegetable oil), 1 tablespoon
Mayonnaise: regular, 1 teaspoon
    reduced fat, 1 tablespoon
Nuts, walnuts, English, 4 halves
Oil (corn, safflower, soybean), 1 teaspoon
Salad dressing, regular*, 1 tablespoon
    reduced-fat, 2 tablespoons
Miracle Whip Salad Dressing*, regular, 2 teaspoons
    reduced-fat, 1 tablespoon
Seeds, pumpkin, sunflower, 1 tablespoon

Saturated fats exchanges with 5 grams of fat and 45 calories include the following items:

Bacon, cooked, 1 slice (20 slices per pound)
Bacon grease, 1 teaspoon
Butter, stick, 1 teaspoon
    whipped, 2 teaspoons
    reduced-fat, 1 tablespoon
Chitterlings, boiled, 2 tablespoons (½ ounce)
Coconut, sweetened, shredded, 2 tablespoons
Cream, half and half, 2 tablespoons

* = 400 mg or more sodium per exchange

Cream cheese, regular, 1 tablespoon (½ ounce)
   reduced-fat, 2 tablespoons (1 ounce)
Fatback or salt pork. Use a piece 1" × 1" × ¼" if you plan
   to eat the fatback cooked with vegetables. Use a piece
   2" × 1" × ½" when eating only the vegetables with the
   fatback removed.
Shortening or lard, 1 teaspoon
Sour cream, regular, 2 tablespoons
   reduced-fat, 3 tablespoons

Free foods list. A free food is any food or drink that contains
less than 20 calories or less than 5 grams carbohydrate per serving. Foods with a serving size listed should be limited to three
servings per day. Be sure to spread them out throughout the day.
If you eat all three servings at one time it could affect your blood
glucose. Foods listed without a serving size can be eaten as often
as you like.

Fat-free or reduced-fat foods include the following items:

Cream cheese, fat-free, 1 tablespoon
Creamers, nondairy, liquid, 1 tablespoon
Creamers, nondairy, powdered, 2 teaspoons
Mayonnaise, fat-free, 1 tablespoon
Mayonnaise, reduced-fat, 1 teaspoon
Margarine, fat-free, 4 tablespoons
Margarine, reduced-fat, 1 teaspoon
Miracle Whip, nonfat, 1 tablespoon
Miracle Whip, reduced-fat, 1 teaspoon
Nonstick cooking spray
Salad dressing, fat-free, 1 tablespoon
Salad dressing, fat-free, Italian, 2 tablespoons
Salsa, ¼ cup
Sour cream, fat-free or reduced-fat, 1 tablespoon
Whipped topping, regular or light, 2 tablespoons

Sugar-free or low-sugar foods include the following items:

Candy, hard, sugar-free, 1 candy
Gelatin dessert, sugar-free

Gelatin, unflavored
Gum, sugar-free
Jam or jelly, low sugar or light, 2 teaspoons
Syrup, sugar-free, 2 tablespoons
Sugar substitutes, alternatives, or replacements that are
    approved by the Food and Drug Administration (FDA)
    are safe to use. Common brand names include:
    Equal (aspartame)
    Sprinkle Sweet (saccharin)
    Splenda No Calorie Sweetener (sucralose)
    Sweet One (acesulfame)
    Sweet-10 (saccharin)
    Sugar Twin (saccharin)
    Sweet'n Low (saccharin)
    Weight Watchers Low Calorie Sweetener (saccharin)

Drinks include the following:

Bouillon, broth, consomme*
Bouillon or broth, low sodium
Carbonated or mineral water
Cocoa powder, unsweetened, 1 tablespoon
Coffee or tea
Club soda
Diet soft drinks, sugar-free
Drink mixes, sugar-free
Tonic water, sugar-free

Condiments include the following:

Ketchup, 1 tablespoon
Horseradish
Lemon juice
Lime juice
Mustard
Pickles, dill*, 1½ large
Soy sauce, regular or light*

* = 400 mg or more sodium per exchange

Taco sauce, 1 tablespoon
Vinegar

Seasonings. Be careful with seasonings that contain sodium or salts, such as garlic or celery salt and lemon pepper. Free seasonings include the following:

Flavoring extracts
Garlic
Herbs, fresh or dried
Pimiento
Spices
Tabasco* or hot pepper sauce
Wine, used in cooking
Worcestershire sauce

Combination foods list. Many of the foods we eat are mixed together in various combinations. These combination foods do not fit into any one exchange list. Often it is hard to tell what is in a casserole dish or prepared food item. This is a list of exchanges for some typical combination foods. The list will help you fit these foods into your meal plan. Ask your dietitian for information about any other combination foods you would like to eat. (If you like, you can calculate the food exchanges in your own recipes, using the information in Chapter 3 "Calculating Food Exchanges.")

Entrées include the following:

Tuna noodle casserole, lasagna, spaghetti with meatballs, chili with beans, macaroni and cheese*, 1 cup (8 ounces), 2 carbohydrates, 2 medium-fat meats
Chow mein (without noodles or rice), 2 cups (16 ounces), 1 carbohydrate, 2 lean meats
Pizza, cheese, thin crust*, ¼ of 10-inch round (5 ounces), 2 carbohydrates, 2 medium-fat meats, 1 fat

---

* = 400 mg or more sodium per exchange

Pizza, meat topping, thin crust*, ¼ of 10-inch round (5
ounces), 2 carbohydrates, 2 medium-fat meats, 2 fats
Pot pie*, 1 (7 ounces), 2 carbohydrates, 1 medium-fat
meat, 4 fats

Frozen entrées include the following:

Salisbury steak with gravy, mashed potato*, 1 (11 ounces),
2 carbohydrates, 3 medium-fat meats, 3–4 fats
Turkey with gravy, mashed potato, dressing*, 1 (11 ounces),
2 carbohydrates, 2 medium-fat meats, 2 fats
Entrée with less than 300 calories*, 1 (8 ounces), 2
carbohydrates, 3 lean meats

Soups include the following:

Bean*, 1 cup, 1 carbohydrate, 1 very lean meat
Cream (made with water)*, 1 cup (8 ounces),
1 carbohydrate, 1 fat
Split pea (made with water)*, ½ cup (4 ounces),
1 carbohydrate
Tomato (made with water)*, 1 cup (8 ounces),
1 carbohydrate
Vegetable beef, chicken noodle, or other broth types*, 1
cup (8 ounces), 1 carbohydrate

Fast foods include the following (ask at your favorite fast
food restaurant for nutrition information about your favorite fast
food):

Burritos with beef*, 2, 4 carbohydrates, 2 medium-fat
meats, 2 fats
Chicken nuggets*, 6, 1 carbohydrate, 2 medium-fat meats,
1 fat
Chicken breast and wing, breaded and fried*, 1 each, 1
carbohydrate, 4 medium-fat meats, 2 fats

* = 400 mg or more sodium per exchange

Fish sandwich/tartar sauce*, 1, 3 carbohydrates, 1 medium-fat meat, 3 fats

French fries, thin, 20–25, 2 carbohydrates, 2 fats

Hamburger, regular, 1, 2 carbohydrates, 2 medium-fat meats

Hamburger, large*, 1, 2 carbohydrates, 3 medium-fat meats, 1 fat

Hog dog with bun*, 1, 1 carbohydrate, 1 high-fat meat, 1 fat

Individual pan pizza*, 1, 5 carbohydrates, 3 medium-fat meats, 3 fats

Soft-serve cone, 1 medium, 2 carbohydrates, 1 fat

Submarine sandwich*, 1 sub (6 inches), 3 carbohydrates, 1 vegetable, 2 medium-fat meats, 1 fat

Taco, hard shell*, 1 (6 ounces), 2 carbohydrates, 2 medium-fat meats, 2 fats

Taco, soft shell*, 1 (3 ounces), 1 carbohydrate, 1 medium-fat meat, 1 fat

You will notice that many of the exchanges listed with the recipes are different from the ones you are accustomed to using. This is because the new exchange system is more precise and descriptive so we can be more accurate. The term "starch exchange" is frequently used when you might be expecting "bread exchange." If there is a doubt in your mind regarding the values of a certain recipe or exchange, consult the listings in this chapter. After you grow accustomed to the new exchange listings, you will appreciate the precise nature of these listings.

---

* = 400 mg or more sodium per exchange

3

Calculating
Food Exchanges

Information about food exchanges is basic to good management
of your diabetic diet. You need to learn as much about them as
possible—what they are and how to use them.

Food exchanges are a method of measuring food values so
that a person with diabetes can control the amount of carbohydrate and other nutrients consumed. The nutritional value of the
exchanges has been determined by the American Dietetic Association. You can't change their values, but you can work with
them better when you understand more about them. They have
been standardized as follows.

The exchanges are established in grams—which are more
familiar to other nationalities than to Americans since we use the
British system of pounds and ounces. Grams are a measure of
weight used in most laboratories and research centers here in our
country as well as abroad. One ounce equals 28.35 grams. Therefore, a 1-ounce slice of bread that contains 15 grams of carbohydrate is about half carbohydrate and the rest water, fiber, fat,
and other ingredients. A vegetable exchange that weighs 3½ to 4
ounces contains only 5 grams of carbohydrate and therefore has
a much smaller percentage of carbohydrate and a larger percentage of fiber, water, and other nutrients. A fruit exchange has
about 15 grams of carbohydrate, and a milk exchange has 12
grams of carbohydrate in 8 ounces of milk. Since the percentage
of carbohydrate in a food is important to us, it is helpful to realize that most vegetables have a much smaller percentage of carbohydrate than bread and some of the starchier vegetables.

COMPOSITION OF FOOD GROUPS OR
EXCHANGES PER SERVING

Food Exchanges	Carbohydrate (grams)	Protein (grams)	Fat (grams)	Calories
Carbohydrate Group				
Starch/bread	15	3	1 or less	80
Fruit	15	–	–	60
Milk				
Skim	12	8	0–3	90
Low-fat	12	8	5	120
Whole	12	8	8	150
Other				
Carbohydrates	15	varies	varies	varies
Vegetables	5	2	–	25
Meat and Meat Substitute Group				
Very lean	–	7	0–1	35
Lean	–	7	3	55
Medium-fat	–	7	5	75
High-fat	–	7	8	100
Fat Group	–	–	5	45

At first most people with diabetes tend to use recipes that have been calculated by someone else—it's often hard enough to get used to thinking in terms of exchanges without worrying about how they were determined. After a while, though, you begin to wonder how to use some of your own recipes. The next step generally is comparing a recipe that has been calculated with one of your own recipes and accepting the exchanges determined for the other recipe for your own recipe. This isn't a bad idea, but it can cause trouble because the recipes aren't exactly alike. Some little ingredient in your recipe can throw the whole calculation off and your estimate may be less accurate than you realize.

The final and best step is learning to calculate your own recipes. Sometimes you may have to adjust them a bit—cutting out some of the flour, reducing the sugar, or substituting a low-carbohydrate vegetable for a high-starch one—but eventually you'll learn how to manage your own recipes after you learn to calculate them.

In order to establish the nutritive values of each portion in a recipe, you must calculate the total nutritive values of the complete recipe, divide by the number of servings the recipe yields, and then compare the nutritive values of each portion with the chart showing the carbohydrate, protein, and fat values of each of the exchanges.

Calculating your own recipes would be more difficult if it weren't for all of the excellent information available to us—thanks to the many dedicated people who have worked hard establishing the nutritive values of foods.

It is helpful to collect information about the nutritive values of foods you use every day. There is an increasing amount of help available from many sources. Now that most cans and packages include nutritive information on the labels, you can collect that information and use it to establish a file of your own. Many of the cereal companies have very complete information available regarding their products, and most companies will send it to you if you are unable to find it on the package. The following books contain information that is invaluable when calculating recipes:

Nutritive Value of American Foods in Common Units, *Agricultural Handbook 456*, U.S. Department of Agriculture. Washington, D.C.: Superintendent of Documents, U.S. Printing Office, 1975, and all current revisions.

Nutritive Value of Foods, *Home and Garden Bulletin 72*, U.S. Department of Agriculture. Washington, D.C.: Superintendent of Documents, U.S. Printing Office, 1977, and all current revisions.

Composition of Foods, Raw, Processed, and Prepared, *Agriculture Handbook No. 8*, U.S. Department of Agriculture. Washington, D.C.: Superintendent of Documents, U.S. Printing Office, 1963, and all current revisions.

Food Values of Portions Commonly Used, Bowes and Church, J. B. Lippincott Company.

The first three books are available in many large cities from the U.S. Government printing office stores, or may be ordered at your local county extension agent office or purchased from the Superintendent of Documents, U.S. Government Printing Office, Washington, DC 20402.

There are several good programs with nutritive information available for your computer that can help you analyze the nutritive values of your recipes.

Nutritive information is also available on the Internet at nal .usda.gov/fnic/cgi-bin/nut_search.pl.

RECIPE ANALYSIS

The nutritive values that concern us most are calories (Cal.), carbohydrate (Carbs.), protein (Pro.), fat, and for some of us, sodium (Na) and cholesterol (Chol.). To calculate a recipe, the simplest procedure is to make a chart showing the list of ingredients and the nutritive values of each. Use the following "Recipe Analysis" form as a model to help you calculate your recipes.

In this form, list the ingredients for each recipe and then look for the appropriate values for each ingredient in one of the references in this book as in the sample form filled in for the Yankee Cornbread recipe (see Index and p. 36).

After you have calculated the total nutritive values of the recipe, divide the total of each of the elements (Cal., Carbs., Pro., Fat, Na, and Chol.) by the total number of portions to get the nutritive values per serving. Then compare it with the table at the beginning of this chapter to decide how many food exchanges you will get from each serving—see the bottom of the sample recipe analysis.

ADJUSTING YOUR RECIPE

Your recipe may not turn out exactly the way you want it to the first time. I have tested most of the recipes in this book several times. The first time I test a recipe, I use the ingredients listed in the basic recipe, cutting down on the sugar or fat or whatever else I think I need to reduce. While some recipes need a little sugar for color and texture, you will be surprised at the

RECIPE ANALYSIS

Name of recipe _____ Date tested _____

Source of recipe _____

Type and number of pans used _____

_____

Temperature _____ Number of servings _____

Baking or cooking time _____

Comments on recipe _____

Ingredient	Amount	Cal.	Carbs. (gm)	Pro. (gm)	Fat (gm)	Na (mg)	Chol. (mg)
Total nutritive values							
Divided by the total number of portions							
Rounded to the nearest number							
Number of food exchanges equal to nutritive value:							

RECIPE ANALYSIS

Name of recipe _Yankee Cornbread_ Date tested _July 25_

Source of recipe _My favorite recipe_

Type and number of pans used _mixer bowl and 9-inch square baking pan_

Temperature _400 degrees_ Number of servings _16_

Baking or cooking time _25 minutes_

Comments on recipe _Chuck's favorite, good texture + color_

Ingredient	Amt.	Cal.	Carbs. (gm)	Pro. (gm)	Fat (gm)	Na (mg)
Corn meal	1 cup	502	108.2	10.9	1.7	1
all-purpose flour	1 cup	455	95.1	13.1	1.3	3
baking powder	4 tsp	20	4	trace	0	1,316
sugar	1/4 cup	193	49.8	—	—	trace
instant dry milk	1/4 cup	61	9	6	trace	93
salt	1/4 tsp	—	—	—	—	533
liquid egg sub.	1/4 cup	25	1	5	0	80
vegetable oil	1/4 cup	482	—	—	54.5	—
Total nutritive values		1,738	267.1	35	57.5	2,026
Divided by the total number of portions	16	108.6	16.7	2.19	3.59	126.6
Rounded to the nearest number		109	17	2	4	127
Number of food exchanges equal to nutritive value:						
1 Starch		80	15	3	4	
1 Fat		45			5	
		125	15	3	9	—

amount of sugar you can take out of a recipe and still get a pretty good product. On the first test of a recipe with the sugar reduced, I add sugar substitute equal to the amount of sugar that I removed. I probably will cut down on the sugar substitute on the next testing because I don't like the taste of an excessive amount of it, but I need to determine how much I want to use in the final recipe. Remember when you are adding sugar substitute that Equal (NutraSweet) breaks down if it is baked or heated too long; if you are using prolonged heat, use some other kind of sugar substitute such as Splenda or Sugar Twin. I try to add Equal after I have taken whatever I'm cooking off the heat, which seems to work very well; or else I use it in things that don't need to be cooked, such as gelatin or fruit.

You can also reduce the fat in a recipe quite a bit, although you do need some fat in baked goods for texture and tenderness.

You can decrease the amount of dietary cholesterol in a recipe by substituting two egg whites or ¼ cup liquid egg substitute for one large egg. (On the other hand, if you would like to use some of your increased allowance of egg yolks in your recipes, substitute one large egg for two egg whites or one large egg for ¼ cup liquid egg subsitute.)

After the first time you test a recipe and calculate its nutritive values, you can decide how much more you need to cut ingredients in order to have a product suitable for your use. Sometimes the calories or fat or carbohydrate are too high and you need to try it again, cutting down on the offending ingredient. It is possible to repeatedly try a recipe and never get it right, but generally, you can work with it and find a variation of the original recipe that you can use. One important thing to remember is to write down exactly what you use when you are testing a recipe. It is so frustrating to get just what you want in a recipe and then forget exactly how much of each ingredient you used.

Another way to control the food exchanges is by dividing a recipe into the size portions that conform to what you can have. In the Breads chapter, you will notice that the number of slices per loaf varies according to the recipe. That is because you need to cut a certain size slice to arrive at a bread exchange for each slice. To find this, divide the total grams of carbohydrate in the recipe by 15, which is the amount allowed for a bread exchange; that tells you how many slices you need from each loaf in order to have each slice equal one bread exchange.

A calculator may be a big help when calculating recipes. It is much faster and gives me more confidence that my totals are correct.

As an aid in developing recipes for my cookbooks, I keep a chart of nutritive values of many ingredients that I use frequently so I don't have to look them up every time. This is very helpful to me, and since it is likely to be helpful for you also, I'm including it in this chapter. I have only included foods that may be used on a low-cholesterol diet. I have not included cream or other high-fat foods. However, I did include chocolate chips because you might like to use them occasionally—and you should have their nutritive value so you will know how many you can use.

When calculating meat recipes, I subtract the values for any fat that cooks out of the meat, using the values for fat in the chart. I chill the fat and then measure it very carefully after it is hardened in the refrigerator.

I have included sugars because research now shows a little can be used as long as it is calculated in the total exchanges for that food. You might discuss this with your doctor; however, most doctors and dietitians concur that a small amount will not upset your sugar count. (See Introduction, page xi.)

The following measures may also help you in your own calculations:

3 teaspoons = 1 tablespoon
4 tablespoons = ¼ cup
5⅓ tablespoons = ⅓ cup
8 tablespoons = ½ cup
10⅔ tablespoons = ⅔ cup
12 tablespoons = ¾ cup
16 tablespoons = 1 cup
2 cups = 1 pint
4 cups = 1 quart

4 quarts = 1 gallon
16 ounces = 1 pound

I have used pound and cup measures for many items in this table so that from them you can calculate your own recipes.

Remember as you are using this information that it is specifically written for the person on a low-cholesterol diabetic diet. All values for fruits and fruit juices are without any added sweetener, and meats that are high in fat are not included—nor are any other products that are not recommended for a low-cholesterol diet.

I hope you will be encouraged to use this information in calculating your own favorite recipes and to devise variations of other recipes that will help to add some spice and variety to your diabetic diet.

NUTRIENT ANALYSIS OF ACCEPTABLE FOODS

Food Item	Amount	Cal.	Carbs. (gm)	Pro. (gm)	Fat (gm)	Sat. Fat (gm)	Chol. (mg)	Fiber (gm)	Na (mg)
VEGETABLES									
Artichoke	1 med	60	13	4	Trace	Trace	0	6.7	120
Asparagus, cooked	½ cup	22	4	2	Trace	Trace	0	3.1	4
Bamboo shoots, canned	1 cup	25	4	2	1	Trace	0	3.9	9
Beans, great northern, cooked	1 cup	209	37	15	1	Trace	0	6	4
Beans, green, cooked	½ cup	22	5	1	Trace	Trace	0	1.1	2
Beans, green, raw	½ cup	17	4	1	Trace	Trace	0	1	3
Beans, lima, dry, cooked	1 cup	216	39	15	1	Trace	0	13.5	4
Beans, lima, green, cooked	1 cup	209	40	12	1	Trace	0	7.1	29
Beans, navy, dry, cooked	1 cup	258	48	15	1	Trace	0	6.6	2
Beans, pinto, dry, cooked	1 cup	234	44	14	1	Trace	0	6.8	3
Bean sprouts, mung, cooked	1 cup	26	5	3	Trace	Trace	0	na	12
Bean sprouts, mung, raw	½ cup	16	3	2	Trace	Trace	0	0.6	3
Beets, cooked	1 cup	26	6	1	Trace	Trace	0	2.2	42
Broccoli, raw	½ cup	12	2	1	Trace	Trace	0	1.2	12
Broccoli, cooked	½ cup	22	4	2	Trace	Trace	0	2	20
Brussels sprouts, raw	½ cup	19	4	1	Trace	Trace	0	2.6	11
Brussels sprouts, cooked	½ cup	30	7	2	Trace	Trace	0	3.4	16
Cabbage, raw	½ cup	8	2	Trace	Trace	Trace	0	0.8	6
Cabbage, cooked	½ cup	16	4	1	Trace	Trace	0	2.1	14
Cabbage, red, raw	½ cup	9	2	Trace	Trace	Trace	0	0.7	4
Cabbage, red, cooked	½ cup	16	3	1	Trace	Trace	0	1.8	4
Carrots, raw	½ cup	24	6	1	Trace	Trace	0	1.8	19

Food	Amount								
Carrots, cooked	½ cup	35	8	1	Trace	Trace	0	1.5	51
Cauliflower, raw	½ cup	12	2	1	Trace	Trace	0	1.2	8
Cauliflower, cooked	½ cup	15	3	1	Trace	Trace	0	1.4	4
Celeriac, raw	½ cup	30	7	Trace	Trace	Trace	0	na	78
Celery, raw	½ cup	10	2	1	Trace	Trace	0	1	52
Celery, cooked	½ cup	14	3	Trace	Trace	Trace	0	1.4	68
Chard, Swiss, raw	½ cup	3	1	2	Trace	Trace	0	0.3	38
Chard, Swiss, cooked	½ cup	18	4	2	Trace	Trace	0	na	158
Chicory leaves, raw	½ cup	21	4	2	Trace	Trace	0	1.4	41
Chives, raw	1 tbsp	1	Trace	Trace	Trace	Trace	0	0.1	Trace
Collards, cooked	½ cup	17	4	1	Trace	Trace	0	na	10
Corn, cream-style, canned	½ cup	92	23	2	1	Trace	0	1.5	365
Corn, sweet, raw	½ cup	66	15	2	1	Trace	0	2.5	12
Corn, sweet, cooked	½ cup	89	21	3	1	Trace	0	3	14
Corn, sweet, canned	½ cup	83	20	3	1	Trace	0	1.5	286
Cowpeas, raw	½ cup	65	14	2	Trace	Trace	0	na	3
Cowpeas, cooked	½ cup	79	17	3	Trace	Trace	0	na	3
Cress, garden, raw	½ cup	8	1	1	Trace	Trace	0	na	4
Cucumber, raw	½ cup	7	2	Trace	Trace	Trace	0	0.5	1
Eggplant, raw	½ cup	11	3	Trace	Trace	Trace	0	0.5	2
Eggplant, cooked	½ cup	13	3	Trace	Trace	Trace	0	1	1
Endive, raw	½ cup	4	1	Trace	Trace	Trace	0	0.6	6
Garlic, raw	1 clove	4	1	Trace	Trace	Trace	0	0.1	1
Gingerroot, raw	¼ cup	17	4	1	Trace	Trace	0	na	3
Kale, raw	½ cup	17	3	1	Trace	Trace	0	2.2	15
Kale, cooked	½ cup	21	4	1	Trace	Trace	0	3.3	15

Food Item	Amount	Cal.	Carbs. (gm)	Pro. (gm)	Fat (gm)	Sat. Fat (gm)	Chol. (mg)	Fiber (gm)	Na (mg)
Kohlrabi, raw	½ cup	19	4	1	Trace	Trace	0	0.8	14
Kohlrabi, cooked	½ cup	24	5	1	Trace	Trace	0	na	17
Leeks, raw	½ cup	32	7	1	Trace	Trace	0	0.6	10
Leeks, cooked	½ cup	16	4	Trace	Trace	Trace	0	na	5
Lettuce, butterhead	½ cup	4	1	Trace	Trace	Trace	0	0.3	1
Lettuce, iceberg	½ cup	5	1	Trace	Trace	Trace	0	0.3	3
Lettuce, romaine	½ cup	4	1	Trace	Trace	Trace	0	0.5	2
Mushrooms, raw	½ cup	9	2	1	Trace	Trace	0	0.5	1
Mushrooms, cooked	½ cup	21	4	2	Trace	Trace	0	1.7	2
Mustard greens, raw	½ cup	7	1	1	Trace	Trace	0	0.2	7
Mustard greens, cooked	½ cup	11	1	2	Trace	Trace	0	1.6	11
Okra, raw	½ cup	19	4	1	Trace	Trace	0	1.6	4
Okra, cooked	½ cup	25	6	1	Trace	Trace	0	na	4
Onion, raw	½ cup	30	7	1	Trace	Trace	0	1.3	2
Onion, cooked	½ cup	46	11	1	Trace	Trace	0	2.2	3
Onion, green, raw	½ cup	16	4	1	Trace	Trace	0	1.2	8
Parsley, raw	¼ cup	5	1	Trace	Trace	Trace	0	0.7	6
Parsnips, raw	½ cup	50	12	1	Trace	Trace	0	3	7
Parsnips, cooked	½ cup	63	15	1	Trace	Trace	0	2.1	8
Peas, green, raw	½ cup	58	10	4	Trace	Trace	0	2.9	4
Peas, green, cooked	½ cup	67	13	4	Trace	Trace	0	3.3	2
Peppers, chili, raw	½ cup	30	7	2	Trace	Trace	0	1.1	5
Peppers, sweet green, raw	½ cup	14	3	Trace	Trace	Trace	0	0.8	1
Peppers, sweet green, cooked	½ cup	19	5	1	Trace	Trace	0	1.2	1

Peppers, sweet yellow, raw	1 large	na	na	na	na	na	na	na	na
Pickle, dill	1 med	12	3	Trace	Trace	Trace	0	0.8	833
Pickle, sweet	1 large	41	11	Trace	Trace	Trace	0	0.4	329
Pickle, relish, sweet	1/4 cup	80	21	Trace	Trace	Trace	0	na	495
Pimiento, canned	1 tbsp	3	1	Trace	Trace	Trace	0	na	2
Potatoes, white, raw	1/2 cup	59	13	2	Trace	Trace	0	1.2	5
Potatoes, white, baked, no skin	1/2 cup	57	13	1	Trace	Trace	0	0.9	3
Potatoes, white, boiled	1/2 cup	67	16	1	Trace	Trace	0	1.2	4
Potatoes, white, mashed	1/2 cup	111	18	2	4	1	2	1.7	310
Pumpkin, cooked	1/2 cup	24	6	1	Trace	Trace	0	na	1
Radicchio, raw	1/2 cup	5	1	Trace	Trace	Trace	0	na	4
Radishes, red, raw	1/2 cup	10	2	Trace	Trace	Trace	0	1.3	14
Radishes, white, raw	1/2 cup	7	1	1	Trace	Trace	0	na	8
Rutabaga, raw	1/2 cup	25	6	1	Trace	Trace	0	1.7	14
Rutabaga, cooked	1/2 cup	29	7	1	Trace	Trace	0	1.7	15
Shallots, raw	1 tbsp	7	2	Trace	Trace	Trace	0	0.1	1
Spinach, raw	1/2 cup	6	1	1	Trace	Trace	0	0.7	22
Spinach, cooked	1/2 cup	21	3	3	Trace	Trace	0	2	63
Squash, summer, raw	1/2 cup	13	3	1	Trace	Trace	0	0.8	1
Squash, summer, cooked	1/2 cup	18	4	1	Trace	Trace	0	1.3	1
Squash, winter, raw	1/2 cup	21	5	1	Trace	Trace	0	1	2
Squash, winter, cooked	1/2 cup	40	9	1	1	Trace	0	2.9	1
Sweet potatoes, raw	1/2 cup	70	16	1	Trace	Trace	0	2	9
Sweet potatoes, cooked	1/2 cup	172	40	3	Trace	Trace	0	4.9	21
Tomatillos, raw	1 med	11	2	Trace	Trace	Trace	0	na	Trace
Tomatoes, red, raw	1 med	26	6	1	Trace	Trace	0	1.6	11

Food Item	Amount	Cal.	Carbs. (gm)	Pro. (gm)	Fat (gm)	Sat. Fat (gm)	Chol. (mg)	Fiber (gm)	Na (mg)
Tomatoes, red, cooked	½ cup	32	7	1	Trace	Trace	0	1	13
Tomato, paste, canned	½ cup	110	25	5	1	Trace	0	5.6	1,035
Tomato, puréed, canned	½ cup	51	13	2	Trace	Trace	0	2.9	499
Tomato, sauce, canned	½ cup	37	9	2	Trace	Trace	0	1.8	738
Turnips, raw	½ cup	18	4	1	Trace	Trace	0	1.2	44
Turnips, cooked	½ cup	14	4	1	Trace	Trace	0	1.6	39
Turnip greens, raw	½ cup	15	3	1	Trace	Trace	0	1.3	22
Turnip greens, cooked	½ cup	14	3	1	Trace	Trace	0	2.2	21
Water chestnuts, canned	½ cup	35	9	1	Trace	Trace	0	3.2	6
Watercress, raw	½ cup	2	Trace	Trace	Trace	Trace	0	0.4	7

LEGUMES

Food Item	Amount	Cal.	Carbs. (gm)	Pro. (gm)	Fat (gm)	Sat. Fat (gm)	Chol. (mg)	Fiber (gm)	Na (mg)
Beans, dry, black	1 cup	662	121	42	3	1	0	25.6	10
Beans, dry, cranberry	1 cup	653	117	45	2	1	0	18.1	12
Beans, dry, great northern	1 cup	621	114	40	2	1	0	73.2	26
Beans, dry, kidney	1 cup	613	110	43	2	Trace	0	19.1	44
Beans, dry, lima	1 cup	602	113	38	1	Trace	0	33.8	32
Beans, dry, navy	1 cup	697	126	46	3	1	0	20.2	29
Beans, dry, pink	1 cup	720	135	44	2	1	0	18.7	17
Beans, dry, pinto	1 cup	656	122	40	2	Trace	0	23.2	19
Carob flour	1 cup	394	92	5	1	Trace	0	41	36
Chickpeas, dry	1 cup	728	121	39	12	1	0	12.8	48
Lentils, dry	1 cup	649	110	54	2	Trace	0	21.9	19
Lentils, cooked	1 cup	230	40	18	1	1	0	7.9	4

Peas, split	1 cup	672	119	48	2	Trace	0	11	30
Tofu, raw firm	½ cup	183	5	20	11	2	0	na	18
Tofu, raw regular	½ cup	94	2	10	6	1	0	1.5	9
FRUIT (JUICE PACK)									
Avocado, puréed	1 cup	370	17	5	35	6	0	4.6	23
Avocado, whole	1	324	15	4	31	5	0	4	20
Apricots, raw	3	51	12	1	Trace	Trace	0	1.4	1
Apricots, canned	½ cup	60	15	1	Trace	0	0	0.6	5
Applesauce, canned, unsweetened	½ cup	52	14	Trace	Trace	Trace	0	1.8	2
Apple, raw	1 med	81	21	Trace	1	Trace	0	3	0
Banana, raw	1 med	105	27	1	1	Trace	0	1.8	1
Blackberries, raw	1 cup	75	18	1	1	Trace	0	6.5	0
Blueberries, raw	1 cup	81	20	1	1	Trace	0	3.3	9
Cherries, sour, red, raw, pitted	1 cup	52	13	1	Trace	Trace	0	1.2	3
Cherries, sour, red, canned	1 cup	87	22	2	Trace	Trace	0	na	17
Cherries, sweet, raw	1 cup	104	24	2	1	Trace	0	2.2	0
Cherries, sweet, canned	1 cup	135	35	2	Trace	0	0	0.6	8
Cranberries, raw	1 cup	54	14	Trace	Trace	Trace	0	4	1
Currant, red, fresh	1 cup	63	15	2	Trace	Trace	0	4.8	1
Dates, dry	1 cup	490	131	4	1	Trace	0	9.1	5
Elderberries, raw	1 cup	105	27	1	1	Trace	0	na	na
Figs, raw	1 med	37	10	Trace	Trace	Trace	0	1.4	1
Figs, canned, unsweetened	1 cup	131	35	1	Trace	Trace	0	na	2
Figs, dried	1 cup	508	130	6	2	Trace	0	18.5	22
Gooseberries, raw	1 cup	66	15	1	1	Trace	0	na	2

Food Item	Amount	Cal.	Carbs. (gm)	Pro. (gm)	Fat (gm)	Sat. Fat (gm)	Chol. (mg)	Fiber (gm)	Na (mg)
Grapefruit, fresh	½	38	10	1	Trace	Trace	0	0.7	0
Grapes, Concord	1 cup	58	16	1	Trace	Trace	0	1.5	2
Grapes, European	1 cup	114	1	28	1	Trace	0	2.6	3
Groundcherries, raw	1 cup	74	16	3	1	Trace	0	na	na
Guava, raw	1 cup	84	20	1	1	Trace	0	8.9	5
Kiwifruit, raw	1 med	46	11	1	Trace	Trace	0	2.6	4
Lemon, raw	1 med	22	12	1	Trace	Trace	0	na	3
Lime, raw	1 med	20	7	Trace	Trace	Trace	0	na	1
Mango, raw	1 med	135	35	1	1	Trace	0	2.2	4
Melon, cantaloupe	1 cup	56	13	1	Trace	Trace	0	1.3	14
Melon, casaba	1 cup	44	11	2	Trace	Trace	0	1.4	20
Melon, honeydew	1 cup	60	16	1	Trace	Trace	0	1.5	17
Melon, watermelon	1 cup	51	11	1	1	Trace	0	0.6	3
Nectarines	1 med	67	16	1	1	Trace	0	2.2	0
Orange, fresh, peeled	1 med	62	15	1	Trace	Trace	0	3.1	0
Papaya, fresh	1 med	119	30	2	Trace	Trace	0	2.8	9
Peaches, raw	1 med	55	14	1	Trace	Trace	0	2.1	0
Pears, raw	1 med	98	25	1	1	Trace	0	4.3	0
Persimmon, raw	1 med	32	8	Trace	Trace	Trace	0	na	Trace
Pineapple, raw	1 cup	76	19	1	1	Trace	0	1.9	2
Pineapple, canned	1 cup	150	39	1	Trace	Trace	0	1.9	3
Plantain, raw	1 med	218	57	2	1	Trace	0	4.1	7
Plantain, cooked	1 cup	179	48	1	Trace	Trace	0	3.5	6

Food	Measure								
Plums, raw	1 cup	91	21	1	1	Trace	0	3.5	0
Plums, purple, canned	1 cup	102	27	1	Trace	0	0	na	2
Pomegranate, raw	1	105	26	1	Trace	Trace	0	0.9	5
Prunes, dry	1 cup	385	102	4	1	Trace	0	11.6	6
Prunes, cooked	1 cup	227	60	2	Trace	Trace	0	14	4
Quince, raw	1 med	52	14	Trace	Trace	Trace	0	1.8	4
Raisins, seedless	1 cup	435	115	5	1	Trace	0	7.7	17
Raspberries, raw	1 cup	60	14	1	1	Trace	0	5.8	0
Rhubarb, raw	1 cup	26	6	1	Trace	Trace	0	2.2	5
Strawberries, raw	1 cup	46	11	1	1	Trace	0	4	2
Tangerine, raw	1 med	37	9	1	Trace	Trace	0	1.7	1

JUICES

Food	Measure								
Apple	1 cup	116	29	Trace	Trace	Trace	0	0.3	7
Apricot nectar	1 cup	141	36	1	Trace	Trace	0	1.5	8
Grape	1 cup	155	38	1	Trace	Trace	0	0	8
Grapefruit, canned, unsweetened	1 cup	94	22	1	Trace	Trace	0	Trace	2
Lemon, bottled	1 tbsp	3	1	Trace	Trace	Trace	0	Trace	3
Lime, bottled	1 tbsp	3	1	Trace	Trace	Trace	0	Trace	2
Orange	1 cup	112	27	2	Trace	Trace	0	0.5	2
Pineapple	1 cup	140	35	1	Trace	Trace	0	Trace	3
Prune	1 cup	182	45	2	Trace	0	0	2.6	3
Tomato	1 cup	41	10	2	Trace	Trace	0	Trace	881

MEATS

Food Item	Amount	Cal.	Carbs. (gm)	Pro. (gm)	Fat (gm)	Sat. Fat (gm)	Chol. (mg)	Fiber (gm)	Na (mg)
Composite of lean beef without fat, raw	1 oz	82	0	5	7	3	19	0	15
Composite of lean beef without fat, cooked	1 oz	91	0	7	7	3	24	0	20
Composite of lean beef without fat, cooked	1 cup	730	0	58	53	22	188	0	140
Beef brisket, without fat, raw	1 oz	75	0	5	6	2	20	0	20
Beef brisket, without fat, cooked	1 oz	88	0	8	6	2	27	0	15
Beef chuck roast, without fat, raw	1 oz	63	0	5	7	2	20	0	15
Beef chuck roast, without fat, cooked	1 oz	92	0	8	3	3	29	0	20
Beef flank steak, without fat, raw	1 oz	45	0	5	5	1	12	0	10
Beef flank steak, without fat, cooked	1 oz	75	0	8	8	2	20	0	10
Beef, ground, regular (27% fat), raw	1 oz	88	0	5	8	3	24	0	15
Beef, ground, extra lean (9% fat), raw	1 oz	48	0	6	3	1	10	0	20
Beef round, without fat, raw	1 oz	38	0	6	1	.50	15	0	15
Beef round, without fat, cooked	1 oz	50	0	8	2	.60	20	0	20
Beef sirloin, without fat, raw	1 oz	44	0	7	2	.70	19	0	15

Beef sirloin, without fat, cooked	1 oz	57	0	9	5	.90	25	0	20
Beef, tenderloin, without fat, raw	1 oz	44	0	6	2	1	18	0	15
Beef, tenderloin, without fat, cooked	1 oz	60	0	8	3	1	24	0	20
Veal, chop, lean, without fat, raw	1 oz	46	0	5	3	1	22	0	20
Veal, chop, lean, without fat, cooked	1 oz	64	0	10	3	.70	35	0	35
Veal, leg, without fat, raw	1 oz	33	0	6	1	.30	22	0	20
Veal, leg, without fat, roasted	1 oz	45	0	8	1	.50	29	0	20
Veal, stew meat, without fat, raw	1 oz	31	0	6	.70	.20	24	0	25
Lamb, composite of lean only, raw	1 oz	75	0	5	6	3	20	0	15
Lamb, composite of lean only, cooked	1 oz	83	0	7	6	3	28	0	20
Lamb, chop, without fat, raw	1 oz	43	0	6	2	.50	20	0	20
Lamb, cubed for stew, without fat	1 oz	38	0	6	1.5	.50	18	0	20
Lamb, ground, raw	1 oz	80	0	5	7	3	20	0	15
Lamb, leg, without fat, raw	1 oz	74	0	5	6	3	20	0	15
Lamb, leg, without fat, cooked	1 oz	80	0	7	6	3	27	0	20
Pork, Canadian bacon, raw	1 oz	33	Trace	4	2	.50	10	0	276
Pork, Canadian bacon, cooked	1 oz	45	Trace	6	2	.60	14	0	399
Pork, center cut chop, without fat, raw	1 oz	43	0	5	2	.60	16	0	13

Food Item	Amount	Cal.	Carbs. (gm)	Pro. (gm)	Fat (gm)	Sat. Fat (gm)	Chol. (mg)	Fiber (gm)	Na (mg)
Pork, center cut chop, without fat, cooked	1 oz	61	0	8	3	1	23	0	18
Pork, fresh ham, without fat, raw	1 oz	33	0	5	1	.40	12	0	339
Pork, fresh ham, without fat, cooked	1 oz	45	0	7	2	.50	16	0	376
Pork, loin, without fat, raw	1 oz	40	0	6	1.5	.50	15	0	15
Pork, loin, without fat, cooked	1 oz	55	0	8	2	.70	22	0	13
Pork, tenderloin, without fat, raw	1 oz	34	0	6	1	.30	18	0	14
Pork, tenderloin, without fat, cooked	1 oz	64	0	8	3	1	22	0	12
Ham, cured, without fat, uncooked	1 oz	46	Trace	5	2	.70	15	0	362
Ham, cured, without fat, cooked	1 oz	47	Trace	6	2	.70	16	0	392
Ham, precooked without fat	1 oz	35	0	6	1	.40	13	0	359
POULTRY									
Chicken, white meat only, raw	1 oz	56	0	8	2	1	25	0	20

50

Food	Serving								
Chicken, white meat only, cooked	1 oz	60	0	8	2	1	25	0	20
Chicken, dark meat only, raw	1 oz	65	0	7	4	1	24	0	25
Chicken, dark meat only, cooked	1 oz	65	0	7	4	1	25	0	20
Chicken, light and dark meat only, raw	1 oz	60	0	5	4	1	21	0	20
Chicken, roasted, light and dark meat only	1 oz	65	0	7	4	1	21	0	20
Chicken, roasted, light and dark meat only	1 cup	560	0	57	35	10	210	0	190
Chicken, stewed, light and dark meat only	1 oz	50	0	8	2	1	24	0	20
Chicken, stewed, light and dark meat only	1 cup	247	0	38	9	3	116	0	100
Turkey, white meat only, raw	1 oz	45	0	6	2	1	18	0	17
Turkey, white meat only, cooked	1 oz	59	0	8	2	1	22	0	18
Turkey, dark meat only, raw	1 oz	45	0	5	3	1	20	0	20
Turkey, dark meat only, cooked	1 oz	63	0	8	3	1	25	0	22
Turkey, light and dark meat only, raw	1 oz	35	0	6	1	.50	16	0	14

Food Item	Amount	Cal.	Carbs. (gm)	Pro. (gm)	Fat (gm)	Sat. Fat (gm)	Chol. (mg)	Fiber (gm)	Na (mg)
Turkey, ground, raw	1 oz	47	0	6	3	1	21	0	22
Turkey, ground, cooked	1 oz	67	0	8	4	1	29	0	30
Turkey, ham	1 oz	36	.10	5	2	.50	16	0	282
Turkey, roasted, light and dark meat only	1 oz	48	0	8	2	.50	22	0	20
Turkey, roasted, light and dark meat only	1 cup	238	0	41	7	2	106	0	98
FISH									
Codfish, raw	1 oz	23	0	5	.20	.04	12	0	15
Flounder, raw	1 oz	34	0	7	.50	.17	20	0	30
Haddock, raw	1 oz	25	0	5	.20	.04	16	0	20
Halibut, raw	1 oz	37	0	8	.70	–	12	0	20
Herring, plain	1 oz	98	0	3	9	–	–	0	180
Salmon, pink, raw	1 oz	33	0	6	1	.20	15	0	20
Salmon, pink, canned, drained, meat only	1 oz	44	0	7	1	.30	24	0	20
Salmon, red, raw	1 oz	48	0	6	2	.40	18	0	15
Salmon, red, canned, drained, meat only	1 oz	43	0	6	2	.50	13	0	150
Sardines, canned	1 oz	46	0	5	3	.60	17	0	190
Trout, raw	1 oz	30	0	5	1	.30	24	0	15
Tuna, canned in water, drained	1 oz	33	0	7	.20	.07	9	0	95
Tuna, canned in oil, drained	1 oz	56	0	8	2	.40	5	0	100

SHELLFISH

Clams, raw, composite of types, drained	1 oz	12	0	2	.11	—	—	0	—
Clams, canned, composite of types, drained	1 oz	42	0	7	.55	.05	15	0	32
Crab, Alaska king, raw	1 oz	24	0	5	.17	.03	12	0	237
Oysters, eastern, raw	1 oz	19	0	2	.70	.20	9	0	60
Scallops, mixture, cooked	1 oz	28	0	5	2	.20	9	0	46
Shellfish, imitation, cooked	1 oz	33	0	4	.20	.03	14	0	17
Shrimp, raw, shelled, mixture of types	1 oz	30	Trace	6	.50	.09	43	0	42
Shrimp, cooked, shelled, mixture of types	1 oz	28	0	6	.30	.08	55	0	64

DAIRY PRODUCTS

Buttermilk, dry	1 cup	464	59	41	7	4	83	0	620
Buttermilk, dry	½ cup	232	29	21	3	2	41	0	310
Buttermilk, dry	¼ cup	116	15	10	2	1	21	0	155
Buttermilk, dry	1 tbsp	29	4	3	Trace	Trace	5	0	39
Egg, large	1	75	1	6	5	2	213	0	63
Egg white, large	1	17	Trace	4	0	0	0	0	55
Egg substitute, liquid	1 cup	100	4	5	0	0	0	0	320
Egg substitute, liquid	⅓ cup	33	1	1	0	0	0	0	106
Egg substitute, liquid	¼ cup	25	1	4	0	0	0	0	80
Egg substitute, liquid	1 tbsp	6	Trace	Trace	0	0	0	0	20

Food Item	Amount	Cal.	Carbs. (gm)	Pro. (gm)	Fat (gm)	Sat. Fat (gm)	Chol. (mg)	Fiber (gm)	Na (mg)
Ice milk, hard	½ cup	92	15	3	3	2	9	0	56
Ice milk, soft serve	½ cup	111	19	4	2	1	10	0	62
Milk, instant, dry nonfat	1 cup	243	35	24	Trace	Trace	12	0	373
Milk, instant, dry nonfat	½ cup	122	18	12	Trace	Trace	6	0	187
Milk, instant, dry nonfat	⅓ cup	80	12	8	Trace	Trace	4	0	123
Milk, instant, dry nonfat	¼ cup	61	9	6	Trace	Trace	3	0	93
Milk, instant, dry nonfat	1 tbsp	15	2	1	Trace	Trace	1	0	23
Milk, skim, fresh	1 cup	86	12	8	Trace	Trace	5	0	127
Milk, skim, evaporated	1 cup	199	29	19	1	Trace	10	0	293
Sherbet, orange	½ cup	132	29	1	2	1	5	0	44
Yogurt, plain, low-fat	½ cup	71	8	6	2	1	7	0	79
Yogurt, plain, fat-free	½ cup	64	9	7	Trace	Trace	2	0	86
Yogurt, frozen, composite of fruit flavors	½ cup	Varies greatly with brand							

CHEESE

Food Item	Amount	Cal.	Carbs. (gm)	Pro. (gm)	Fat (gm)	Sat. Fat (gm)	Chol. (mg)	Fiber (gm)	Na (mg)
Cheddar, low-fat	1 oz	50	1	6	2	na	na	0	na
Cheese food	1 oz	93	2	6	7	4	18	0	337
Cottage with 2% milk	1 cup	203	8	31	4	3	18	0	918
Cottage with 1% milk	1 cup	163	6	28	2	1	9	0	918
Mozzarella, with part skim milk	1 oz	72	1	7	5	3	16	0	132
Neufchâtel	1 oz	9	1	3	7	4	22	0	113
Parmesan, grated	1 oz	111	1	10	7	5	19	0	454
Ricotta with part skim milk	1 cup	339	13	28	19	12	76	0	308

NUTS AND SEEDS (unsalted)

	Serving								
Almonds, dry roasted	1 oz	167	7	5	15	1	0	3.2	3
Brazil nuts	1 oz	186	4	4	19	5	0	5.7	1
Cashews, dry roasted	1 oz	163	9	4	13	3	0	0.9	5
Chestnuts, European, raw, peeled	1 oz	64	14	1	Trace	Trace	0	na	Trace
Filberts, dry roasted	1 oz	188	5	3	19	1	0	1.7	1
Macadamia nuts, dried	1 oz	199	4	2	21	3	0	2.6	1
Peanut butter, chunky, salted	2 tbsp	190	7	8	16	3	0	2.1	157
Peanut butter, smooth, salted	2 tbsp	191	5	9	16	2.8	0	1.9	151
Peanuts, dry roasted	1 oz	166	6	7	14	2	0	2.3	2
Peanuts, oil roasted	1 oz	165	5	7	14	2	0	2.5	2
Pecans, dry roasted	1 oz	187	6	2	18	1	0	na	Trace
Pine nuts, dry, pignolia	1 oz	146	4	7	14	2	0	3	1
Pine nuts, piñon	1 oz	161	5	3	17	3	0	3	20
Pistachio nuts, dry roasted	1 oz	172	8	4	15	2	0	3.1	2
Pumpkin and squash seeds, shelled, roasted	1 oz	148	4	9	12	2	0	1.9	5
Sesame seeds, whole, roasted	1 oz	161	7	5	14	2	0	3.3	3
Sunflower seed kernels, dried	1 oz	162	5	6	14	1	0	3	1
Walnuts, black, dry	1 oz	172	3	7	16	1	0	1.4	Trace
Walnuts, English, dry	1 oz	182	5	4	18	2	0	1.4	3

FATS

	Serving								
Corn oil	1 cup	1,927	0	0	218	28	0	0	0
Corn oil	1 tbsp	120	0	0	14	2	0	0	0

Food Item	Amount	Cal.	Carbs. (gm)	Pro. (gm)	Fat (gm)	Sat. Fat (gm)	Chol. (mg)	Fiber (gm)	Na (mg)
Margarine—corn oil, stick	½ cup	815	1	1	91	15	0	0	1,070
Margarine—corn oil, stick	1 tbsp	102	Trace	Trace	11	2	0	0	134
SUGARS									
Chocolate chips, semisweet	1 cup	811	108	7	50	30	0	na	19
Chocolate chips, semisweet	1 tbsp	51	7	Trace	3	2	0	na	1
Cocoa	1 tbsp	12	3	1	1	Trace	0	1.6	1
Honey	1 cup	1,031	279	1	0	0	0	0	14
Marshmallows	1 oz	90	23	1	Trace	0	0	0	13
Sugar, brown, packed	1 cup	827	214	0	0	0	0	0	86
Sugar, granulated	1 cup	770	199	0	0	0	0	0	Trace
Sugar, powdered	1 cup	467	119	0	Trace	0	0	0	1
Syrup, corn, light	1 cup	925	251	0	0	0	0	0	397
Syrup, maple	1 cup	825	212	0	1	Trace	0	0	28
Syrup, molasses, light	1 cup	872	226	0	Trace	Trace	0	0	121
Syrup, sorghum	1 cup	957	247	0	0	0	0	0	26
CEREAL AND STARCHES									
Barley, pearl, light	1 cup	704	155	20	2	Trace	0	31.2	18
Bran, wheat	1 cup	130	39	9	3	Trace	0	25.4	1
Breads, commercial									
rye	1 oz	73	14	2	1	Trace	0	1.8	187
white	1 oz	76	14	2	1	Trace	Trace	0.7	153
whole wheat	1 oz	70	13	3	1	Trace	Trace	2	149
Bread crumbs, dry	1 cup	427	78	14	6	1	Trace	4.5	931

Food	Measure							
Bulgur, dry, cracked wheat	1 cup	479	106	17	2	Trace	0	25.6	24
Cornmeal	1 cup	505	107	12	2	Trace	0	7.2	4
Flour								
all-purpose	1 cup	455	95	13	1	Trace	0	3.4	3
bread	1 cup	495	99	16	2	Trace	0	2.3	3
cake	1 cup	395	85	9	1	Trace	0	na	2
rye, light	1 cup	374	82	9	1	Trace	0	14.9	2
soybean, low-fat	1 cup	286	33	41	6	1	0	9	16
whole wheat or graham	1 cup	407	87	16	2	Trace	0	15.1	6
Graham crackers	1 dble	59	11	1	1	Trace	0	0.4	85
crumb	1 cup	480	88	8	8	na	na	3.6	720
Macaroni, dry	1 lb	1,684	339	58	7	1	0	10.9	32
cooked	1 cup	197	40	7	1	Trace	0	2.2	1
Noodles, dry, commercial	1 lb	1,730	323	64	19	4	431	12.3	95
cooked	1 cup	213	40	8	2	1	53	3.5	11
chow mein, canned	1 cup	237	26	4	14	2	0	1.8	197
Oat bran	1 cup	231	62	16	7	1	0	15	4
Oatmeal, dry	1 cup	311	54	13	5	1	0	8.4	3
Oats, rolled, dry	1 cup	311	54	13	5	1	0	8.4	3
Rice								
brown, raw	1 cup	685	143	15	5	1	0	6.5	13
brown, cooked	1 cup	216	45	5	2	Trace	0	3.3	10
white, instant, dry	1 cup	360	79	7	Trace	Trace	0	1.5	6
white, long-grain, raw	1 cup	675	148	13	1	Trace	0	1.9	9
white, long-grain, cooked	1 cup	265	57	6	1	Trace	0	0.7	4
wild, raw	1 cup	571	120	24	2	Trace	0	8.3	11
Tapioca, dry, pearl	1 tbsp	35	9	Trace	Trace	Trace	0	na	45

Food Item	Amount	Cal.	Carbs. (gm)	Pro. (gm)	Fat (gm)	Sat. Fat (gm)	Chol. (mg)	Fiber (gm)	Na (mg)
CONDIMENTS									
Baking powder	1 tsp	2	1	0	0	0	0	0	489
Baking soda	1 tsp	0	0	0	0	0	0	0	1,261
Cream of tartar	1 tsp	8	2	0	0	0	0	na	2
Chicken bouillon concentrate	1 cube	6	1	1	Trace	0	0	0	960
Ketchup	1 tbsp	16	4	Trace	Trace	Trace	0	0.2	178
Mustard, prepared	1 tsp	4	Trace	Trace	Trace	Trace	0	na	65
Olives, green	1 oz	33	Trace	Trace	4	Trace	0	0.7	680
Olives, ripe	1 oz	33	2	Trace	3	Trace	0	0.9	247
Salt	1 tsp	0	0	0	0	0	0	0	2,200
Sesame butter (tahini)	1 tbsp	89	3	3	8	1	0	1.4	17
Soy sauce	1 tbsp	10	2	1	Trace	0	0	0	1,029
Vinegar	1 tbsp	2	1	0	0	0	0	0	Trace
Worcestershire sauce	1 tbsp	15	3	1	0	0	0	0	165
Yeast, active dry	1 pkt	21	3	3	Trace	Trace	0	1.9	4

Notes

1. "na" means the information was not available.
2. Trace means a very small amount.

This information is an average of many samples of the item. If a can or package you want to use has a different nutritive analysis, substitute that information for this, but check the portion sizes carefully for the product you want to use.

4

Carbohydrate Counting*

Carbohydrate counting is another meal-planning approach that many people have found to be successful in controlling blood glucose levels. Scientific evidence and clinical observation have shown that carbohydrate in foods is the primary nutrient that affects blood glucose levels. Carbohydrate counting has been used at some medical centers in the United States since 1935 and in Europe for even longer. It is within the last three to five years that it has gained increased popularity for controlling blood glucose levels in persons with diabetes.

When you eat, your blood glucose level goes up; however, your blood glucose level does not always rise the same amount. This is because different types and amounts of foods affect your blood glucose differently. Knowing how certain foods affect your blood sugar can help you control it and keep it at a healthy level.

The type and amount of food that you eat will determine how high and how fast your blood glucose level goes up. Carbohydrate in food affects your blood glucose the most. Carbohydrates are found mainly in breads/starches, cereals, fruits, fruit juices, milk and milk products, carbonated beverages, and desserts. When you know how much carbohydrate you are eating, you can predict what your blood glucose level will be. This is why carbohydrate counting can help you plan the foods you eat.

Eating only small amounts of carbohydrate will cause your blood glucose level to go up. Eating large amounts of carbohy-

---

* This chapter was written by Anne K. Blocker, R.D./L.D., a dietitian friend of mine from Waukon, Iowa.

drate will cause it to go up more. For example, eating two apples will make your blood sugar go higher than eating one apple. In the same way, eating three apples will cause your blood sugar to be higher than if you ate two apples.

Liquid beverages rich in carbohydrate may make your blood glucose rise faster than solid foods. As an example, drinking orange juice will cause your blood sugar to go up more quickly than eating an orange. This happens because solid foods take longer to digest in the body than liquids.

Carbohydrate is found primarily in starches and sugars. Sugars may be natural in foods like fruits or added to foods such as desserts and sauces. Foods that contain carbohydrate include:

- Breads, crackers, and cereals
- Pasta, rice, grains, beans, and legumes
- Vegetables
- Milk and yogurt
- Fruit and juice
- Table sugar, honey, syrup, molasses, jellies and jams, carbonated beverages, etc.

Additionally, many foods contain both carbohydrate and fat. This includes foods like peanut butter, sauces, and salad dressing; sweets, such as cakes, pies, cookies, ice cream, chocolate, and candy; and snack foods such as crackers and chips. Some foods like pizza, casseroles, stews, and soups are a combination of carbohydrate, protein, and fat.

Carbohydrate counting makes it easier for you to eat sugar and sugary foods. However, sugar and sweets contain few vitamins and minerals. Even in small servings they tend to have high amounts of carbohydrate and calories. This means that when these types of foods are used, the portion size should be small.

Carbohydrate information can be found in a variety of places. Carbohydrate is measured in grams. You can use the exchange lists to estimate the carbohydrate content of many foods. Foods listed in the bread/starch exchange contain about 15 grams of carbohydrate per serving, as do foods in the fruit group. Foods in the milk and dairy group contain 12 grams of carbohydrate per serving, and most vegetables have approximately 5 grams of carbohydrate per serving. The starchy vegetables such as corn, peas, squash, and potatoes have 15 grams per serving.

The food label on prepared foods is another way to obtain carbohydrate information. The Nutrition Facts panel on the food label lists the amount of carbohydrate per serving of food. The label will also list the amount of sugar in a food. This information can help you identify a food that may be high in sugar content and low in nutritional value. However, for carbohydrate counting purposes focus on the total grams of carbohydrate in each serving of a food.

In addition to exchange lists and food labels, bookstores and libraries have books that list the carbohydrate in restaurant foods, fast foods, convenience foods, and fresh foods. These books will list the amount of carbohydrate in a serving of food. Many times they will also include other information like calories, sodium, fat, and cholesterol. Two helpful books are *The Complete Book of Food Counts* by Corinne T. Netzer and *The Diabetes Carbohydrate and Fat Gram Guide, 2nd Edition* by Lea Ann Holzmeister.

No matter which carbohydrate-counting system you may choose to use, it is still important to know the portion size of the food you are eating. To do this, you may need to weigh or measure the amount of food you are going to eat.

Your registered dietitian or diabetes educator can help you figure out how much carbohydrate you need to eat at meals and snacks each day. About half of the calories you eat should come from carbohydrate. Keeping carbohydrate intake consistent during the day helps to normalize blood glucose levels.

As much as possible, it is best to spread your carbohydrate foods over the day. This means you should have carbohydrate-containing foods at each meal and/or snack. Spacing your intake of carbohydrates makes it easier for the insulin in your body, or the diabetic medication that you take, to work best.

Carbohydrate counting focuses on keeping the intake of these carbohydrate-containing foods even during the day. Foods with protein and fat such as meat, poultry, fish, nuts, butter, mayonnaise, and margarine do not raise your blood glucose levels as high as carbohydrates do. That is why you do not actually count them in your meal plan. These foods, however, still contain calories and fat and can affect both weight and cholesterol levels. Therefore, these foods must also be used in moderation. Your dietitian or health-care provider can help you determine an amount that is best for you.

As in the exchange system, the carbohydrate-counting meal plan also allows you to use "free" foods. A free food is any food or drink that contains less than 20 calories and 5 grams or less of carbohydrate per serving. Typically, these foods do not need to be counted. However, if you have three servings of a "free" food at one time, then you should count the carbohydrate as this will have an effect on your blood glucose level.

Some people like to count the total amount of carbohydrate consumed during the day. This means that if you need 200 grams of carbohydrate per day, you would count the carbohydrate in all the foods you choose to eat. Ideally, you would divide the 200 grams into three meals and one to two snacks. This would give you about 45 to 60 grams of carbohydrate at each meal and 15 grams at snack time.

While some people like to keep track of all the carbohydrate they eat during the day, others prefer to count servings of food that contain carbohydrate. In this method, a single portion of food is equal to approximately 15 grams of carbohydrate or one carbohydrate choice. People who like the exchange system often find this system simple to use because one serving of bread/starch, fruit, or milk equals one carbohydrate choice. Other foods like meats and fats are recommended in moderation, but total servings are not counted. See Chapter 5, "Planning for Special Menus," for ideas.

Keep in mind that beverages like carbonated soda, fruit drinks, and alcohol also contain carbohydrate. A typical 12-ounce can of soda contains an average of 45 grams of carbohydrate or three carbohydrate choices. As for alcohol, you may have an alcoholic drink occasionally. If you take insulin or an oral diabetic medication, be sure to eat food with your drink. Ask your physician, dietitian, or diabetic educator about a safe amount of alcohol for you and how to successfully work it into your meal plan. The carbohydrate of some typical alcoholic beverages follows.

Beer (12 ounces)
Miller Lite = 12.5 grams carbohydrate
Michelob Lite = 12.5 grams carbohydrate
Regular beer = 15 grams carbohydrate

Mixed Drinks
Bloody Mary (6 ounces) = 6 grams carbohydrate
Screwdriver (6 ounces) = 16 grams carbohydrate
Margarita (8 ounces) = 30 grams carbohydrate

Wines
Chardonnay (6 ounces) = 0 grams carbohydrate
Red wine (6 ounces) = 0 grams carbohydrate
Champagne, brut (4 ounces) = 3.5 grams carbohydrate
Zinfandel (6 ounces) = 4.5 grams carbohydrate
Dessert wines (6 ounces) = 18 grams carbohydrate

When counting carbohydrate choices, try to stay within 5 grams (plus or minus) of your carbohydrate goal at each meal or snack. For example, a person needing 200 grams of carbohydrate each day could have three to four carbohydrate servings at each meal and one carbohydrate serving at each snack.

For some people, carbohydrate counting gives them more flexibility in meal planning. This method is often helpful for those who need to adjust their insulin frequently due to growth, such as children, teenagers, or pregnant women, for persons using an insulin pump or intensive insulin management, for athletes, or for persons whose routines change frequently. As with any health issue, it is recommended that you discuss potential changes with your personal diabetes educator first.

All the recipes in this book contain information on both the exchange system and grams of carbohydrate. If you prefer to count carbohydrate choices, remember that one carbohydrate choice equals 15 grams of carbohydrate. Dividing the total amount of carbohydrate in a portion by 15 will give you the number of carbohydrate choices per recipe portion. I recommend counting 7 to 11 grams as a half carbohydrate choice, 12 to 20 grams as one carbohydrate choice, 21 to 25 grams as one-and-a-half choices, and 26 to 35 grams as two carbohydrate choices. The information listed with each recipe allows you to use the system that works best for you.

5

Planning for Special Menus

Menus can be very helpful when you plan your diabetic diet. Writing down the foods you will use helps clarify the relationship of menu items and makes it easier to see the whole thing in perspective.

It is important to eat everything listed in a diabetic daily meal plan. Changes should not be made without first checking with your doctor. You can sometimes save something from a meal for a snack or eat a little earlier or later than scheduled, but even that must be planned in advance.

When planning menus you may want to try to include the following:

- Six or more servings of whole grains and legumes (beans) daily
- A varied diet with selections from the major food groups, including fat-free and low-fat dairy products, lean meats, and poultry
- At least two servings weekly of fatty fish such as tuna or salmon

Desserts and other less necessary extras are included only after all other nutritional needs have been met. Because fiber is helpful to most people, you should try to include as many foods rich in fiber as possible.

All of the necessary ingredients for a well-balanced menu are included in the diabetic daily food plan, so if you are following your food plan you needn't worry about having a balanced diet.

The following guidelines will help you plan your menus. However, your own doctor, dietitian, or nutritionist may develop a different plan for you depending on your age, sex, and physical activity.

I hope you will find the following menus useful and that they will help you find ways to include new items—especially the recipes in this book—in your own diet plans.

BASIC DAILY FOOD EXCHANGE ALLOWANCE AT DIFFERENT CALORIC LEVELS

Exchanges	1,200	1,400	1,600	1,800	2,000
Breakfast					
Carbohydrate group					
Starch	2	2	2	2	2
Fruit	1	1	1	1	1
Skim milk	1	1	1	1	1
Meat group	–	–	–	–	–
Fat group	1	1	1	1	1
Lunch or dinner at noon					
Carbohydrate group					
Starch	2	2	2	2	3
Fruit	1	1	1	1	1
Skim milk	–	–	–	½	½
Meat group (lean)	3	3	3	3	3
Vegetables	1	1	1	1	1
Fat group	1	1	1	2	2
Dinner or supper in the evening					
Carbohydrate group					
Starch	1	2	2	3	3
Fruit	1	1	1	1	1
Skim milk	–	–	–	½	½
Meat group (lean)	2	2	3	3	3
Vegetables	1	2	2	2	2
Fat group	–	1	1	1	1

Exchanges	1,200	1,400	1,600	1,800	2,000
Evening snack					
Carbohydrate group					
Starch	–	–	1	1	1
Fruit	1	1	1	1	2
Skim milk	1	1	1	1	1
Fat group	–	–	–	–	1

For persons who wish to count carbohydrate choices, total the food items from the carbohydrate group to determine the total number of carbohydrate choices recommended per meal. For example, at breakfast, a person eating 1,200 calories could have four carbohydrate choices, a total of the two starches, one fruit, and one milk.

For someone counting grams of carbohydrate per meal, multiply the total carbohydrate choices by 15. The 1,200 calorie breakfast with four carbohydrate choices would allow 60 grams of carbohydrate (4 servings × 15 grams/serving choice = 60 grams).

When counting carbohydrate, choices of carbohydrate can come from any combination of milk, bread/starch, fruit, or sugary foods. The exchange system provides guidelines for a balanced distribution of nutrients and carbohydrate for the day.

The menu plan is based on the groups in the new exchange lists. Please remember that not all of your starch exchanges need to be used for bread. Starch exchanges can also be used for starchy vegetables and items from the other food groups such as the "other carbohydrates" group or high-fiber bran muffins; of course, you can use part of them for some simple desserts such as ice milk, frozen yogurt, or angel food cake.

The number of exchanges for each diet is based on the following table, which lists the number of exchanges for different caloric levels and the percentages of carbohydrate, protein, and fat included at the different levels. As you see, the table follows the high-carbohydrate, low-fat, and moderate-protein diet recommended by the American Diabetes Association, Inc., and the American Dietetic Association.

After the basic menu is planned, it must be extended to provide a diet modification at each level of the diabetic diet. The following menus have been extended with a column for each of the levels of the diet. To read the menu, find the diet heading that you need and then plan to use everything in that column for your diet for that meal. Some foods are free and you can use as much of them as you like—that is indicated, as well as the portion size for each item.

MENU PLAN FOR DIABETIC DIETS

Exchanges	1,200	1,400	1,600	1,800	2,000
Carbohydrate group					
Starch	5	6	7	8	9
Fruit	4	4	5	5	6
Skim milk	2	2	2	3	3
Meat group (lean)	5	5	6	6	6
Fat group	2	3	3	4	5
Vegetables	2	3	3	3	3
Total calories	1,235	1,385	1,580	1,795	1,980
Percentages					
Carbohydrate	57	57	55	58	58
Protein	24	23	23	22	21
Fat	19	20	22	20	21
Total percent	100	100	100	100	100

For persons counting carbohydrate grams or choices, the following conversions from the exchange table can be used:

Caloric level	1,200	1,400	1,600	1,800	2,000
Carbohydrate grams	165	180	210	240	270
Carbohydrate choices	11	12	14	16	18

You should also be aware that many doctors, dietitians, and nutritionists are counseling their patients to count the total amount of carbohydrate they consume at each meal rather than follow the diet plan we have just discussed. This has been very successful in many cases and you should try it if you are advised to do so. This table can be used for carbohydrate counting or the exchange system. Because it gives you good advice and follows a healthy meal plan based on the Food Guide pyramid with choices from all areas, it is a suggested healthy eating model. Most commercial food products give you the carbohydrate value per serving, and the recipes in this book also give you the carbohydrate content per portion for each recipe.

Breakfast

Orange or grapefruit juice
Cereal
Skim milk
Hard boiled egg
Bran Muffin*
Coffee or tea

Food Item	1,200	1,400	1,600	1,800	2,000
Orange or grapefruit juice	4 ounces at all levels of the diet				
½ cup cooked or ¾ cup unsweetened prepared cereal	1 serving at all levels of the diet				
Skim milk	8 ounces at all levels of the diet				
Hard boiled egg	1 egg at all levels of the diet				
Bran Muffin	1 at all levels of the diet				
Coffee or tea	as desired at all levels of the diet				
Fruit exchange for morning snack			1	1	1

Menu notes: The Bran Muffin may also be saved for a morning snack, if desired. If you choose a bran muffin that includes only a half fat exchange, the remaining half fat exchange could be margarine or a half serving of Cinnamon Spread.*

Carbohydrate information:
(not counting the morning snack)

Caloric level	1,200–1,600	1,800	2,000
Carbohydrate grams	57	57	57
Carbohydrate choices	4	4	4

*See Index.

Breakfast

Orange juice
Sliced fresh peaches
Shredded wheat
Ham
Cinnamon Roll*
Margarine
Skim milk
Coffee or tea

Food Item	1,200	1,400	1,600	1,800	2,000
Orange juice			4 oz	4 oz	4 oz
Sliced unsweetened fresh, frozen, or canned peaches	½ cup at all levels of the diet				
Shredded wheat	1 large biscuit at all levels of the diet				
Ham slice	1 ounce at all levels of the diet				
Cinnamon Roll	1 at all levels of the diet				
Margarine	½ teaspoon at all levels of the diet				
Skim milk	8 ounces at all levels of the diet				
Coffee or tea	as desired at all levels of the diet				

Menu notes: One slice whole wheat toast and 1 teaspoon margarine may be substituted for the Cinnamon Roll and ½ teaspoon margarine.

Carbohydrate information:

Caloric level	1,200–1,400	1,600–2,000
Carbohydrate grams	59	74
Carbohydrate choices	4	5

*See Index.

Breakfast

Orange juice
Cereal
Skim milk
Coffee or tea

Morning Coffee with Friends

Chocolate Nut Bread*
Pastel Cookie*
Fresh fruit cup with Orange Liqueur*
Coffee or tea

Food Item	1,200	1,400	1,600	1,800	2,000
Breakfast					
Orange juice	4 oz	4 oz	4 oz	4 oz	4 oz
½ cup cooked or ¾ cup unsweetened prepared cereal	1 serving 1,200 to 1,400–calorie level; 2 servings at 1,600 to 2,000–calorie level				
Skim milk	8 oz at all levels of the diet				
Coffee or tea	as desired at all levels of the diet				

Carbohydrate information:

Caloric level	1,200–1,400	1,600–2,000
Carbohydrate grams	42	57
Carbohydrate choices	3	4

*See Index.

Morning Coffee with Friends

Chocolate Nut Bread	½ slice at all levels of the diet
Pastel Cookie	1 at all levels of the diet
Fresh fruit cup with Orange Liqueur	½ cup fruit with ½ teaspoon Orange Liqueur at all levels of the diet
Coffee or tea	as desired at all levels of the diet

Menu notes: The Chocolate Nut Bread and one Pastel Cookie give you one starch and one fat exchange. You can substitute any other foods that total one starch and one fat exchange for your morning coffee, if desired.

Carbohydrate information:
All caloric levels

Carbohydrate grams	32
Carbohydrate choices	2

The purpose of the Morning Coffee with Friends and the Lunch or Dinner (and) Afternoon Tea menus is to show that you can save food from a meal to use as a snack in the morning, afternoon, or evening. However, this is meant to be a guide and should be changed according to your own schedule. Non-insulin-dependent persons have more leeway in their diet than do insulin-dependent persons. If you are insulin dependent, you should check with your doctor or dietitian before attempting any drastic reduction in any of your menus.

Salad Luncheon

at noon

Hot Beef Bouillon* with melba toast rounds
Chef's Salad*
Raisin Bread*
Cinnamon Spread*
Coleslaw*
Skim milk
Pineapple Gelatin*
Whipped Topping*
Coffee or tea

Food Item	1,200	1,400	1,600	1,800	2,000
Hot Beef Bouillon	as desired at all levels of the diet				
Melba toast rounds					5
Chef's Salad with 1 extra ounce meat or chicken	1 serving at all levels of the diet				
Raisin Bread	1 slice at all levels of the diet				
Cinnamon Spread	2 tsp	2 tsp	2 tsp	1½ T	1½ T
or					
Margarine	1 tsp	1 tsp	1 tsp	2 tsp	2 tsp
Coleslaw	½ cup at all levels of the diet				
Skim milk				4 oz	4 oz
Pineapple Gelatin	1 serving at all levels of the diet				
Whipped Topping	2 tablespoons at all levels of the diet				
Coffee or tea	as desired at all levels of the diet				

*See Index.

Menu notes: Prepare Pineapple Gelatin using ½ cup crushed, canned unsweetened pineapple per serving in Fruit-Flavored Gelatin* or sugar-free gelatin. As much gelatin as desired may be used per serving.

Use recipe for Beef Broth* to prepare Hot Beef Bouillon.

Raisin Bread may be toasted or served at room temperature.

Carbohydrate information:

Caloric level	1,200–1,600	1,800	2,000
Carbohydrate grams	46	52	64
Carbohydrate choices	3	3.5	4

*See Index.

Lunch or Dinner

at noon

Broiled round steak
Stir-Fry Tomatoes*
Lettuce salad with Creamy Garlic Dressing*
Unsweetened applesauce
Skim milk, coffee, or tea

Afternoon Tea

Devil's Food Cake* with Fluffy Frosting*
High-Fiber Cookies*
Graham crackers
Sparkling Punch*
Coffee or tea

Food Item	1,200	1,400	1,600	1,800	2,000
Lunch or Dinner at Noon					
Broiled round steak	3 ounces cooked weight at all levels of the diet				
Stir-Fry Tomatoes	about ¾ cup at all levels of the diet				
Lettuce salad	as desired at all levels of the diet				
Creamy Garlic Dressing	up to 2 tablespoons at all levels of the diet				
Unsweetened applesauce	½ cup at all levels of the diet				
Skim milk				4 oz	4 oz
Coffee or tea	as desired at all levels of the diet				

Carbohydrate information:

Caloric level	1,200–1,600	1,800–2,000
Carbohydrate grams	23	29
Carbohydrate choices	1.5	2

*See Index.

Food Item	1,200	1,400	1,600	1,800	2,000
Afternoon Tea					
Devil's Food Cake	1 square at all levels of the diet				
Fluffy Frosting	1½ tablespoons at all levels of the diet				
High-Fiber Cookies				1	1
Graham crackers	3	3	3	3	3
Sparkling Punch	as desired at all levels of the diet				
Coffee or tea	as desired at all levels of the diet				

Menu notes: This menu does not have to be followed exactly but can serve as a guide. You can substitute other foods with the same exchange values for any food in the menu or you can add free foods such as a relish plate of free food in the afternoon as long as you stay within the guidelines for your diet.

It is easier to control the menu when you serve it in your own home, but you can remember food exchanges and maintain your own diet if you are careful when you go to parties.

If finger sandwiches are served, pick ones with a plain filling and consider each finger sandwich as a half bread exchange if it is a double sandwich with the crusts trimmed off and with a plain filling.

Carbohydrate information:

Caloric level	1,200–1,600	1,800	2,000
Carbohydrate grams	37	39	54
Carbohydrate choices	2.5	2.5	3.5

Vegetable Beef Soup

evening

Vegetable Beef Soup* with melba toast rounds
Lettuce salad with Spicy Tomato Dressing*
Mrs. Riley's Pickles*
Plain roll
Vanilla ice milk
Chocolate Sauce*
Unsweetened pineapple
Skim milk
Coffee or tea

Food Item	1,200	1,400	1,600	1,800	2,000
Vegetable Beef Soup	¾ cup	¾ cup	1 cup	1 cup	1 cup
Melba toast rounds	5	8	8	8	8
Lettuce salad	as desired at all levels of the diet				
Spicy Tomato Dressing	2 tablespoons at all levels of the diet				
Mrs. Riley's Pickles	up to ¼ cup at all levels of the diet				
Small plain roll				1	1
Vanilla ice milk		½ cup	½ cup	½ cup	½ cup
Chocolate Sauce		2 tbsp	2 tbsp	2 tbsp	2 tbsp
Unsweetened pineapple	½ cup at all levels of the diet				
Skim milk				4 oz	4 oz
Coffee or tea	as desired at all levels of the diet				

Carbohydrate information:

Caloric level	1,200	1,400	1,600	1,800–2,000
Carbohydrate grams	35	64	66	87
Carbohydrate choices	2	4	4	6

*See Index.

Soup and Sandwich

at noon

Tomato Bouillon* with melba toast rounds
Chicken Sandwich Spread* on Rich Whole Wheat Bread*
with Miracle Whip and lettuce
Relish plate (sliced dill pickles,
green pepper sticks, radishes)
Three-Bean Salad*
Fresh pear
Skim milk, coffee, or tea

Food Item	1,200	1,400	1,600	1,800	2,000
Tomato Bouillon	1 cup at all levels of the diet				
Melba toast rounds					5
Chicken Sandwich Spread	⅓ cup at all levels of the diet				
Rich Whole Wheat Bread	2 slices at all levels of the diet				
Miracle Whip salad dressing	2 tsp	2 tsp	2 tsp	4 tsp	4 tsp
Lettuce for sandwich	as desired at all levels of the diet				
Relish plate	as desired at all levels of the diet				
Three-Bean Salad	½ cup at all levels of the diet				
Pear	1 small fresh or canned at all levels of the diet				
Skim milk				4 oz	4 oz
Coffee or tea	as desired at all levels of the diet				

Menu notes: Three ounces of sliced turkey or chicken with fat and gristle removed may be substituted for the Chicken Sandwich Spread, if desired. Two teaspoons of Miracle Whip salad dressing is equal to 1 teaspoon margarine; margarine may be substituted, if desired.

Carbohydrate information:

Caloric level	1,200–1,600	1,800	2,000
Carbohydrate grams	63	66	81
Carbohydrate choices	4	4	5

*See Index.

Minestrone Soup

evening

Minestrone Soup* with melba toast rounds
Coleslaw*
Unsweetened blueberries or blackberries
Plain roll
Key Lime Pie*
Skim milk, coffee, or tea

Food Item	1,200	1,400	1,600	1,800	2,000
Minestrone Soup	1 cup at all levels of the diet				
Melba toast rounds	2	5	5	5	5
Extra ounce(s) of lean meat to be added to each serving of soup	1 oz	1 oz	2 oz	2 oz	2 oz
Coleslaw	½ cup at all levels of the diet				
Unsweetened fresh or frozen blueberries or blackberries	¾ cup at all levels of the diet				
Small plain roll				1	1
Key Lime Pie		⅛ pie	⅛ pie	⅛ pie	⅛ pie
Skim milk				4 oz	4 oz
Coffee or tea	as desired at all levels of the diet				

Carbohydrate information:

Caloric level	1,200	1,400–1,600	1,800–2,000
Carbohydrate grams	41	63	84
Carbohydrate choices	3	4	5.5

*See Index.

Fish for Dinner or Supper

evening

Baked Halibut Steak* with Tartar Sauce*
Broccoli Rice Casserole*
Steamed carrots
Baked potato
Plain roll
Unsweetened fresh or frozen strawberries
Skim milk, coffee, or tea

Food Item	1,200	1,400	1,600	1,800	2,000
Baked Halibut Steak, cooked weight	2 oz	2 oz	3 oz	3 oz	3 oz
Tartar Sauce	up to 2 tablespoons at all levels of the diet				
Broccoli Rice Casserole		½ cup	½ cup	½ cup	½ cup
Steamed carrots	½ cup				
Baked potato	1 sm	1 med	1 med	1 med	1 med
Small plain roll				1	1
Unsweetened fresh or frozen strawberries	1¼ cups at all levels of the diet				
Skim milk				4 oz	4 oz
Coffee or tea	as desired at all levels of the diet				

Menu notes: Strawberries may be molded in unsweetened fruit gelatin, if desired, at all levels of the diet.

Use recipe for Baked Fish Steak* to prepare Baked Halibut Steak.

Carbohydrate information:

Caloric level	1,200	1,400–1,600	1,800–2,000
Carbohydrate grams	37	47	64
Carbohydrate choices	2.5	3	4.5

*See Index.

Labor Day Picnic

at noon

Hamburger on a bun with lettuce, ketchup,
mustard, and pickle relish
Potato Salad*
Pickled Vegetables*
Tossed vegetable salad with Vinaigrette Dressing*
Cubed fresh watermelon
Skim milk, coffee, tea, or Sparkling Punch*
Buttermilk Cookies*

Food Item	1,200	1,400	1,600	1,800	2,000
Hamburger, raw weight	4 ounces at all levels of the diet				
Hamburger bun	1 small at all levels of the diet				
Margarine				1 tsp	1 tsp
Lettuce	as desired at all levels of the diet				
Ketchup	1 tablespoon at all levels of the diet				
Mustard	1 teaspoon at all levels of the diet				
Pickle relish	1 teaspoon at all levels of the diet				
Potato Salad	½ cup at all levels of the diet				
Pickled Vegetables	½ cup at all levels of the diet				
Tossed vegetable salad	as desired at all levels of the diet				
Vinaigrette Dressing	2 tablespoons at all levels of the diet				
Cubed watermelon	1 cup at all levels of the diet				
Skim milk				4 oz	4 oz
Buttermilk cookies					2
Coffee, tea, or Sparkling Punch	as desired at all levels of the diet				

*See Index.

Menu notes: The tossed salad should be something beautiful, with fresh vegetables that are low in carbohydrate so everyone can eat all they want of it. It might include broccoli spears, cauliflower slices, mushrooms, green peppers julienne, a little red cabbage—anything that is colorful, fresh, and low in calories—along with fresh crisp lettuce or other greens such as escarole or spinach.

Carbohydrate information:

Caloric level	1,200–1,600	1,800	2,000
Carbohydrate grams	67	73	85
Carbohydrate choices	4	5	5.5

Thanksgiving

Dinner at noon

Tomato Bouillon*
Roast turkey
Bread Dressing*
Turkey Gravy*
Baked sweet potato
Broccoli
Cranberry Gelatin Salad* with Kay's Cooked Dressing*
Relish plate (green pepper strips, dill pickles,
carrot and celery strips)
Margarine
Skim milk, coffee, or tea
Pumpkin Scotch Pie* with Whipped Topping*

Food Item	1,200	1,400	1,600	1,800	2,000
Tomato Bouillon	1 cup at all levels of the diet				
Roast Turkey	3 ounces cooked weight at all levels of the diet				
Bread Dressing	1 square at all levels of the diet				
Turkey Gravy	¼ cup at all levels of the diet				
Baked sweet potato	1 small at 1,200 to 1,800–calorie level; 1 medium at 2,000–calorie level				
Broccoli	½ cup at all levels of the diet				
Cranberry Gelatin Salad	1 square at all levels of the diet				
Kay's Cooked Dressing	1 tablespoon at all levels of the diet				
Relish plate	as desired at all levels of the diet				
Margarine			1 tsp		
Skim milk				4 oz	8 oz
Pumpkin Scotch Pie	⅛ pie at all levels of the diet				
Whipped Topping	2 tablespoons at all levels of the diet				
Coffee or tea	as desired at all levels of the diet				

*See Index.

Carbohydrate information:

Caloric level	1,200–1,600	1,800	2,000
Carbohydrate grams	47	53	68
Carbohydrate choices	3	3.5	4

Christmas Day

Dinner at noon

Hot Beef Bouillon*
Roast Beef
Mashed potatoes
Brown Gravy*
Stewed Cranberries*
Cauliflower
Relish plate (Mrs. Riley's Pickles,*
carrot and celery sticks)
Banana gelatin with Kay's Cooked Dressing*
Small plain roll
Margarine
Skim milk, coffee, or tea
Strawberry Chiffon Pie*

Food Item	1,200	1,400	1,600	1,800	2,000
Hot Beef Bouillon	1 cup at all levels of the diet				
Roast Beef	3 ounces at all levels of the diet				
Mashed potatoes	½ cup at all levels of the diet				
Brown Gravy	¼ cup at all levels of the diet				
Stewed Cranberries	½ cup at all levels of the diet				
Cauliflower	½ cup at all levels of the diet				
Relish plate	as desired at all levels of the diet				
Banana gelatin	1 serving at all levels of the diet				
Kay's Cooked Dressing	1 tablespoon at all levels of the diet				
Small plain roll					1
Margarine				1 tsp	1 tsp
Skim milk				4 oz	4 oz
Strawberry Chiffon Pie	⅛ pie at all levels of the diet				
Coffee or tea	as desired at all levels of the diet				

*See Index.

Menu notes: Prepare banana gelatin by using ½ banana per person in Fruit-Flavored Gelatin.*

Use recipe for Beef Broth* to prepare Hot Beef Bouillon.

Carbohydrate information:

Caloric level	1,200–1,600	1,800	2,000
Carbohydrate grams	56	62	77
Carbohydrate choices	4	4	5

New Year's Day

Dinner at noon

Fruit Soup* with melba toast rounds
Baked ham
Escalloped potatoes
Creole Green Beans*
Tossed vegetable salad with Vinaigrette Dressing*
Stewed Cranberries*
Relish tray (dill pickles, celery, and carrot sticks)
Skim milk, coffee, or tea
Lemon Pie*

Food Item	1,200	1,400	1,600	1,800	2,000
Fruit Soup	½ cup at all levels of the diet				
Melba toast rounds					5
Baked ham	3 ounces at all levels of the diet				
Escalloped potatoes	½ cup at all levels of the diet				
Creole Green Beans	½ cup at all levels of the diet				
Tossed vegetable salad	as desired at all levels of the diet				
Vinaigrette Dressing	2 tablespoons at all levels of the diet				
Stewed Cranberries	½ cup at all levels of the diet				
Relish tray	as desired at all levels of the diet				
Skim milk				4 oz	4 oz
Margarine				1 tsp	1 tsp
Lemon Pie	⅛ pie at all levels of the diet				
Coffee or tea	as desired at all levels of the diet				

Carbohydrate information:

Caloric level	1,200–1,600	1,800	2,000
Carbohydrate grams	67	73	85
Carbohydrate choices	4	5	5.5

*See Index.

6

Cholesterol

Research indicates that the majority of all persons with diabetes die of atherosclerosis or related diseases. Therefore, the American Medical Association, the American Diabetes Association, and the American Heart Association all stress the importance of keeping your cholesterol count below 200 mg/dl. Regular exercise and a sensible diet is a good way to maintain and/or lower your blood cholesterol level. This includes eating less saturated fatty acids and controlling your weight. Some very good medications have been developed to help lower your blood cholesterol level, but it is still a good idea to avoid foods high in fat, which are known to elevate blood cholesterol levels.

It isn't hard to follow a low-cholesterol diet, and it is simple to plan your diabetic diet using low-cholesterol guidelines. Both ways of eating emphasize decreased sugar and fat intake with a moderate amount of meat, fruits, and vegetables, and a moderate amount of complex carbohydrates.

I have been following low-cholesterol guidelines for years since our doctor put my husband Chuck on a low-cholesterol diet when we were first married. Since I liked the food prepared that way, I always ate what I had already prepared for him and didn't need to change to a low-cholesterol diet after I was diagnosed with diabetes.

Because it is important for anyone with diabetes to follow a low-cholesterol diet, the following information based on the American Heart Association's guidelines will help you do so.

AMERICAN HEART ASSOCIATION
DIETARY GUIDELINES 2000

General Information

New focus has been placed on an overall dietary pattern based on foods, rather than nutrient components. For example, the recommendations suggest individuals eat:

- At least five servings of fruits and vegetables daily
- Six or more servings of whole grains and legumes (beans) daily
- A varied diet with selections from the major food groups, including fat-free and low-fat dairy products, lean meats, and poultry
- At least two servings weekly of fatty fish such as tuna or salmon

By following this eating plan, most people will be able to focus on the positive message of selecting healthy foods, rather than trying to follow a diet based on percentages. However, the recommended percentages of food components remain the same.

The guidelines emphasize the importance of attaining and maintaining healthy body weight, and for the first time, the association emphasizes the prevention of obesity.

Additionally, specific dietary recommendations are now included that address lipid disorders, the elderly, children, diabetes, congestive heart failure, and kidney disease.

Body Weight

Balancing food intake with physical activity is still recommended as a means to achieve and maintain a healthy body weight. However, because weight gain often accompanies aging, and children and adolescents are getting heavier overall, prevention of weight gain is a high priority because it is very difficult to lose and then maintain a lower body weight. At least 30 minutes of brisk walking is recommended daily to help balance calorie intakes. The walking can be done in segments or all at once. (The *American*

Diabetes Association 2001 Clinical Practice Recommendations suggest persons with diabetes strive for an HDL cholesterol level of greater than 45 mg/dl in men and greater than 55 mg/dl in women to lower the risk of cardiovascular disease.)

LDL Cholesterol

LDL cholesterol is low-density lipoprotein, the "bad" cholesterol. The major components that raise LDL cholesterol are saturated fats, trans fatty acids, and to a lesser extent, dietary cholesterol—the cholesterol found in food, rather than manufactured by the body. Based on limited information, the American Heart Association recommends limiting trans fatty acid intake by substituting soft margarines for hard. (The *American Diabetes Association 2001 Clinical Practice Recommendations* suggest persons with diabetes strive to maintain an LDL cholesterol level of less than 100 mg/dl.)

Trans Fatty Acids and Saturated Fat

The association recommends that healthy adults minimize the intake of foods containing high levels of saturated fats (found in animal products and tropical oils) and substantially reduce the intake of trans fatty acids (the hydrogenated oil found in commercially prepared foods and some hard margarines). If an individual eats a diet low in saturated fats, in all likelihood he or she will also be eating a diet low in dietary cholesterol. For individuals with risk factors for heart disease or existing heart disease, a further reduction in saturated fats is recommended. The Food and Drug Administration is considering the labeling of foods for trans fatty acids. At that time, the American Heart Association will issue an update on the subject.

Dietary Cholesterol

The recommended intake of dietary cholesterol remains the same—however, individuals may choose to eat one egg yolk daily, if the amount of foods high in dietary cholesterol in the rest of the diet is very limited.

Triglycerides and Sugar

Choose a diet moderate in sugar. High levels of triglycerides—blood fats—may be a risk factor for heart disease, and triglycerides react with other factors, such as LDL. For individuals with elevated triglycerides, attaining a healthy body weight is important, as is reducing the intake of sugar and refined carbohydrates, especially if the individual is also insulin resistant. In addition, drinking alcoholic beverages can elevate triglyceride levels. (The *American Diabetes Association 2001 Clinical Practice Recommendations* recommend persons with diabetes try to maintain a triglyceride level of less than 200 mg/dl to lower the risk of cardiovascular disease.)

Salt

It is recommended that the general public consume no more than 6 grams of sodium daily. This recommendation is unchanged from previous guidelines. The guidelines note that the high-quality evidence provided by the landmark study *DASH (Dietary Approach to Stop Hypertension)*, which showed that a dietary pattern such as the one recommended by the American Heart Association can result in a substantial decrease in blood pressure for both people with elevated blood pressure and those with normal blood pressure.

Alcohol

Alcohol intake should be limited to no more than one drink a day for women and two drinks a day for men, in individuals who already drink alcoholic beverages. If you drink, do so in moderation. Some studies have shown a lower incidence in heart disease in moderate drinkers, but add the important caveat that increased consumption of alcohol can lead to hypertension, obesity, stroke, and other extremely serious health and social issues.

Fish

Because a growing body of evidence indicates that foods rich in omega-3 fatty acids confer cardioprotective effects, the association specifically recommends eating at least two servings of fish each week. The association continues to recommend getting omega-3 fatty acids from fish, not fish oil capsules.

Considerations for Special Populations

Specific guidelines are suggested for the elderly, children, and those with specific medical conditions such as elevated LDL cholesterol with cardiovascular disease, diabetes, congestive heart failure, kidney disease, and a cluster of metabolic factors that include insulin resistance, high blood pressure, and elevated cholesterol. See your health-care provider if you have any of these conditions.

High Unsaturated Fat Diets

A diet high in unsaturated fats and low in saturated fat can be a viable alternative to a diet that is very low in saturated fat.

Ancillary Lifestyle and Dietary Issues

Smoking   The guidelines cite the "overwhelming evidence for the adverse effects of smoking," and counsel that concern about weight gain should not be a reason to continue to smoke.

Very Low Fat Diets   "Although in certain individuals under physician supervision, very low fat diets may lead to a weight loss and improved lipid profiles, they are not recommended for the general population." Diets with less than 15 percent of calories derived from fat have been advocated by some. There is little evidence about the potential value of such diets. At present, a diet of 25 to 30 percent fat is adequate for the general population.

High Protein Diets   There is at present no scientific evidence to support the concept that high protein diets result in sustained weight loss, significant changes in metabolism, or improved health.

Persons with diabetes often have little trouble following the low-cholesterol diet because it fits into our meal plan perfectly.

A balanced meal plan will almost automatically give us the right amount of meat, fish, or poultry each day, as well as include the right amount of fruits, vegetables, and breads. Our diabetic diet wouldn't eliminate coconut, coconut oil, or palm oil, but since that is part of the low-cholesterol diet, we only have to read labels carefully to be sure we avoid foods containing these ingredients.

If you choose meats from the lean meat exchanges shown in Chapter 2, you will have no trouble choosing the right meat, fish, or poultry entrées. The high-fat or even the medium-fat exchanges contain too much fat for a good low-cholesterol diet.

Some Eating Plan Tips

The American Heart Association, the American Dietetic Association, and the American Diabetes Association have all contributed background information for the following guidelines to help you keep the fat and cholesterol content of your diabetic diet at a manageable level.

1. Trim all visible fat off the meat before cooking.

2. Place browned ground beef in a colander and rinse with one to two quarts of very hot water to wash away as much fat as possible. Drain well and proceed with your recipe.

3. Use cooking methods that do not use much fat such as baking, broiling, roasting, grilling, steaming, poaching, stir-frying, sautéing, or using a microwave.

4. Use skim, 1 percent, or non-fat dry milk and low-fat yogurt and cheese.

5. Save your fat exchanges for fried or baked items.

6. Chill soups, broths, and stews so you can remove the hardened fat from them before you use them.

7. Use low-fat recipes featuring vegetables, fruits, and pastas.

8. Use a nonstick cooking spray or a nonstick pan to brown or fry foods.

9. Do not add flour, breadcrumbs, coating mixes, or fat to the foods when preparing them.

10. Weigh meat after removing bones and fat and after it is cooked. Three ounces of cooked meat is about equal to 4 ounces of raw meat.

11. Organ meats such as liver, brains, chitterlings, heart, gizzards, and sweetbreads are very high in cholesterol. However, liver is rich in iron and vitamins, and a 3-ounce serving once a month is okay.

12. Use whole turkeys that have not been injected with fat or broth. Remove the fat and skin from poultry before it is cooked. If you are roasting a chicken or turkey the skin can be left on during baking to help keep the meat from getting dry while it is cooking. The skin should be removed before the meat is carved.

13. When dried beans, peas, or lentils are used as a meat substitute, l cup cooked dried beans, peas, or lentils provides two starches and one lean meat exchange and 3 grams of fiber.

14. Shrimp and crayfish are higher in cholesterol than most meat and poultry. I suggest that you restrict yourself to one serving of them per month.

Some examples of meat portions are as follows: Two ounces (two meat exchanges) are equal to one small chicken leg or thigh or ½ cup cottage cheese or tuna. Three ounces (three meat exchanges) are equal to one medium pork chop, one small hamburger patty, half of a whole chicken breast, one unbreaded 4-ounce fish fillet, or cooked meat about the size of a deck of cards.

Remember to count any egg yolks used in cooking or in purchased, prepared baked items. None of the recipes in this book require egg yolks. Instead, you'll use egg whites and liquid egg substitute. You can feel free to use your egg allowance as you see fit. If you want to use your egg allowance in baked goods, substitute one large whole egg for ¼ cup liquid egg substitute or two large egg whites.

You should also watch the fat content of dairy products. It is best to choose 1 percent milk or nonfat fluid milk, low-fat powdered dry milk, evaporated skim milk, buttermilk made from skim milk, and low-fat or nonfat fresh or frozen yogurt. There are also some low-fat cheeses such as dry-curd, skim, or low-fat cottage cheese and natural or processed cheese with no more than 5 grams of fat per ounce.

Vegetables and fruits are high in vitamins and fiber and low in fat, sodium, and calories. You should include at least one serving high in vitamin C such as orange, grapefruit, or tomato juice, citrus fruits or tomatoes every day and one serving of foods high in vitamin A such as broccoli, squash, or dark-colored vegetables several times weekly according to your meal plan.

Breads, cereals, pasta, and starchy vegetables are high in complex carbohydrates and low in fat and cholesterol. They are also a good source of vitamin B, iron, and fiber and tend to be moderate in calories. It's the fatty sauces we add to them that make them high in calories. Good choices in this group include:

1. Low-fat breads such as whole wheat, rye, raisin, and white bread. Italian and French breads are traditionally made with very little fat.

2. Low-fat rolls such as English muffins, pita breads, frankfurter and hamburger rolls, and bagels, except for egg bagels.

3. Low-fat crackers and snacks such as saltines, matzos, bread sticks, melba toast, flat bread, and pretzels.

4. Yeast or quick breads made at home using approved ingredients such as nonfat dry milk, egg whites or liquid egg substitutes, vegetable oil or margarine.

5. Hot or cold cereals, all kinds except granola-type cereals with coconut, coconut oil, or palm oil. (Persons with diabetes should also limit the use of cereals sweetened with sugar.)

6. Rice and pasta of all kinds except those made with egg yolks. Read the labels when purchasing these foods to make sure

they include only approved ingredients. Try to buy those items made with whole-wheat flour, if possible, and without egg yolks.

Fats and oils are high in vitamin A and E but are also high in fat and calories. (There are 9 calories per gram of fat and only 4 calories per gram of carbohydrates and protein.) Remember to include the hidden fat in bakery products and snack foods, in cooking, and in desserts and breads. Try to use preparation methods that use little or no fat. Using a nonstick pan or a vegetable pan spray are two ways to do this. The following guidelines should help you choose the best sources of fat for your diet. Keep in mind that you do need some fat in your diet. A completely fat-free diet is not healthy or well balanced.

1. Avoid solid fats and shortening, butter, bacon fat, lard, salt pork, ham hocks, meat fat and drippings, shortenings, and margarine made with lard or other unacceptable fats.

2. Avoid chocolate (cocoa is OK), coconut, coconut oil, palm oil, and palm kernel oil, which are often used in bakery products, nondairy creamers, whipped toppings, candy, and commercially fried foods. Read all labels carefully to see if any of those ingredients are present in the products.

3. Use light, tub, or soft margarine made with safflower, sunflower, corn, or soybean oil. Partially hydrogenated soybean or cottonseed oils may also be used.

Oils in order of their increasing saturated fatty acid content are safflower, sunflower, corn, and partially hydrogenated soybean and cottonseed oils.

Seeds and nuts may be used except for cashews, macadamia, and pistachio. Peanut butter may be used within the limits of your diabetic diet, but remember that nut butters are very high in fat.

Most of our diabetic diets allow for some snacks, but we should follow our low-cholesterol diet as well as our diabetic diet when we are eating those snacks. The following list, based on information from the American Heart Association, can help you choose your snacks wisely.

1. First choice items that are low in calories include raw vegetables, fresh fruit, fruit canned or frozen without sugar, sugar-free gelatin, tea, coffee, cocoa powder, and sugar-free soft drinks.

2. Second choice foods that are low in saturated fats and fairly low in calories include dried fruits; seeds; approved nuts; plain popcorn; pretzels, crackers, cookies, or cake without egg yolks; sherbet; ice milk; low-fat frozen yogurt; and angel food cake.

3. Other choices include diabetic desserts made with little or no sugar (see Introduction) and low-fat milk products.

4. Alcoholic beverages should be consumed in moderation within the framework of your meal plan.

5. Limit foods not recommended in your diabetic diet including baked goods and mixes that you think might include hidden ingredients high in fat and/or sugar, fructose, high fructose corn syrup, etc. (Always read the ingredient list, if available.) Limit foods containing coconut, high-fat items such as cream or whole milk, snacks that have been fried, and high-fat cheeses.

If you are on a low-cholesterol diet, you may use any of the recipes in this book, secure in the knowledge that they are suitable for a low-cholesterol diet. These recipes can also be helpful for anyone on a low-cholesterol diet who is interested in cutting calories to lose weight.

7

Equipment and Ingredients

EQUIPMENT

Having and using the right equipment is a plus when you are preparing your low-cholesterol diabetic diet.

Knives

Sharp knives to prepare fruits and vegetables and to cut away all visible fat from meat and chicken are important. Kitchen scissors are also very helpful for removing fat from meat. A good chopping knife and a knife with a serrated edge for slicing bread will prove useful in the kitchen. One knife that has a specialized use is a rather round, thin, serrated knife, which is excellent for cutting fresh tomatoes. A good boning knife and a knife for slicing are also important. If you have any doubt about the kinds of knives that you want, any good hardware store can recommend the types of knives that would be helpful to you.

Scales

You may need two different scales—a small one for weighing diabetic portions and a large one for weighing pounds and ounces. Persons with diabetes should not have to weigh everything they eat, but it is a good idea to weigh out portions occasionally to keep the feel of what is correct. So many times people will give themselves smaller portions than they are allowed because they think that something weighs more than it actually does.

Measuring Cups and Spoons

Standardized measuring cups and spoons are also essential equipment. Keeping several sets of measuring cups and spoons on hand will allow you to cook without stopping to wash them. It is not a good idea to use regular kitchen spoons for measuring. Most teaspoons hold about 1½ times the amount that measuring teaspoons hold and can wreak havoc with a cake or other baked item when substituted for a measuring spoon. Two-cup and quart measures are also helpful. A large glass measure for use in the microwave is also a must—you can use it for so many things in the microwave as well as using it for measuring liquids.

Pots and Pans

There is such a variety of pots and pans that it is hard to recommend any one kind to the exclusion of the others, for example, stainless steel with a copper bottom or core or glass pots and pans. Nonstick pans can be used for baking as well as frying. They need very little fat for frying and are so easy to clean that it is a pleasure to use them. You may want a special pan for crepes and blintzes, several large pans for soups and spaghetti sauce, and an old standard iron frying pan, which cooks have used for years. If you are happy with the pans you have now, don't feel you need to change them, but if you don't have nonstick frying and baking pans, do try them.

Casseroles

Casseroles are important, and you may want to use a variety of them such as Corning Ware and Pyrex, although there are some beautiful ones in enamelware these days. Casserole dishes come in a wide variety of shapes, styles, materials, and price ranges. Undoubtedly, you will want to stock your kitchen with a variety of dishes so that you'll be sure to have the perfect one on hand no matter what kind of dish you want to prepare. High quality, relatively inexpensive casserole dishes can be found in any department store, kitchen supply store, or even online at any one of a number of culinary websites.

Thermometers

Several kinds of thermometers are useful in the kitchen. A good meat thermometer for testing roasts and turkey, a candy thermometer for making candy for family and friends, and a yeast thermometer for testing the liquid in which you dissolve yeast when baking bread are all handy instruments to have.

Mixers

Several recipes in this book use the dough hook attachment on a mixer. If you don't have a dough hook on your mixer, use the mixer as long as you can and then pour the batter into a mixing bowl and do the rest of the bread mixing by hand. I suggest getting a mixer with a dough hook if you don't have one, however; you'll never be sorry that you did because it makes bread baking at home so much easier.

Food Processors

A food processor is also a big help. A low-cholesterol diabetic diet includes a lot of vegetables and fruits, and the food processor saves so much time preparing them. I don't use it for a table-spoonful of chopped onions or other small quantities of food. However, I do use it to chop a cup or so of onions or celery to keep on hand in the refrigerator, because I use them so often.

Chopping Boards

A good chopping board is a must. There are some very good plastic ones that don't dull the knife when you use them. They should be dishwasher-safe, easy to wipe off, and large enough to be efficient. Wooden chopping boards are hard to keep clean but sometimes they are worth it.

Steamers

I like to use a stainless-steel steamer with a double-boiler top and a steamer basket. Steamers help preserve vitamins and minerals in vegetables. Find a handy-sized one that will hold a bunch of broccoli or enough carrots for two meals, hot the first meal and cold with diabetic dressing the second meal. It is best to get one that will steam only the amount of food you need. There is no sense using a big one and wasting the extra heat and water.

Bread Makers or Machines

Bread machines can be a mixed blessing. It is hard to resist that extra slice of fresh baked bread. However, the machines are easy to use and will allow you to bake your own bread and analyze the recipe so you know the exact nutritive values in each slice. You can also make specialty breads, which you shouldn't buy at a bakery because you might not know the exact ingredients and nutritive values.

Ice Cream Dippers

You can buy and use ice-cream dippers for many things, including muffins, cupcakes, and cookies. A level No. 16 dipper provides ¼ cup batter, which is used for larger muffins, and a level No. 20, 3 tablespoons of batter, which is used for regular-size muffins. A level No. 60 dipper provides 1 tablespoon cookie dough while a level No. 40 dipper is just right for 1½ tablespoons dough. I have indicated the right size dipper to use in recipes for muffins, cupcakes, and cookies. You may be able to get them in your hardware store, but if you can't get them there a good specialty kitchen shop will have them or can get them for you.

The numbers on the inside of the dipper tell you the capacity of a level dipper, e.g., a No. 16 dipper is ¼ cup because the yields are based on that portion of a quart.

No. 8 . . . . ½ cup
No. 12 . . . . ⅓ cup
No. 16 . . . . ¼ cup
No. 20 . . . . 3 tablespoons
No. 40 . . . . 1½ tablespoons
No. 60 . . . . 1 tablespoon

INGREDIENTS

It is important to understand which foods have cholesterol and which are cholesterol-free, as well as the cholesterol count of the foods that do contain cholesterol. The following table includes average cholesterol counts for various foods. The information is based on that found in the following references:

Nutritive Value of Foods. Home and Garden Bulletin no. 72. U.S. Department of Agriculture, Washington, D.C., 1981.

Composition of Foods, Raw, Processed, and Prepared. Agriculture Handbook no. 8. U.S. Department of Agriculture, Washington, D.C., 1963 and all current revisions.

Information on the cholesterol counts of many more foods can be found in Chapter 3.

INGREDIENTS

Item	Milligrams of Cholesterol
Dairy Products	
1 cup whole milk	33
2 tablespoons sour cream	12
½ cup ice cream	29
½ cup soft-serve ice cream or ice milk	10
½ cup sherbet	5
Cheese (per ounce)	
Brie	28
Cheddar	30
Cheese spread	16
Colby	27
Cream	31
Feta	25
Gouda	32
Mozzarella made with part-skim milk	16
Neufchâtel or Parmesan	22
Romano	29
Roquefort or Swiss	26
Eggs	
1 egg yolk	213
Fats	
1 tablespoon butter	31
¼ cup lard	49

Item	Milligrams of Cholesterol
Meats (30 grams, about 1 ounce)	
Beef, T-bone steak, lean only, broiled	24
Beef, ground, extra lean, cooked	25
Beef, ground, regular, cooked	26
Beef brains, cooked, simmered	622
Beef heart, cooked, simmered	58
Beef kidneys, cooked, simmered	117
Beef liver, pan cooked, fried	146
Beef tongue, cooked, simmered	32
Beef tripe, raw	29
Lamb liver, cooked	152
Lamb tongue, cooked	57
Veal liver, cooked	170
Veal kidneys, cooked	240
Pork, fresh, Italian sausage, cooked	24
Pork, fresh, country-style sausage, cooked	25
Pork liver, cooked	108
Pork, cured, bacon, raw	20
Pork, braunschweiger	47
Pork ham, cured, boneless, cooked	18
Buffalo, composite of cuts, cooked, roasted	18
Deer, cooked, roasted	34
Rabbit, domestic, composite of cuts, cooked	25
Squirrel, cooked, roasted	37
Poultry (30 grams, about 1 ounce)	
Chicken giblets, cooked	108
Duck, domestic, flesh only, cooked	27
Goose, domestic, flesh only, cooked	29
Turkey giblets, cooked	127
Turkey bologna	30
Turkey frankfurter	18
Turkey salami	25
Fish (30 grams, about 1 ounce)	
Sardines in oil	43

Item	Milligrams of Cholesterol
Shellfish (30 grams, about 1 ounce)	
Crab, blue, cooked	30
Lobster, northern, cooked	22
Shrimp, mixed species, cooked	59
Shrimp, mixed species, canned	52
Abalone, mixed species, cooked	29
Squid, mixed species, cooked	61

Which foods should and shouldn't be used in the low-cholesterol diet has been discussed in detail in Chapter 6.

Sugar Substitutes

Even though you can now use a small amount of sugar, you might still want to use sugar substitutes in many of your recipes. The sugar improves texture, and adding sugar substitutes will make it taste sweeter, if necessary. If you would like to do so, feel free to increase or decrease the amount of sugar substitute if you think you'd like it better that way. You don't generally need to worry about changing the food exchange values if you add sugar substitute because there would need to be a big increase in sweetness to add enough carbohydrate to change any of the values.

You may use a variety of sugar substitutes. Most of the recipes have been tested using dry rather than liquid sugar substitutes, and mainly Equal and other NutraSweet sweeteners. For baking, Weight Watchers Low Calorie Sweetener or Splenda No Calorie Sweetener is the preferred choice, unless you want a brown sugar substitute, in which case you should use Sugar Twin Brown Sugar Replacement. Of course, you should always follow your taste buds and experiment with the sweeteners that you prefer.

Sugar Substitute	Amount	Carbohydrate (gm)	Calories	Sugar Equivalent
Equal Measure	½ teaspoon	2	8	1 tablespoon
	1¾ teaspoons	7	28	¼ cup
	2½ teaspoons	10	40	⅓ cup

Sugar Substitute	Amount	Carbohydrate (gm)	Calories	Sugar Equivalent
	3½ teaspoons	14	56	½ cup
Equal Packets	1½ packets	1	6	1 tablespoon
	6 packets	4	24	¼ cup
	8 packets	6	32	⅓ cup
Equal Tablets	1	0	0	1 teaspoon
	10	1	4	3 tablespoons
Weight Watchers Low Calorie Sweetener	¼ teaspoon	1	5	1 teaspoon
	1 teaspoon	4	20	4 teaspoons
	1½ teaspoons	6	30	2 tablespoons
	1 tablespoon	12	60	¼ cup
	¼ cup	48	240	1 cup
Splenda No Calorie Sweetener	Use an equal measure as a sugar substitute.			
Sprinkle Sweet	Use an equal measure as a sugar substitute.			
Sugar Twin	Use an equal measure as a sugar substitute.			
Sweet'n Low and Liquid Sucaryl	⅓ teaspoon			1 tablespoon
	1⅓ teaspoons			¼ cup
	1¾ teaspoons			⅓ cup
Adolph's Sugar Substitute	1 teaspoon			¼ cup
	1⅓ teaspoons			⅓ cup
	2 teaspoons			½ cup

One thing to remember is that most of the sugar substitutes have some carbohydrate in them, so you need to include their values in your daily diet plan. Don't worry about a couple of packets of sweetener, but count them if you are going to use several of them at a time. You may find the above table handy.

Milk Products and Substitutes

Instant nonfat dry milk is also used frequently in these recipes. Dry milk is good because it has all of the nutrients of whole milk except for the fat. It keeps well without refrigeration, is easy to store, is low in calories, and costs about the same as fresh milk. You may also use dry buttermilk because it is simpler to keep a can of dry buttermilk in the refrigerator than to keep liquid buttermilk on hand. The regular instant dry milk whips easily with an equal measure of milk or fruit juice, partially set gelatin, or egg whites to add more variety to the diet.

Instant nonfat dry milk is particularly good in yeast breads—when using it you no longer need to scald the milk, it helps form a good brown crust, and it yields bread with a softer texture. Dry milk can be reconstituted and used as a beverage or in a recipe that needs liquid milk, or it can be used dry along with the flour or other ingredients.

Most packages of instant nonfat dry milk direct you to use ⅓ cup of instant nonfat dry milk to 1 cup of water, but you will find that some recipes in this book have only ¼ cup of instant dry milk to 1 cup of water. That is because when working on a diabetic recipe, you want to cut down on the carbohydrate as much as possible and therefore should use only as much of the milk as necessary to get good results.

You can also use soy milk or rice milk as a dairy-free substitute. Use in recipes exactly as you would use regular skim milk.

Low-fat cottage cheese is usually available in most grocery stores. If it isn't available, buy the regular cottage cheese and wash it off with lukewarm water to get rid of the cream, then put it back in the container with a little skim milk if you like it creamy.

If you are accustomed to using cream in your coffee, you can use instant nonfat dry milk or one of the coffee whiteners that list a vegetable oil as their main ingredient. Be careful not to buy a coffee whitener that includes palm oil, coconut oil, or hydrogenated vegetable oil as an ingredient. Better yet, drink your coffee black—or best of all, stop drinking coffee. Tests and research seem to be telling us that too much coffee isn't good for us.

Vegetable Oils and Margarine

Learning to use vegetable oil and margarine instead of lard and butter seems to be one of the hardest things for most cooks to do when they start following a low-cholesterol diet plan. You don't really need all of that butter in a frying pan anyway, especially if it is a nonstick pan. A tablespoon of fat is generally enough to fry almost anything and the oil doesn't burn and turn brown quickly like butter does. If you think you absolutely have to have that butter flavor in baked goods, try adding some butter flavoring.

The type of fat used makes a difference in the texture and flavor of baked goods. You can substitute margarine for butter in baked goods, but use the regular stick margarine, not the soft or "lite" margarine. You can use vegetable oil as a substitute for melted fat in recipes, but if the recipe directs you to cream the fat with sugar, it is always best to use stick margarine.

Vegetable oil should be kept in a cool spot, out of sunlight, because you don't want it to get rancid. It shouldn't be refrigerated unless you expect to keep it for a long time, and then it should be brought back to room temperature before it is used.

It is always a good idea to read the ingredient list of any item, and it is particularly important when you are buying margarine. You need to know what kind of fat has been used in the margarine. Vegetable oil should be the first ingredient in the margarine. Fat is fat in a diabetic diet but the type of fat is very important to anyone on a low-cholesterol diet. You don't want to even consider margarine that contains lard or other animal fat, palm oil, cocoa butter, or coconut oil. If you are in doubt about your local brands, call your Heart Association and ask them to recommend the best ones available. Remember, a fat exchange is a fat exchange, no matter what brand of margarine you use, although you may get more volume for your exchange with the new soft and/or light margarines.

Eggs and Egg Substitutes

Liquid egg substitute is based on egg whites and is a wonderful substitute for whole eggs. It is more expensive than egg whites, so try to use egg whites whenever possible; however, there are certain recipes that need whole eggs, and liquid egg substitute works very well when you aren't supposed to be using egg yolks.

If you like, you can buy dehydrated egg whites and then you won't have to toss away the yolks. It costs about the same over a period of time.

Oat Bran

Oat bran has proved to be a very valuable source of water-soluble fiber, which helps reduce sugar and cholesterol in the blood. I am convinced that oat bran should be a part of every diabetic's diet. Oat bran can be used alone or you can use half oat bran and half oatmeal as a cooked cereal. Either way, cook them as you would oatmeal (add the cereal to boiling water, using twice as much water as cereal. Cook and stir for 1 minute, cover the cereal, remove it from the heat, and let stand for 5 minutes). You can serve it hot with skim milk and sugar substitute. You can also use half oat bran and half bread flour in most baked recipes. You need the bread flour because it has more gluten than all-purpose flour and oat bran doesn't have an appreciable amount of gluten. You can also add 2 teaspoons of wheat gluten for each cup of oat bran if you want to use it in equal proportions with all-purpose flour for most recipes. Wheat gluten is available at health food stores and many supermarkets. If your store doesn't have it, you can ask them to order it for you. It can also be used to add gluten to flours like whole wheat and rye when you want to use them for baking.

Fiber

We have known for a long time that a high-fiber diet with plenty of liquid will help control constipation, and now research has shown that a high-fiber diet with a generous proportion of water-soluble fiber will also help control blood sugar and cholesterol.

Dietary fiber is a general term for the indigestible carbohydrates including pectin, cellulose, hemicellulose, and lignin, which make up the cell walls of plants. Many foods contain fiber but it is found most abundantly in raw leafy, root, and tough-skinned vegetables; edible seeds; nuts; fruits; and the outer layer of grains. Because our digestive system does not contain the essential bacteria that breaks down this fiber, it remains more or less unchanged and is passed out of the body through the gastrointestinal system. Dietary fibers have a large capacity to hold water, which gives bulk and softness to the stool and enables food to pass more quickly through the digestive system.

There are two main types of fiber, water-soluble and water-insoluble. Water-soluble fiber forms a gel in water and is found in oats, beans, seeds, and fruits, especially apples and citrus fruits. Water-soluble dietary fiber helps control cholesterol and blood sugar. Water-insoluble dietary fiber is the kind we generally associate with the word *fiber* and is found in wheat, corn and oat bran, whole grains, and vegetables. It, along with liquid, forms bulky stools that travel faster through the intestines and help prevent constipation.

Most doctors agree you need 30 to 40 grams of dietary fiber each day for the best results, but the average is about 20 grams per day. Many diabetics are on a moderately high-fiber diet already because of all of the vegetables and fruit we eat. If you eat whole grain bread and at least five servings of fruits and vegetables each day, you are probably getting most of your fiber already, but it is a good idea to check on your consumption of fiber because of the very positive results achieved from eating it. Also don't forget to drink six to eight glasses of water every day because fiber needs a lot of water to expand.

Please be cautious when adding more fiber to your diet if you aren't using much of it now. Although it helps lower cholesterol and blood sugar and aids in relieving diverticulitis and preventing cancer of the lower bowel, it is best to add fiber gradually until you are up to 30 to 40 grams per day. Cereal boxes and food packages are a good source of information about the fiber content of foods not found in Chapter 3.

Dr. James Anderson, professor of medicine and clinical nutrition at the University of Kentucky and chief of the metabolic-endocrine section of the Veteran's Administrative Medical Center in Lexington, Kentucky, has pioneered new avenues of research using the High-Carbohydrate High-Fiber (HCF) diet for diabetics and others. If you want further information, you can write to HCF Nutrition Research Foundation, Inc., Box 22124, Lexington, Kentucky, 40522. Information on fiber in this book is based on the work of Dr. Anderson and the USDA.

Other Ingredients

There is only one ingredient used in this book that doesn't fit into a low-cholesterol diabetic diet. All of the other ingredients are acceptable on the diet, but you will find a recipe for chocolate chip cookies. There isn't that much cholesterol in the chips, and they can be fit into the typical doctor-recommended limit of 300 milligrams of cholesterol per day. After all, chocolate chip cookies are a part of the American way—we would hate to have to get along without them completely! Many supermarkets and health-food stores now carry dairy-free chocolate chips, which contain no cholesterol. You can also use chips made from carob, a widely used substitute for chocolate that is made from the seeds of the carob tree. One tablespoon of carob powder has 60 calories, 0 grams fat, 0 milligrams cholesterol, 27 grams carbohydrate, and 1 gram protein.

If you have a question about an ingredient that isn't used in a recipe, check the tables of nutritive values in Chapter 3, "Calculating Food Exchanges," and if the ingredient is listed you will know that it is acceptable for your diet.

Fruits, vegetables, and cereals are all free of cholesterol and are mostly complex carbohydrates that are recognized to be good for us. Vegetables and fruits should be used as much as possible because they are high in fiber and most of them are low in carbohydrate. A vegetable plate has most of the nutrients we need for a well-balanced meal along with a little cottage cheese, lean meat, or fish.

Since fiber is so good for us, I have used oat bran, whole wheat flour, and other whole grains as often as possible in these recipes. Whole wheat flour and graham flour have the same nutrients except that graham flour has been ground to yield a finer texture and therefore is more suitable in some recipes. When using white flour, be sure to purchase the "unbleached" variety, which contains more of the original nutrients that were present in the wheat kernel.

Bread flour is also used several times. Bread flour has a higher gluten content than all-purpose flour and helps make really good bread. It takes more liquid than all-purpose flour, but the final product has a finer texture and greater strength.

Since you will no longer be buying commercial mixes because of the fat and sugar in them, you can make your own or mix up a fresh batch each time. Angel food cake mix or mixes to which you add the egg and fat are acceptable if you add oil and liquid egg substitute to them; however, beware of using most mixes because they usually have ingredients that you shouldn't use.

Cocoa is used in these recipes instead of chocolate because chocolate contains cocoa butter, which isn't good for a low-cholesterol diet. Three tablespoons of cocoa plus one tablespoon of fat is equal to 1 ounce of baking chocolate. The cocoa can also be mixed with boiling water without any fat and used as a chocolate substitute with very good results. (Use only enough boiling water to make a smooth paste.)

Low-sodium variations are included for the recipes whenever practical. You won't find many salt substitutes in these recipes because not all doctors approve of them for all patients. If you want to use them, it is best to discuss them with your doctor. Each patient is different and no doctor will make a blanket statement that everyone can use salt substitutes.

The low-sodium diet notes in these recipes are planned for low-sodium diets, not salt-free diets. Mary Agnes Jones, R.D., formerly of Holy Cross Hospital in Chicago, and Muriel Urbashich, R.D., former head of the dietary department of South Chicago Community Hospital, both agreed that the low-sodium diet is more liberal than it used to be. Therefore I have used regular milk on the low-sodium diet, rather than salt-free milk. Salt-free margarine is available in most stores now and several packagers are now offering low-sodium canned vegetables that also may be used. Low-sodium soups are also available. Anyone on a "no added salt" diet can use the basic recipes in this book by deleting the salt when salt is specified. Some recipes that contain soy sauce or other highly salted ingredients cannot be changed successfully so they are not recommended for use on a low-sodium diet.

Ice milk, fruit ices, and sherbet can be used on the low-cholesterol diet, so feel free to use them within the limits of your diabetic diet. Lemon sorbet topped with raspberries or blueberries is a delicious and totally cholesterol-free dessert.

The most important thing to remember when planning your low-cholesterol diabetic diet is that you have many food items left that you can use. It is best to work with those and see what interesting and tasty dishes you can develop rather than mourning the loss of those few foods that are no longer available to you.

8
Understanding Food Labels

Food labels are a big help for anyone who is concerned about the contents of cans or packages, as we are. However, they can be hard to understand if you aren't used to reading them.

The following discussion of the label is based on information from the American Heart Association, the American Dietetic Association, and the Food and Drug Administration.

Nutrition Facts: If the label is titled "Nutrition Facts," it meets the 1993 government nutrition labeling requirements.

Serving Size: Is the serving size on the label the one you use? If you use twice as much, double the calories and other information for your size serving. If you only use half as much as the serving listed, divide the calories and other information by 2 to fit your serving.

Calories from Fat: Try to limit your calories from fat. Most people need to cut back on their total fat intake. Try to choose foods that don't get their main percentage of calories from fat.

Calories: This lists the total calories for the size serving shown on the label. If you need to cut your calories, consider cutting the serving size or buying another item that would fit into your meal plan more easily.

% Daily Value: The percentage of the total amount you need daily of each of the items listed.

Total Fat: The total amount of fat in each serving and the percentage of the daily amounts needed for a normal diet. (A 5'4", 138-pound active woman needs about 2,200 calories each day. A

Nutrition Facts

Serving Size ¹/₂ cup (114g)

Servings Per Container 4

Amount Per Serving

Calories 90   Calories from Fat 30

% Daily Value*

Total Fat 3g	**5%**
Saturated Fat 0g	**0%**
Cholesterol 0mg	**0%**
Sodium 300mg	**13%**
Total Carbohydrate 13g	**4%**
Dietary Fiber 3g	**12%**
Sugars 3g	
Protein 3g	

Vitamin A	80%	•	Vitamin C	60%
Calcium	4%	•	Iron	4%

* Percent Daily Values are based on a 2,000 calorie diet. Your daily values may be higher or lower depending on your calorie needs:

	Calories	2,000	2,500
Total Fat	Less than	65g	80g
Sat Fat	Less than	20g	25g
Cholesterol	Less than	300mg	300mg
Sodium	Less than	2,400mg	2,400mg
Total Carbohydrate		300g	375g
Fiber		25g	30g

Calories per gram:

Fat 9   •   Carbohydrate 4   •   Protein 4

More nutrients may be listed on some labels.

5'10", 174-pound active man needs about 2,900 calories per day. You will know how many you need according to your diet.) Each fat exchange contains 5 grams of fat (see table, Composition of Food Groups or Exchanges per Serving, in Chapter 3, "Calculating Food Exchanges.")

Saturated Fat: This is the kind of fat that helps raise your blood cholesterol. Avoiding it whenever you can is an important part of your low-cholesterol diet.

Cholesterol: Too much cholesterol can lead to heart problems. Try to eat less than 300 milligrams a day. (See table, Ingredients, in Chapter 7, "Equipment and Ingredients.")

Sodium: An excess amount of sodium can aggravate high blood pressure for some people. Try to keep your sodium intake below 2,400 to 3,000 milligrams (mg) of salt per day.

Total Carbohydrates: The amount of carbohydrate per serving is very important to anyone on a diabetic diet. We must count our carbohydrate, so it is important to know how much carbohydrate we would get in a serving of food. (There are 15 grams of carbohydrate, 3 grams of protein, and a trace of fat in a bread/starch exchange.)

Dietary Fiber: We need both soluble and insoluble fiber in our diets. Fruits, vegetables, whole-grain cereals, beans, and peas are all high in fiber and can help reduce the risk of cancer, heart trouble, and constipation. Thirty to 40 grams of fiber per day is about the right amount for most of us. However, we must remember that it is also important to drink enough liquid, preferably water, to rehydrate the fiber. Six to eight glasses of water per day should be your goal. Another important thing to remember is to start increasing, if necessary, your fiber, gradually adding a little more every few days until you have reached your goal.

Sugars: You will notice there is no percentage of Daily Value for sugar. We are now allowed a little sugar, but it isn't considered a necessary part of our diet.

Protein: It is important to have enough protein in our diet to maintain our bodily structure. However, we don't need as much protein as many people think we need. You will know how much protein you need for your diet from the number of meat exchanges you are allowed. Each meat exchange contains 7 grams of protein and 3 to 8 grams of fat depending upon whether you choose lean meat (3 grams of fat and 7 grams of protein), medium-fat meat (5 grams of fat and 7 grams of protein), or high-fat meat (8 grams of fat and 7 grams of protein). It is advisable to choose the lean meat with less fat because it will also have less cholesterol in it.

Vitamins and Minerals: Our goal here is to reach 100 percent of the daily requirements.

Daily Values: Let the daily values be your guide to what you need but always concentrate on your own food plan. Daily values are listed for people with a 2,000- or 2,500-calorie intake. Your daily values will be determined by your own food plan.

There are some key words used on labels that are important to us. They have been defined by the government, and you can be confident that if the label uses the following phrases, it can be proved to the government's satisfaction that the phrase is justified:

Fat Free: Less than 0.5 gram of fat per serving.

Low Fat: 3 grams or less of fat per serving.

Reduced Fat: At least 25 percent less fat when compared with a similar food.

Lean: Less than 10 grams of fat, 4 grams of saturated fat, and 95 milligrams of cholesterol per serving.

Light or Lite: One-third less calories or no more than half the fat of the higher-calorie, higher-fat version, or no more than half the sodium of the higher sodium version.

Low Saturated Fat: 1 gram or less saturated fat per serving and no more than 15 percent calories from saturated fat.

Cholesterol Free: Less than 2 milligrams cholesterol per serving and 2 grams or less saturated fat per serving.

Low Cholesterol: Less than 20 milligrams cholesterol per serving and 2 grams or less saturated fat per serving.

Reduced Cholesterol: At least 25 percent less cholesterol when compared with a similar food, and 2 grams or less saturated fat per serving.

Sodium or Salt Free: Less than 5 milligrams sodium in each serving.

Very Low Sodium: 35 milligrams or less sodium per serving.

Low Sodium: 140 milligrams or less sodium per serving.

Reduced Sodium: At least 25 percent less sodium when compared with a similar food.

Light in Sodium: 50 percent less sodium per serving; restricted to foods with more than 40 calories or 3 grams of fat per serving.

Excellent Source of: Contains more than 20 percent of the Daily Value per serving.

9

Soups

Soup is always a good addition to a low-cholesterol diabetic diet. For the diabetic diet you are interested only in the amount of carbohydrate, protein, and fat that is in the soup; however, for the low-cholesterol diet you also want to substitute polyunsaturated fats for animal fats, so you need to find substitutes for the animal fat, egg yolks, cream, whole milk, or butter often used in soup recipes.

There are all sorts of tricks you can use for changing a high-cholesterol soup into one suitable for a low-cholesterol diet. Liquid egg substitute can be used instead of egg yolks, margarine or oil instead of butter, a double amount of instant dry milk instead of evaporated milk, and a little more margarine in the soup along with the milk instead of cream. Of course this changes the flavor a little bit (but not too much) and the soups are still good in their own right.

You won't find many soups in this chapter based on dried peas, beans, and lentils, since they are so high in carbohydrate that one bowl of soup takes up most of a meal's allowance. Therefore, I concentrated on vegetable soups that provide fiber with less carbohydrate.

Because many soups are based on a good, rich chicken or beef broth, and because a low-cholesterol diet needs broth without any animal fat in it, I use a great deal of the fat-free chicken and beef broth concentrates available in the stores. These concentrates generally have a large amount of salt in them so the sodium count is very high when they are used. If you are on a low-sodium diet, you can handle this by buying low-sodium bouillon cubes or by preparing your own low-sodium, fat-free broth. When buying low-sodium soup concentrates, check the list of ingredients carefully, because several of them are based on animal fats instead of salt, and these concentrates aren't acceptable on a low-cholesterol diet.

If you decide to make your own low-sodium, fat-free broth, start by buying (if you don't have one) a heavy stainless steel or aluminum stock pot with a 2- or 3-gallon capacity and a tight-fitting lid. The broth needs to cook for a long time to develop flavor and it isn't worth doing unless you can cook a large amount. The broth freezes well and can be frozen in containers holding the right amount for future soups or casseroles.

There is very little added salt in most of the soup recipes containing broth because I used the commercial bouillon cubes that are high in salt in making the broth. If you use your own broth you will probably have to add salt (if you can) or a salt substitute if your doctor approves.

Fat-Free, Low-Sodium Beef Broth

Although we class it as beef broth, veal bones are also very good and may be used whenever available.

Any beef or veal bones are acceptable. You can get soup bones or soup meat from your butcher, save any bones from roasts, and collect any available bones from your family until you have enough to make a good, big pot of broth. It just isn't worthwhile unless you save enough bones.

Beef or veal bones, any kind
1 onion
2 carrots
1–2 celery stalks
Water to cover, at room temperature

The broth will have a better flavor if you roast the bones and trimmings in an open roaster in the oven at 350°F until they are well browned. Place the bones in a stock pot. Add onion, a couple of carrots, and a stalk or so of celery. Add water. Cover and simmer for 4–6 hours. Scum will rise to the top when the liquid first begins to simmer and it is a good idea to skim most of this off. (It is almost impossible to get it all off; I know, I've tried it often enough.) The broth may look done to you long before the cooking time is ended, but it won't have the flavor and body it will have if cooked the full length of time.

Remove from heat. Strain well, putting the broth in a pan and leaving the bones out. Refrigerate the broth until the fat has risen to the top and solidified. Remove the fat, place the clear broth in another container, and freeze or refrigerate until needed. At this stage add any broth, with the fat removed, that you have gathered from roasts. The broth from the roasts also has a good flavor and seems to add something to the broth. (Throw away the murky part at the bottom of the broth.)

As soon as the bones are cool enough to handle, remove any meat from them and refrigerate or freeze until needed. This meat is excellent for future use in soups. Discard the bones and any bits of overcooked vegetables with them.

Since this broth is considered free on a diabetic diet, it may be used for soups or other recipes without adding any nutritive values that need to be counted.

Fat-Free, Low-Sodium Chicken or Turkey Broth

Chicken or turkey bones, necks, wings
1 quart cold water for each pound of
    bones
1 onion
2 carrots, small
2 celery stalks
A little parsley

Weigh the chicken or turkey bones, necks, and wings, place in a stock pot, and add 1 quart cold water for each pound of bones. Don't add any giblets, skin, or fat because they are all forbidden on a low-cholesterol diet. Bring the water to a boil, reduce heat, and simmer 5 minutes. Drain well. Replace with the same amount of cold water. Add one onion, two small carrots, a couple of stalks of celery, and a little parsley. Cover tightly and simmer for 2½–3 hours. If you are using a precooked carcass of a turkey or chicken with no raw bones, it isn't necessary to discard the first liquid. Just cover with cold water and simmer an hour or so or until the meat is falling off the bones. If the carcass is still whole, you will get a richer broth if you crush the bones or separate them so they won't need as much water to cover them.

After the cooking period, strain the broth, setting aside the chicken or turkey bones to cool. Chill the broth until the fat has risen to the top and solidified. Discard the fat. Remove the clear broth to another container and freeze or refrigerate until used. (Throw away the murky part at the bottom of the pot.)

Pick any chicken or turkey meat off the bones as soon as they are cool enough to handle and refrigerate or freeze it for future use in soups, discarding the bones.

Since this broth is considered free on a diabetic diet, it may be used for soups or other recipes without adding any nutritive values that need to be counted.

Chunky Split Pea Soup

This soup has little bits of vegetable in it. If you want a smoother soup, it can be puréed in the blender or food processor before it is served.

1 cup dried split peas
6 cups water
6 chicken bouillon cubes
1 cup finely chopped onions
¼ cup finely chopped celery
¼ cup finely chopped fresh green peppers
¼ cup finely chopped fresh carrots
2 tablespoons margarine
¼ teaspoon ground thyme
Salt and pepper to taste

Wash split peas and put in a saucepan. Add water and bouillon cubes; cover and simmer 1½ hours, stirring frequently.

Add onions, celery, peppers, and carrots to split peas; cover and simmer ½ hour, stirring frequently.

Add margarine and seasonings to soup and continue to simmer for 10 minutes. Remove from heat and serve hot. Serve ¾ cup per serving. (The amount of salt needed will depend upon the saltiness of the bouillon cubes. The recipe is calculated using chicken bouillon cubes instead of low-sodium chicken broth.)

Yields 6 cups—8 servings

Nutritive Values Per Serving

CAL	CARBS (g)	PRO (g)	TOTAL FAT (g)	SAT. FAT (g)	CHOL (mg)	FIBER (g)	NA (mg)
125	18	7	3	.5	0	2	762

Food exchanges per serving: 1 starch, 1 lean meat.
Low-sodium diets: Use low-sodium broth instead of the water and chicken bouillon cubes or delete the chicken bouillon cubes and use only water. Use salt-free margarine and don't add any salt to the soup.
Sugar content per serving: None.

Barley Mushroom Soup

"Chef Dave" Hutchins gave me this recipe. It is kosher as long as you use vegetable stock, which you can buy in a health food store or some supermarkets. I'm happy to say that Chef Dave is very careful to follow low-cholesterol guidelines when cooking or planning menus. This low-cholesterol food is greatly appreciated by his many older patrons who are attempting to keep their cholesterol count under 200.

> ³/₄ cup pearl barley
> ¹/₄ cup vegetable oil
> 2 pounds sliced fresh mushrooms
> 2 cups diced celery
> 2 cups julienned onions
> 4 minced garlic cloves
> 3 quarts vegetable stock
> Salt to taste
> ¹/₈–¹/₄ teaspoon freshly ground black pepper
> ¹/₂ cup plain yogurt
> ¹/₄ cup soy sauce

Put barley in a food processor, preferably a small one, and give it a couple of pulses to chop the barley into grits. Set aside.

Preheat a 4- or 6-quart heavy pot on medium heat for 1 minute. Swirl oil around the bottom of pot. Add mushrooms and cook, stirring frequently, until mushrooms are well browned. Add celery, onions, and garlic and continue to cook and stir until onions are soft. Add vegetable stock and barley and bring to a rolling boil. (If you don't have vegetable stock, you can use fat-free beef stock, in which case the soup will no longer be kosher.) Decrease heat, cover, and simmer until barley is tender. Add salt and pepper (the amount of salt you need will depend upon the saltiness of the stock).

Remove soup from heat and stir ½ cup of it into yogurt. Add yogurt mixture and soy sauce to soup. Serve hot, but don't boil after adding yogurt. Use 1 cup per serving.

Yields 3 quarts—12 servings

Nutritive Values Per Serving

CAL	CARBS (g)	PRO (g)	TOTAL FAT (g)	SAT. FAT (g)	CHOL (mg)	FIBER (g)	NA (mg)
147	21	4	6	.8	1	4	1,370

Food exchanges per serving: 1 starch, 1 vegetable, 1 fat.
Low-sodium diets: Omit salt and use low-sodium vegetable or beef broth and soy sauce.
Sugar content per serving: None.

Cabbage and Rice Soup

1 tablespoon vegetable oil
1 pound (about 5 cups) shredded cabbage
1 cup thinly sliced onions
4 cups fat-free beef broth
4 cups fat-free chicken broth
Sprinkle of pepper
¼ teaspoon grated nutmeg
½ cup long-grain rice

Preheat a heavy saucepan on medium heat for 1 minute. Swirl oil around bottom of pan. Add cabbage and onions and cook, stirring frequently, over medium heat until cabbage and onions are soft. Add broths, pepper, nutmeg, and rice. Cover and simmer about 20 minutes, or until rice is tender. Do not overcook. Serve hot, using 1 cup soup per serving.

Yields 2 quarts—8 servings

Nutritive Values Per Serving

CAL	CARBS (g)	PRO (g)	TOTAL FAT (g)	SAT. FAT (g)	CHOL (mg)	FIBER (g)	NA (mg)
96	15	5	2	.3	0	2	648

Food exchanges per serving: 1 starch, 1 vegetable.
Low-sodium diets: Omit salt. Use salt-free broth.
Sugar content per serving: None.

Cream of Tomato Soup

This recipe came from Vera Wilson, a friend of mine from Wadena. She made it with home-canned tomato juice, but it is also good made with commercially canned tomato juice.

> **1 tablespoon finely chopped onions**
> **3 tablespoons margarine**
> **3 tablespoons all-purpose flour**
> **1 teaspoon salt**
> **1/8 teaspoon pepper**
> **2 cups tomato juice**
> **2 cups skim milk at room temperature**
> **1 1-gram packet Equal (aspartame) sugar
> substitute**

Fry onions in margarine in a saucepan, stirring constantly, until soft but not brown. Add flour and seasonings to onion and cook and stir over moderate heat until bubbly but not browned.

Add tomato juice to flour mixture. Bring to a boil, stirring constantly, for 1 minute. Stir tomato mixture into milk. Place soup in the top of a double boiler. Return to heat and heat to serving temperature. Remove from heat.

Stir Equal into soup and serve hot, 3/4 cup per serving.

Yields about 4 cups—6 servings

Nutritive Values Per Serving

CAL	CARBS (g)	PRO (g)	TOTAL FAT (g)	SAT. FAT (g)	CHOL (mg)	FIBER (g)	NA (mg)
130	11	4	8	2.6	11	1	767

Food exchanges per serving: 1 skim milk, 1 fat.
Low-sodium diets: Omit salt. Use salt-free margarine and tomato juice canned without salt.
Sugar content per serving: None.

Gazpacho

This is refreshing on a warm summer day—a good way to celebrate the first ripe tomatoes in summer, although it is equally tasty later in the fall.

> **3 cups fat-free beef broth**
> **3/4 cup tomato juice**
> **2 tablespoons lemon juice**
> **3 tablespoons Spicy Tomato Dressing (see Index)**
> **1/3 cup finely chopped onions**
> **1/3 cup finely chopped fresh green peppers**
> **2 tablespoons finely chopped celery**
> **1 cup diced, peeled, and cored fresh tomatoes**
> **1/4 teaspoon garlic powder**
> **1 teaspoon salt**
> **1 tablespoon chopped parsley**
> **1/4–1/2 cup thinly sliced or diced cucumbers**

Combine all ingredients except cucumbers; mix lightly and refrigerate overnight or at least 4 hours.

Serve soup in chilled cups garnished with cucumbers, using ³/₄ cup soup per serving.

Yields about 4¹/₂ cups—6 servings

Nutritive Values Per Serving

CAL	CARBS (g)	PRO (g)	TOTAL FAT (g)	SAT. FAT (g)	CHOL (mg)	FIBER (g)	NA (mg)
30	6	2	trace	0	0	1	842

Food exchanges per serving: 1 vegetable.
Low-sodium diets: Omit salt. Use low-sodium broth and low-sodium version of the salad dressing.
Sugar content per serving: None.

Goulash Soup

Muriel Urbashich, a dietitian who was the head of the Dietary Department at South Chicago Community Hospital, tells me that this soup was a great favorite in its employees' cafeteria. The cafeteria sold gallons of it whenever it was on the menu.

> 2 cups chopped onions
> 3 tablespoons vegetable oil, divided
> 1 pound beef round
> 8 cups fat-free broth
> ¹/₄ teaspoon garlic powder
> 2 teaspoons paprika
> ¹/₂ cup drained, crushed, canned tomatoes
> Salt to taste
> 1¹/₂ cups diced fresh white potatoes

Brown onions in 2 tablespoons vegetable oil in a heavy frying pan over moderate heat, stirring occasionally. Transfer onions with a slotted spoon to a heavy saucepan.

Add remaining tablespoon of oil to frying pan. Trim all visible fat from the beef and cut it into ¾-inch cubes. (This is easier if the meat is slightly frozen.) Brown beef in the frying pan over moderate heat, stirring occasionally. Transfer meat with a slotted spoon into saucepan with the onions. Discard as much fat as possible from the frying pan.

Add broth to frying pan and cook and stir over low heat to get as many of the brown particles in the pan as possible into the broth. Pour the hot broth into the saucepan with the onions and meat.

Add seasonings and tomatoes to meat and broth. Cover and simmer over low heat until meat is tender. Remove from heat. Cool to room temperature. Refrigerate until thoroughly chilled and the fat has risen to the top. Remove the fat and discard it. Return the soup to heat. Taste for seasoning and add salt, if it seems necessary.

Add potatoes to soup. Cover and simmer 15–20 minutes or until the potatoes are tender. Serve 1 cup hot soup per serving.

Yields 2 quarts—8 servings

Nutritive Values Per Serving

CAL	CARBS (g)	PRO (g)	TOTAL FAT (g)	SAT. FAT (g)	CHOL (mg)	FIBER (g)	NA (mg)
183	11	17	8	1.6	33	1	688

Food exchanges per serving: 2 lean meat, ⅓ starch, 1 vegetable, ½ fat.
Low-sodium diets: Use low-sodium broth and fresh tomatoes or tomatoes canned without salt.
Sugar content per serving: None.

Fruit Soup

I can never decide if this is a soup or a fruit. I generally serve it as a dessert, so I calculated it using a ½-cup serving. If you want to serve it chilled or hot as a soup, it would be 2 fruit exchanges for a 1-cup portion.

> **4 cups water**
> **2 whole cinnamon sticks**
> **1 teaspoon whole cloves**
> **3 tablespoons instant tapioca**
> **⅓ cup golden raisins**
> **1 cup drained, canned unsweetened mandarin oranges**
> **1 cup drained, canned unsweetened pineapple tidbits**
> **1 cup drained, canned unsweetened diced peaches**
> **Sugar substitute equal to ⅔ cup sugar**

Combine water, cinnamon, and cloves in a saucepan. Cover and bring to a boil. Reduce heat and simmer for 5 minutes. Remove from heat and allow to marinate overnight. Drain spices from the liquid and discard spices.

Add tapioca and raisins to liquid and let stand at room temperature for 5 minutes. Place in saucepan, cover, and simmer until clear. Remove from heat.

Add fruits and sweetener to soup and refrigerate at least overnight before serving. If you want to serve it warm, it can be reheated after it has marinated. Serve ½ cup per serving.

Yields 6 cups—12 servings

Nutritive Values Per Serving

CAL	CARBS (g)	PRO (g)	TOTAL FAT (g)	SAT. FAT (g)	CHOL (mg)	FIBER (g)	NA (mg)
56	15	trace	trace	trace	0	.5	54

Food exchanges per serving: 1 fruit.
Low-sodium diets: May be served as written.
Sugar content per serving: None.

Golden Squash Soup

This recipe is a memento of my trip to Argentina. They use squash much more frequently than we do as a vegetable as well as in soups and stews.

> 2 tablespoons margarine
> 3/4 cup finely chopped onions
> 1/3 cup all-purpose flour
> 1/2 cup instant nonfat dry milk
> 2 cups hot water
> 6 cups fat-free chicken broth at room
>   temperature
> 2 cups cooked, puréed winter squash
> 1/8 teaspoon white pepper
> 1/2 teaspoon celery salt
> 1/4–1 teaspoon curry powder
> 1/2 teaspoon salt
> 2 tablespoons chopped chives or parsley

Preheat a heavy saucepan over medium heat for 1 minute. Melt margarine in pan, add onions, and cook and stir over medium heat until onions are soft and lightly browned. Sprinkle flour evenly over onions and continue to cook and stir until flour is lightly browned. Dissolve milk in hot water, combine with broth (combined liquid should be lukewarm), and add to onions and flour. Cook and stir over medium heat until smooth and thickened. Add puréed squash, pepper, celery salt, curry powder, and salt. Simmer 5 minutes. Serve hot, garnished with chives or parsley, using 1 cup soup per serving.

Yields 2 quarts—8 servings

Nutritive Values Per Serving

CAL	CARBS (g)	PRO (g)	TOTAL FAT (g)	SAT. FAT (g)	CHOL (mg)	FIBER (g)	NA (mg)
99	13	5	3	.5	1	2	718

Food exchanges per serving: 1 starch, 1/2 fat.
Low-sodium diets: Omit salt and use salt-free broth.
Sugar content per serving: None.

Minestrone Soup

This is a hearty Italian vegetable soup that is high in fiber. I think it is my favorite soup. I generally make a double batch and freeze most of it in containers to use later. It is high in sodium because I calculated it with commercial beef concentrate for the beef broth. If you are watching your salt, you should prepare it with home-made or low-sodium beef broth. Most minestrone contains pasta in some form but I leave that out because I want to use my bread exchanges for crackers with my soup.

3 quarts fat-free beef broth
1 cup peeled, diced fresh white potatoes
1/2 cup chopped onions
1/2 cup chopped carrots
1/4 cup diced celery
1/4 cup diced fresh green peppers
1 tablespoon chopped parsley
1 cup diced canned tomatoes and juice
1/2 cup coarsely chopped cabbage
2 cups (16-ounce can) cooked navy or
   great northern beans
1/2 teaspoon garlic powder
Salt to taste
1/4 teaspoon pepper
1 1/2 teaspoons Italian seasoning
1 teaspoon leaf oregano
1/2 teaspoon basil
1 1/2 cups diced cooked beef without visible
   fat
Water as necessary

Place first six ingredients in a large soup kettle, at least 6 quarts; cover and simmer for 15 minutes.

Add all remaining ingredients except meat to soup, cover, and simmer for another 15 minutes.

Add meat to soup. Add enough water, if necessary, to make 3 quarts soup. Serve hot, 1 cup per serving.

Yields 3 quarts—12 servings

Nutritive Values Per Serving

CAL	CARBS (g)	PRO (g)	TOTAL FAT (g)	SAT. FAT (g)	CHOL (mg)	FIBER (g)	NA (mg)
121	14	12	2	.6	18	3	682

Food exchanges per serving: 1/2 starch, 1 lean meat, 1 vegetable.
Low-sodium diets: Use salt-free broth. Omit salt.
Sugar content per serving: None.

Tomato Bouillon

1 cup chopped celery
1 cup chopped onions
2 cups fat-free chicken broth
3 cups fat-free beef broth
3 cups tomato juice
1 teaspoon Worcestershire sauce
1/4 teaspoon basil
Whisper of black pepper

Place celery, onions, and chicken broth in saucepan. Cover and simmer 30 minutes. Drain well, reserving the broth. Discard vegetables and return broth to saucepan.

Add beef broth, tomato juice, and seasonings to chicken broth. Cover and simmer for about 5 minutes. Taste for seasoning and add more, if necessary. Serve 3/4 cup hot or cold bouillon per serving.

Yields 2 quarts—10 servings

Nutritive Values Per Serving

CAL	CARBS (g)	PRO (g)	TOTAL FAT (g)	SAT. FAT (g)	CHOL (mg)	FIBER (g)	NA (mg)
30	6	3	trace	0	0	1	598

Food exchanges per serving: 1 vegetable.
Low-sodium diets: Use low-sodium broths and tomato juice. Delete
   Worcestershire sauce and add 1/4 teaspoon ground thyme or dried oregano.
Sugar content per serving: None.

Green and Gold Cream Soup

This is a basic cream soup. Other vegetables in the same vegetable food group may be substituted for the carrots and broccoli. The vegetables may also be puréed before they are added to the soup.

> 1 cup frozen or fresh broccoli stems and
>   pieces
> 1 cup finely chopped carrots
> 3 tablespoons flour
> 2 tablespoons margarine
> 4 cups fat-free chicken broth
> 2 tablespoons instant nonfat dry milk
> ¼ teaspoon salt

Chop broccoli into small pieces. They should be large enough to have a little texture but not very large. Place in a small container, cover, and cook for 2 minutes on high in the microwave or cook until barely tender in a small amount of water. Drain well and set aside.

Place carrots in a small container. Add 1 tablespoon water, cover, and cook on high in the microwave for 6–8 minutes or until tender, or cook until barely tender in a small amount of water. Drain well and set aside.

Place flour and margarine in a 1½- or 2-quart saucepan over moderate heat. Cook and stir until smooth. Stir broth, dry milk, and salt together and add to flour mixture. Cook and stir over moderate heat until smooth and thickened. Continue to cook, stirring frequently, over low heat for 1 more minute. Add vegetables and reheat to serving temperature. Serve ¾ cup per serving.

Yields 4 cups—6 servings

Nutritive Values Per Serving

CAL	CARBS (g)	PRO (g)	TOTAL FAT (g)	SAT. FAT (g)	CHOL (mg)	FIBER (g)	NA (mg)
76	7	4	4	.6	trace	1	582

Food exchanges per serving: 1 vegetable, 1 fat.
Low-sodium diets: Omit salt. Use salt-free margarine and low-sodium broth.
Sugar content per serving: None.

Potage Pierre

This luscious soup is from Beverly Wolfrum of Ennis, Montana. She and I share a crusading fervor aimed at helping people lower their cholesterol counts. Don't change a thing in this recipe; it is wonderful just as it is written. You may think it is ready after 2 hours, but please simmer it for at least 4 hours because the flavor continues to improve.

1 pound lean beef with fat and gristle removed
1 29-ounce can whole tomatoes and juice
¾ cup finely chopped onions
¾ cup finely chopped celery
¾ cup finely chopped carrots
4 cups fat-free beef broth
1 teaspoon thyme
10 whole peppercorns

Place meat in a 4-quart pot. Chop tomatoes and add with their juice to meat. Add onions, celery, carrots, broth, thyme, and peppercorns. Cover and simmer 4 to 5 hours. Add hot water if necessary to keep yield at 10½ cups. Serve hot, using 1½ cups per serving.

Yields 10½ cups—7 servings

Nutritive Values Per Serving

CAL	CARBS (g)	PRO (g)	TOTAL FAT (g)	SAT. FAT (g)	CHOL (mg)	FIBER (g)	NA (mg)
132	9	17	3	1	39	2	610

Food exchanges per serving: 2 very lean meat, 2 vegetable.
Low-sodium diets: Use low-sodium canned tomatoes and salt-free broth.
Sugar content per serving: None.

Mulligatawny Soup

This soup is delicious and I think it is well worth the bread exchange it costs me.

> ¹/₄ cup chopped onions
> ¹/₄ cup chopped fresh green peppers
> ¹/₄ cup diced celery
> 2 tablespoons vegetable oil
> ¹/₃ cup flour
> 5 cups fat-free chicken broth at room
>   temperature
> 1 small (4 to the pound) tart apple
> ³/₄ cup drained, crushed canned tomatoes
> ¹/₄ teaspoon curry powder
> ¹/₈ teaspoon ground cloves
> Whisper of white pepper
> 1 cup diced cooked chicken with fat and
>   skin removed
> 1 cup cooked rice

Fry onions, peppers, and celery in oil in a heavy saucepan over moderate heat, stirring frequently, until the onions are limp but not browned. Remove vegetables from the pan with a slotted spoon and reserve for later use.

Add flour to oil in pan and stir over moderate heat until smooth and lightly browned. Add broth to flour mixture and stir over moderate heat until thickened. Add the reserved vegetables.

Wash and core apple and cut into small pieces as though you were going to make Waldorf salad. Add to soup. Add tomatoes and seasonings to soup. Cover and simmer for 45 minutes or until the vegetables are tender.

Add chicken and rice to the soup just before it is served. Reheat soup if necessary and serve 1 cup hot soup per serving.

Yields 7 cups—7 servings

Nutritive Values Per Serving

CAL	CARBS (g)	PRO (g)	TOTAL FAT (g)	SAT. FAT (g)	CHOL (mg)	FIBER (g)	NA (mg)
163	18	10	6	1	18	1	524

Food exchanges per serving: 1 starch, 1 lean meat.
Low-sodium diets: Use low-sodium broth and rice cooked without salt.
Sugar content per serving: None.

Swiss Soup

I like having a soup that is only one vegetable exchange. You can place 1–2 ounces of lean, cubed cooked beef in a soup bowl and add this soup for a good vegetable-beef soup that only costs you the meat and one vegetable exchange.

> **1 tablespoon margarine**
> **¼ cup chopped onions**
> **½ cup chopped celery**
> **¼ cup chopped carrots**
> **¼ cup chopped fresh green peppers**
> **6 cups fat-free beef broth**
> **2 cups shredded cabbage**
> **¹⁄₁₆ teaspoon black pepper (optional)**
> **Salt to taste**
> **¼ teaspoon ground nutmeg**

Melt the margarine in the bottom of a saucepan. Add onions, celery, carrots, and peppers and stir over moderate heat about 4 minutes or until the vegetables are limp but not browned.

Add broth to vegetables; cover and simmer 15 minutes.

Add cabbage and seasonings to soup. Cover and simmer another 5 minutes. Serve soup hot, 1 cup per serving.

Yields 7 cups—7 servings

Nutritive Values Per Serving

CAL	CARBS (g)	PRO (g)	TOTAL FAT (g)	SAT. FAT (g)	CHOL (mg)	FIBER (g)	NA (mg)
41	4	3	2	.3	0	1	571

Food exchanges per serving: 1 vegetable.
Low-sodium diets: Do not add salt. Use salt-free margarine.
Sugar content per serving: None.

Vegetable Beef Soup

1½ pounds beef stew meat
Cold water as necessary
2 quarts cold water
1½ teaspoons salt
⅛ teaspoon black pepper
1 cup diced fresh white potatoes
½ cup diced carrots
1 cup coarsely chopped onions
½ cup shredded cabbage
1 cup canned tomatoes and juice
½ cup fresh or frozen green string beans
    cut into ½-inch pieces

Trim any gristle and visible fat from meat with a sharp knife. Place meat in a saucepan. Cover with cold water, bring to a boil, and boil 1 minute. Discard liquid.

Add 2 quarts cold water, salt, and pepper to meat. Bring to a boil. Reduce heat, cover, and simmer for about 1½ hours or until meat is tender. Drain the broth from the meat. Strain the broth, cover, and refrigerate meat and broth separately. After the broth is chilled, remove the hard fat from the top of the broth.

Measure the broth and add cold water to the broth to equal 7 cups of liquid. Add vegetables to stock. Cover and simmer 30–45 minutes or until vegetables are tender. Taste for seasoning and add more if desired. (Nutritive values are calculated using 1½ teaspoons salt.) Add meat to soup. Reheat to serving temperature, if necessary, and serve hot using 1 cup per serving.

Yields 2 quarts—8 servings

Nutritive Values Per Serving

CAL	CARBS (g)	PRO (g)	TOTAL FAT (g)	SAT. FAT (g)	CHOL (mg)	FIBER (g)	NA (mg)
145	8	19	4	1.4	51	1	523

Food exchanges per serving: 2 very lean meat, 1½ vegetable, 1 fat.
Low-sodium diets: Omit salt. Use fresh tomatoes or salt-free canned tomatoes.
Sugar content per serving: None.

Vegetable Chowder

---

2 tablespoons margarine
½ cup chopped onions
¼ cup chopped carrots
¼ cup chopped fresh green peppers
1 cup diced fresh white potatoes
1 cup cream-style corn
1 teaspoon salt
1/16 teaspoon black pepper
3 cups water
4 ounces sliced fresh or frozen Brussels
  sprouts
⅓ cup instant nonfat dry milk
2 tablespoons flour
1 cup cold water

Melt margarine in the bottom of a saucepan. Add onions, carrots, and peppers and cook and stir over moderate heat until onions are soft but not browned.

Add potatoes, corn, seasonings, and water to vegetables. Bring to a boil. Reduce heat and simmer 20 minutes. Add Brussels sprouts to soup. Cover and simmer 10 minutes.

Stir milk, flour, and cold water together until smooth. Add to soup and stir to mix. Simmer, stirring frequently, for 3 minutes. Remove from heat and serve hot, 1 cup per serving.

Yields 7 cups—7 servings

Nutritive Values Per Serving

CAL	CARBS (g)	PRO (g)	TOTAL FAT (g)	SAT. FAT (g)	CHOL (mg)	FIBER (g)	NA (mg)
106	17	3	4	.6	1	2	482

Food exchanges per serving: 1 starch, ½ fat.
Low-sodium diets: Omit salt. Use salt-free margarine.
Sugar content per serving: None.

10

Fish

Fish is a wonderful food. It is low in calories and saturated fat and easy and quick to prepare. With so many different kinds of fish available and so many different ways to prepare them, it is easy to have fish two or three times a week (as doctors and dietitians recommend) without repeating yourself very often. If you live along the coasts or in the Great Lakes area, you are probably used to serving a great deal of fish. If you live inland and aren't used to using all that much fish, you are going to be very pleasantly surprised as you try the various recipes and different kinds of fish available across the country.

Fish is available in the following forms:

- *Whole fish* are fish as they are caught. The fish needs to be scaled, eviscerated, and cut into portions, if necessary. The head and tail are generally removed although they may be left on some of the smaller fish.
- *Dressed fish* have had the scales and entrails removed. The head, tail, and fins are generally also removed although the head and tail may be left on smaller fish. These are called pan-dressed fish, such as trout or catfish. The fish may also be cut into fillets, steaks, or chunks.
- *Fillets* are ready to be cooked when they are purchased. They are the sides of fish cut from the backbone.
- *Steaks* are generally cut ⅝ to 1 inch thick and are cross sections cut from larger fish. The only bone in them is the

cross section of the backbone. They are ready to be cooked when purchased.

- *Chunks* are cross section pieces of larger fish. The only bone that might be in them would be a cross section of the backbone, but most of the pieces are without bone. They are ready to be cooked when they are purchased.
- *Sticks and squares* are generally cut from frozen fish blocks. They are coated with a batter or breading. They are not recommended for a low-cholesterol diabetic diet unless you are sure the batter does not include whole eggs and the package includes nutritive information to help you determine the exchanges for them.
- *Fish portions* are generally individual pieces of fish that have been dipped in batter or breading and frozen so they can be cooked or reheated without further preparation. They, too, are not recommended for a low-cholesterol diabetic diet unless you are sure the batter does not contain whole eggs and the package includes nutritive information to help you determine the exchanges for them.
- *Canned fish* includes many varieties of fish. They are ready to be used as purchased. The ones packed in water are lower in calories than the ones packed in oil. The most readily available canned fish are salmon, tuna, mackerel, and sardines. Several species of fish are marketed as tuna and all of them are equally desirable.

When you are buying fresh fish, it should be really fresh. Fresh fish should have the following characteristics:

- *Flesh* should be firm and not separated from the bones.
- *Odor* should be fresh and mild. Fish with a strong odor is probably older since the fish odor becomes more apparent with age.
- *Eyes* should be bright and clear. The eyes become sunken as the fish becomes stale.
- *Gills* should be red and free of slime.
- *Skin* should be shiny with the color unfaded. Older fish lose their iridescence and the color is faded.

- *Fish steaks or fillets* should be firm and have a fresh-cut appearance. There should be no trace of brown or drying around the edges.

When you are buying frozen fish, the following points are important:

- *Flesh* should be frozen solid when purchased. There should not be any discoloration or freezer burn.
- *Odor* should not be apparent. Fish that is frozen properly should have little or no odor. A strong fish odor indicates poor quality.
- *Wrappings* should be of moisture- and vapor-retardant materials. There should be little or no space between the fish and the wrappings. Wrappings should not be torn, dirty, or discolored.

After fish are purchased, they must be stored correctly to avoid loss of quality and possible food spoilage or poisoning.

- *Fresh fish* should be placed in the refrigerator immediately after they are purchased. They should be stored in the refrigerator at 35–40°F and should be used within 48 hours after they are purchased.
- *Frozen fish* should be placed in the freezer in their original wrappings and stored at zero degrees or below. Fish should always be dated so you can use the oldest fish first and not have to contend with freezer burn on some package that got shoved to the back of the freezer. It is important to thaw fish correctly. A 1-pound package of fish should thaw in the refrigerator in about 24 hours, or in 1–2 hours under cold running water. I thaw fish in the microwave, placing it at defrost for 5–10 minutes for a 1-pound package. Fish should never be defrosted at room temperature because of the danger of food spoilage or food poisoning. Frozen fillets or steaks may be cooked without thawing if you allow a little more cooking time, but if they are to be breaded or baked, they should always be thawed before they are prepared.

Fish is cooked to develop flavor, soften the small amount of connective tissue, and make it easier to digest. Fish cooked at too high a temperature or for too long will be tough and dry and the flavor will be poor.

Deep-fat-fried fish is a favorite with many people, but it isn't all that good on a low-cholesterol diabetic diet—you can't be sure exactly how much fat the fish has absorbed or what ingredients are in the batter. If you are eating in a restaurant, it is a good idea to order plain broiled or baked fish, and if it is served with a sauce ask them to serve the fish with the sauce on the side. If you can, you should ask what they have used to baste the fish; it might be an oil-based marinade, but then again it might be lemon butter, which you wouldn't want to eat.

I have tried to include recipes in this chapter to illustrate the various methods for preparing fish. If you have a favorite recipe you want to use that doesn't contain cholesterol, you can calculate the exchanges from the information in Chapter 3.

Some fish do contain some fat, although most of the different kinds of fish are very lean. Fish that are considered lean include the following: catfish, cod, flounder, haddock, halibut, lake perch, ocean perch, pike, red snapper, sole, swordfish, and whiting.

Some recipes for preparing fish are methods more than individual recipes. These include the following:

Broiled fish. This is a form of dry heat cooking but the heat is more direct and intense than when fish is baked. It is best to use steaks, fillets, or pan-dressed fish about 1 inch thick because the intense heat will dry out thinner fish. The fish should be thawed and patted dry with a paper towel and should be brushed with an oil-based marinade or sauce while it is being broiled. The directions for your own broiler should be followed; however, it is a general rule that fish should be broiled about 3–4 inches from the source of heat. Thicker cuts should be broiled farther from the heat than thinner cuts. The length of time for broiling depends upon the thickness of the fish to be broiled and the distance from the heat. It generally takes about 10–15 minutes before the fish flakes easily when tested with a fork. Fish do not generally need to be turned while they are being broiled, but thicker pieces such as whole fish should be turned and brushed with more marinade when they are about half-cooked. Always serve broiled fish very hot.

Charcoal-broiled fish. Fish are good for this type of cooking because they cook so quickly. Pan-dressed fish, fillets, and steaks are all suitable for broiling. The fish should be thawed and patted dry before it is broiled; and because it flakes easily, it is a good idea to use a well-greased, long-handled, hinged wire grill for your fish. Thicker cuts of fish are best because they will dry out less than the thinner cuts, but all of them should be basted generously before and during the cooking period. Fish are generally cooked about 4 inches from moderately hot coals for 15–20 minutes depending upon the thickness of the fish. French or Italian style dressings that are based on oil are good for basting the fish. It is not a good idea to baste fish with a sauce high in sugar because it burns easily—but since we would never do that anyway we won't need to worry about that type of marinade. Marinades used for both types of broiling should be calculated when food exchanges for the fish are calculated.

Poached fish. Poaching means to cook in a simmering liquid. The fish should be placed in a single layer in a shallow, wide pan such as a large frying pan and barely covered with liquid. The liquid can be fish stock, lightly salted water, white wine and water, or water with various herbs in it. It is important not to let the water boil and not to overcook the fish. The fish should cook in a simmering liquid, in a covered pan, about 10–15 minutes or until the fish flakes easily when tested with a fork. It can then be served warm or cold with a sauce, in a salad, or used as the main ingredient in a casserole.

Steamed fish. Steamed fish is generally cooked with steam from hot water although some people like to add herbs to the water. It is a good way to cook fish to retain its natural flavor and juices. A steamer is best, but any deep pan with a tight cover may be used if you have a rack that fits in the pan. The rack is to keep the fish out of the water. The fish is placed on a rack over rapidly boiling water and allowed to steam for 10–15 minutes or until the fish flakes easily when tested with a fork. Steamed fish is generally served the same way as poached fish.

Fish cooked in foil. Individual fish portions may be baked in the oven or prepared on an outside grill in foil. Put a single portion of fish in a foil packet along with some sauce or margarine and thinly sliced vegetables. It cooks beautifully this way without getting any pans dirty and tastes delicious when it is finished. It takes longer on the grill than in the oven but either method is satisfactory. The fish should be cooked until it flakes easily when tested with a fork.

Of course, all of the above methods yield fish that should be calculated using 1 ounce of the cooked fish as 1 lean meat exchange plus whatever sauce you use on the fish.

The sauces served in restaurants with fish can add unwanted fat to your diet. If the sauce is based on sour cream or is high in egg yolks or some other forbidden ingredient, ask for lemon juice—or if all else fails, ask for just plain vinegar. You would be surprised at the difference between those sauces and flavored vinegar or lemon juice when you are calculating the exchanges for a fish recipe.

I first discovered the advantages of vinegar with fish when I was eating fish and chips in Great Britain. When I came home, I tried it again and liked it as well as I did over there. I guess I had thought that maybe it was the atmosphere over there that made me like it; however, it worked just as well here, so I experimented with different types of vinegar and discovered I could make my own herb vinegar very easily. I steep about a tablespoon of herbs (fresh if possible) in a cup of vinegar for a few days or until it is as strong as I like it. Then I strain off the herbs, put my vinegar in a cruet, and keep it for the next time we have fish. I even like to use the pickle juice from Mrs. Riley's Pickles (see Index) on fish.

Baked Fish with Mustard Sauce

***

6 3-ounce fillets of codfish, haddock,
    perch, flounder, or whiting
1 tablespoon lemon juice
1 tablespoon vegetable oil
1 teaspoon paprika
1 teaspoon salt
¼ cup all-purpose flour
2 tablespoons margarine
2 tablespoons instant nonfat dry milk
2 cups cool water
1 tablespoon chopped parsley
2 teaspoons prepared mustard
Whisper of white pepper

Defrost fish if necessary. Pat dry with paper towels and place in a shallow baking pan lined with aluminum foil and greased with margarine.

In a small cup mix together lemon juice, oil, paprika, and ½ teaspoon of the salt. Using a pastry brush, brush the tops and sides of the fillets with the mixture. Bake at 350°F for 30–40 minutes depending upon the thickness of the fillets, or until the fish flakes easily when tested with a fork.

While the fish is baking, in a small saucepan cook the flour, margarine, dry milk, and remaining ½ teaspoon salt. Stir over low heat until smooth. Add 2 cups water to the flour mixture and cook and stir until smooth and thickened.

Add remaining seasonings to the sauce and stir to mix well. Serve ⅓ cup hot sauce over one hot fish fillet per serving.

Yields 6 fillets—6 servings

Nutritive Values Per Serving

CAL	CARBS (g)	PRO (g)	TOTAL FAT (g)	SAT. FAT (g)	CHOL (mg)	FIBER (g)	NA (mg)
157	5	16	7	1	37	trace	495

Food exchanges per serving: 2 very lean meat, 1 vegetable, 1¹/₂ fat.
Low-sodium diets: Omit salt and use salt-free margarine.
Sugar content per serving: None.

Baked Fish Steak

**1 pound halibut or salmon steak cut ⁵/₈–1
    inch thick**
¹/₃ cup Spicy Tomato Dressing (see Index)

Defrost fish if necessary. Pat dry with paper towels. Line a small pan with aluminum foil. Grease the foil with margarine and place the steak on the pan. The steak can be cut into 4 equal portions at this time or after it is baked.

Brush steak generously with dressing using a pastry brush. Bake 25–35 minutes at 350°F or until fish flakes easily when tested with a fork. Cut into four equal portions, if not already cut, and serve hot using one portion per serving.

Yields 1 pound—4 servings

Nutritive Values Per Serving

CAL	CARBS (g)	PRO (g)	TOTAL FAT (g)	SAT. FAT (g)	CHOL (mg)	FIBER (g)	NA (mg)
107	1	19	2	trace	29	trace	167

Food exchanges per serving: 3 very lean meat.
Low-sodium diets: Use low-sodium variation of the salad dressing.
Sugar content per serving: None.

Oven-Fried Fish Fillets

3 tablespoons margarine at room
    temperature
½ cup dry bread crumbs
1 teaspoon paprika
¼ teaspoon garlic powder
½ teaspoon salt
2 tablespoons Parmesan cheese
8 4-ounce codfish fillets
½ cup skim milk

Line a 9″ × 13″ cake pan with aluminum foil. Grease the foil using part of the margarine. Set the remaining margarine aside to be used later.

Place bread crumbs, seasonings, and Parmesan in a pie pan. Mix well to blend and set aside for later use.

Defrost fish if necessary. Pat dry with a paper towel. Place milk in an individual salad bowl. Dip fish fillets in milk and then in the bread crumb mixture. Place evenly on the foil in the pan.

Using all the remaining margarine, spread a small amount of the margarine on top of each of the fillets. Bake at 500°F for 10–15 minutes or until lightly browned and firm. (The length of time will depend upon the thickness of the fillets.) Let stand 5 minutes and serve hot, using one fillet per serving.

Yields 8 fillets—8 servings

Nutritive Values Per Serving

CAL	CARBS (g)	PRO (g)	TOTAL FAT (g)	SAT. FAT (g)	CHOL (mg)	FIBER (g)	NA (mg)
170	6	22	6	1	50	trace	338

Food exchanges per serving: 3 very lean meat, ⅓ starch, 1 fat.
Low-sodium diets: Omit salt. Use salt-free margarine.
Sugar content per serving: None.

Shrimp Etouffée

This is a Cajun recipe I developed, with the help of Della Andreassen, R.D., from Lafayette, Louisiana, for a magazine article about Cajun cooking.

1 tablespoon vegetable oil
³/₄ cup chopped onions
¹/₂ cup chopped fresh green peppers
¹/₂ cup chopped celery
¹/₂ cup tomato sauce
¹/₄ cup water
2 teaspoons cornstarch
¹/₈–¹/₄ teaspoon cayenne pepper
¹/₄ teaspoon salt
8 ounces cooked, cleaned shrimp
¹/₄ cup chopped fresh green onion tops

Preheat ¹/₂-quart saucepan over medium heat for 1 minute. Swirl oil in bottom of pan. Add onions, green peppers, and celery and cook, stirring frequently, over medium heat until onions are soft but not browned.

In a separate bowl combine tomato sauce, water, cornstarch, cayenne pepper, and salt and stir until smooth. Add tomato sauce mixture to vegetables and cook and stir until sauce is clear. Add shrimp and heat to serving temperature. Stir chopped onion tops into mixture and serve hot using 1 cup per serving.

Note: This is good over rice, but rice is not included in the nutritive analysis.

Yields 3 cups—3 servings

Nutritive Values Per Serving

CAL	CARBS (g)	PRO (g)	TOTAL FAT (g)	SAT. FAT (g)	CHOL (mg)	FIBER (g)	NA (mg)
158	10	17	6	.8	147	2	615

Food exchanges per serving: 2 very lean meat, 2 vegetable, 1 fat.
Low-sodium diets: Omit salt. Use low-sodium tomato sauce.
Sugar content per serving: None.

Grecian Shrimp and Baby Artichoke Brochette

Since shrimp is not permitted every day on a low-cholesterol diet, I like to use a really good recipe when I prepare it, especially when I'm in Arizona and can pick fresh lemons off the tree.

12 baby artichokes
½ cup olive or vegetable oil
¼ cup fresh lemon juice
1 clove garlic, minced
1 teaspoon oregano
1 teaspoon Dijon mustard
½ teaspoon rosemary
⅛–¼ teaspoon crushed red pepper flakes
¼ teaspoon salt
Whisper of freshly ground black pepper
16 peeled, raw jumbo shrimp with tails left intact
1 fresh lemon, cut into wedges

Cook artichokes in boiling, salted water just until tender, 8–12 minutes, depending on their size. Drain well and hold under cold running water until cool to the touch. They can be cooked a day in advance and refrigerated until needed, if desired.

Combine oil, lemon juice, garlic, oregano, mustard, rosemary, red pepper flakes, salt, and pepper in a large plastic food bag. Add shrimp, seal tightly, and refrigerate 1 hour or longer before cooking.

If artichokes are very small, leave them whole. Larger ones should be cut in half lengthwise and the choke removed. Trim pointed tips of leaves if they are sharp. Thread artichokes and shrimp alternately onto four metal or wooden skewers, using four shrimp and three artichokes for each skewer. (If you are using wooden skewers, soak them in water for 10 minutes before using them.) Brush the shrimp and artichokes with any marinade that remains.

Grill brochettes over a hot fire, turning once, for 7–9 minutes or until shrimp is cooked through. Garnish with lemon wedges. Serve hot, using one brochette per serving.

Note: Baby artichokes, which are about 2 inches long, are too young to have developed the prickly inside choke, so you can eat the whole artichoke. If they are not available, use the smallest mature ones you can find.

Yields 4 brochettes—4 servings

Nutritive Values Per Serving

CAL	CARBS (g)	PRO (g)	TOTAL FAT (g)	SAT. FAT (g)	CHOL (mg)	FIBER (g)	NA (mg)
410	19	23	29	4	140	7	423

Food exchanges per serving: 3 very lean meat, 4 fat, 4 vegetable.
Low-sodium diets: Omit salt.
Sugar content per serving: None.

Tuna Fish, Mushrooms, and Celery

Mushrooms and celery add bulk and flavor to a recipe without adding much carbohydrate or many calories.

> 2 6½-ounce cans of chunk-style tuna fish
>   packed in water
> 3 tablespoons margarine
> 1 cup thinly sliced celery
> 1 4-ounce can mushroom stems and pieces,
>   drained
> 3 tablespoons all-purpose flour
> 2 cups water at room temperature
> ½ cup instant nonfat dry milk
> ½ teaspoon salt
> Whisper of white pepper

Drain tuna well. Discard liquid. Set tuna aside for later use.

Place margarine in a 1½-quart saucepan. Melt over moderate heat. Add celery and mushrooms and cook, stirring occasionally, over moderate heat until celery is limp. Add flour to vegetables and cook and stir until flour is absorbed.

With a fork, mix water, dry milk, salt, and pepper to blend. Add to vegetables and cook and stir over moderate heat until smooth and thickened. Add tuna fish. Mix very lightly and serve hot using ¾ cup per serving.

Yields 4 cups—6 servings

Nutritive Values Per Serving

CAL	CARBS (g)	PRO (g)	TOTAL FAT (g)	SAT. FAT (g)	CHOL (mg)	FIBER (g)	NA (mg)
163	7	19	6	1	24	trace	536

Food exchanges per serving: 3 lean meat, 1 vegetable.
Low-sodium diets: Omit salt. Use salt-free margarine.
Sugar content per serving: None.

Fish Creole

**4 4-ounce fillets of codfish, haddock,
   perch, flounder, or whiting
2 tablespoons vegetable oil
¼ cup chopped fresh green peppers
¼ cup chopped onions
1 tablespoon all-purpose flour
1 cup chopped canned tomatoes and juice
½ teaspoon salt
½ teaspoon sugar
⅛ teaspoon ground cloves
Whisper of pepper**

Defrost fish, if necessary. Pat dry with paper towels and place in a shallow 1-quart casserole.

Place oil in a small saucepan. Bring to a cooking temperature. Add peppers and onions and cook, stirring frequently, over moderate heat until onions are soft but not browned. Add the tablespoon of flour to vegetables. Cook and stir until flour is absorbed by the vegetables.

Add tomatoes and seasonings to vegetables. Cook and stir over moderate heat for 2 minutes. Pour the hot sauce over the fish. Bake, uncovered, at 350°F for 35–40 minutes or until the fish flakes easily when tested with a fork. Serve hot using one fillet and a quarter of the sauce per serving.

Yields 4 fillets—4 servings

Nutritive Values Per Serving

CAL	CARBS (g)	PRO (g)	TOTAL FAT (g)	SAT. FAT (g)	CHOL (mg)	FIBER (g)	NA (mg)
180	6	21	8	1	49	1	433

Food exchanges per serving: 3 lean meat, 1 vegetable.
Low-sodium diets: Omit salt. Use fresh tomatoes or low-sodium canned
    tomatoes.
Sugar content per serving: .1 teaspoon.

Salmon Patties with Creamed Peas

1 1-pound can red salmon
2 large egg whites
1 tablespoon finely chopped onions
¼ teaspoon salt
Whisper of pepper
1 cup crushed white soda crackers or
    saltines
1 cup fat-free chicken broth
1 tablespoon cornstarch
1 tablespoon margarine
1½ cups drained canned peas

Drain salmon and place the juice in a mixing bowl. Remove bones and dark skin from the salmon and set aside. Add egg whites, onions, salt, and pepper to the salmon juice and mix together with a fork.

Crush the crackers with your hands. Don't substitute cracker crumbs. Add to the egg white mixture along with the salmon. Mix well with a fork to blend. (The cracker pieces and small chunks of salmon should still be visible.) Shape into patties about ¾ inch thick using about ⅓ cup of the mixture per patty. Place patties on a small cookie sheet that has been greased with margarine. Bake, uncovered, at 350°F for 35–40 minutes or until firm and lightly browned.

Stir broth and cornstarch together until smooth. Cook and stir over moderate heat in a small saucepan until thickened and smooth. Continue to cook and stir for another minute. Add margarine and peas to sauce and mix lightly. Reheat to serving temperature. Serve one patty with a sixth of the sauce (about ⅓ cup) per serving.

Yields 6 patties—6 servings

Nutritive Values Per Serving

CAL	CARBS (g)	PRO (g)	TOTAL FAT (g)	SAT. FAT (g)	CHOL (mg)	FIBER (g)	NA (mg)
211	15	18	8	4	29	2	833

Food exchanges per serving: 1 starch, 2 lean meat.
Low-sodium diets: Omit salt. Use salt-free margarine, low-sodium crackers, and fresh or frozen peas. Discard salmon juice and substitute an equal amount of water.
Sugar content per serving: None.

Codfish with Mushroom Sauce

1 4-ounce can mushroom stems and pieces
2 tablespoons margarine
2 tablespoons all-purpose flour
¼ teaspoon salt

Whisper of white pepper
1 cup fat-free chicken broth
4 4-ounce codfish fillets

Drain mushrooms. Discard juice. Chop mushrooms into small pieces. Place in small saucepan. Add margarine, flour, and seasonings to mushrooms and cook and stir over moderate heat until lightly browned. Add broth to mushrooms. Cook and stir over moderate heat until smooth and thickened.

Thaw fish if necessary. Pat dry with a paper towel and place in a 1½-quart casserole. Cover with the hot sauce, using a fork to ease the sauce around the fish. Bake uncovered at 350°F for 30–35 minutes or until the fish flakes easily when tested with a fork. Serve one fillet and a quarter of the sauce per serving.

Yields 4 fillets—4 servings

Nutritive Values Per Serving

CAL	CARBS (g)	PRO (g)	TOTAL FAT (g)	SAT. FAT (g)	CHOL (mg)	FIBER (g)	NA (mg)
167	4	22	7	1	49	.5	490

Food exchanges per serving: 3 lean meat, 1 vegetable.
Low-sodium diets: Omit salt. Use salt-free margarine, low-sodium broth, and fresh mushrooms.
Sugar content per serving: None.

Tartar Sauce

---

1 cup Kay's Cooked Dressing (see Index)
2 tablespoons finely chopped Mrs. Riley's
    Pickles (see Index)
1 tablespoon finely chopped onions
1 tablespoon chopped pimientos
1 tablespoon chopped parsley

Mix all ingredients well to blend. Refrigerate until served, using 2 tablespoons per serving.

Yields 1¼ cups—10 servings

Nutritive Values Per Serving

CAL	CARBS (g)	PRO (g)	TOTAL FAT (g)	SAT. FAT (g)	CHOL (mg)	FIBER (g)	NA (mg)
24	2	1	1	trace	0	trace	117

Food exchanges per serving: 2 tablespoons may be considered free. ¼ cup is 1 vegetable exchange.

Low-sodium diets: Use low-sodium variation of salad dressing.

Sugar content per serving: None.

11

Poultry

Chicken and turkey are both important in the low-cholesterol diabetic diet because they are low in calories, easily available, and comparatively inexpensive. It is also relatively simple to remove the skin and fat from them before they are cooked. Goose is a little too fat and I never use it, but I depend upon chicken and turkey for many of our meals.

Chicken and turkey are interchangeable in many recipes and especially so when you are using cubed or diced, raw or cooked chicken or turkey with the fat and skin removed. When they are used interchangeably in recipes the nutritive values are based upon the first one listed. However, the food exchanges do not vary when one or the other is used.

Giblets should be avoided on a low-cholesterol diet. If you don't have someone in your family who can use them, save them for a friend or neighbor who doesn't have to worry about cholesterol, or give them to your cat or dog—they'll probably love them.

All poultry is perishable and you should be careful when you are buying or storing it. It is a good idea to always observe the following precautions:

1. Buy frozen or chilled poultry only from freezers or refrigerated cases.

2. Inspect the wrappers to be sure they are not torn or damaged.

161

3. Keep fresh poultry in the coldest part of your refrigerator; use it within two days after it is purchased or freeze it for later use.

Chicken or turkey parts may be purchased and they are often a better buy than the whole chicken or turkey. Turkey breast makes a very good roast and has less waste than the whole turkey. One ounce of the cooked turkey roast, without any skin, is of course one lean meat exchange. You can also buy turkey legs or thighs. Turkey frankfurters are available in most stores, but they still aren't all that good for you because they do have fat in them. Turkey ham is lean and it is generally lower in fat than is regular ham.

You won't find directions for roasting a turkey because most of the turkeys you buy include that information on the wrapper. Do not cook the dressing inside the chicken or turkey for a low-cholesterol diet. It picks up too much fat that way—saturated fat that is not acceptable on a low-cholesterol diet. I know it is good that way, and that is probably how your grandmother did it, but it is better to cook the dressing in a separate pan where you can control the amount and kind of fat in the dressing.

You should remove the skin from a chicken before you roast it, but you don't have to when roasting a turkey. It is simple to serve a slice of the turkey breast with very little of the fat from the skin on it, but it isn't all that easy on the smaller chicken.

The following are sanitary measures that should be taken when preparing poultry:

1. *Be careful that everything is scrubbed* including table tops, chopping boards, knives, pans, and anything that might touch the poultry—both before and after you work with raw poultry.

2. *Do not defrost poultry at room temperature.* It should be defrosted in the refrigerator even if it does take several days for a large turkey. If you don't have refrigerator space sufficient to keep a large turkey in the refrigerator for that long, it can be defrosted, still in its plastic bag, in the sink in cold running

water. This will take several hours but can be done the day before you want to cook the turkey.

3. *Do not stuff chicken or turkey the night before it is to be cooked,* or stuff it and cook it partially one day and finish cooking it the next day. Prestuffing gives bacteria a chance to multiply and could cause food poisoning.

4. *As soon as possible after dinner, refrigerate leftover chicken or turkey, dressing, and gravy in a shallow pan.* Food stored in a deep pan takes too long to cool to the correct temperature and bacteria can develop while it is chilling. Don't let chicken or turkey, dressing, or gravy stay on the table at room temperature for nibbling after dinner. Refrigerate everything as soon as possible and if anyone wants a snack, let him or her go to the refrigerator for it, or set it out for guests to help themselves later.

5. *Leftover chicken or turkey should be frozen if it is not to be used within the next couple of days.* Divide it into serving-size portions and freeze it for future use. It is a big help when you have unexpected company or want to make yourself a different entrée than you are serving to others in the family. I don't like to carry a chicken or turkey sandwich for lunch because of the danger of bacterial contamination, but if you freeze the sandwich and wrap it in foil it will be cold enough to be safe several hours later when you need it.

I hope you will enjoy the recipes in this chapter. Chicken and turkey are a very special treat in many parts of the world and you can make them a special treat in your home, too. If you have a recipe of your own that you want to use, calculate the nutritive values in the recipe using the information in Chapter 3, and then go on from there. Remember to remove the skin and fat before the chicken is cooked and don't use any butter, cream, eggs, or other no-nos in your recipe.

Roast Chicken

It is almost impossible these days to get an old-fashioned roasting chicken, which is good because those heavier chickens have a very high percentage of the fat we are trying to avoid on a low-cholesterol diabetic diet. Look for the heavier broiler-fryers and you should be able to find one weighing 3½ pounds, big enough for roasting.

1 3½-pound broiler-fryer chicken

Wash chicken well. Remove all skin and visible fat with a sharp knife or kitchen scissors. (Give the giblets to your cat or cook them for someone who isn't on a low-cholesterol diet.) Place the chicken on a rack in a small roaster, breast side down. Cover and roast at 325°F for 1½–1¾ hours or until tender and lightly browned. Remove from the oven and let set 15 minutes before it is carved into portions. (*Note:* If you want to serve a quarter of a chicken, start out with a 2½-pound broiler-fryer and roast it about 1½ hours, cut it into four equal portions, and serve a quarter of the chicken per serving.) Serve 3 ounces of boneless cooked chicken per serving.

Yields 6 3-ounce servings plus leftovers

Nutritive Values Per Serving

CAL	CARBS (g)	PRO (g)	TOTAL FAT (g)	SAT. FAT (g)	CHOL (mg)	FIBER (g)	NA (mg)
162	0	25	6	1.7	76	0	73

Food exchanges per serving: 3 lean meat.
Low-sodium diets: May be used as written.
Sugar content per serving: None.

Oven-Browned Chicken

---

1 2½-pound broiler-fryer chicken
¾ cup dry bread crumbs
1 teaspoon salt
2 teaspoons paprika
1/16 teaspoon black pepper
½ teaspoon rubbed sage or thyme
1 large egg white
½ cup water
1 tablespoon margarine
1 tablespoon vegetable oil

Wash chicken well. Remove skin and all visible fat with a sharp knife and cut into serving-size pieces. You should have two breast halves, two thighs, and two legs. (Freeze the neck, wings, and back to use later to make chicken broth.)

Mix bread crumbs and seasonings well and place in a pie pan. (You won't need but about half of this amount, but you need a certain amount in order to be able to dredge the chicken in it successfully. Discard the remainder. Nutritive values are calculated using half of the bread crumb mixture.)

Mix egg white and water well and put into an individual salad bowl. Spread a small rimmed cookie sheet with aluminum foil and spread the margarine on the aluminum foil. Dip each piece of chicken in the egg white mixture and then dredge it in the bread crumb mixture and place on the aluminum foil.

Dribble ½ teaspoon oil on the top of each piece of chicken. Bake at 350°F for 30 minutes. Remove the chicken from the oven. Turn it over and continue to bake for another 30 minutes. Serve hot or cold using one breast half or one leg and one thigh per serving—about 4 ounces of meat per serving.

Yields 1 chicken—4 servings

Nutritive Values Per Serving

CAL	CARBS (g)	PRO (g)	TOTAL FAT (g)	SAT. FAT (g)	CHOL (mg)	FIBER (g)	NA (mg)
238	9	28	11	2	79	1	773

Food exchanges per serving: 4 lean meat, ¹/₂ starch.
Low-sodium diets: Omit salt. Use salt-free margarine.
Sugar content per serving: None.

Poached Chicken

*The poaching liquid can be changed to suit your favorite season-
ings without changing the nutritive values, as long as it is based
on chicken broth and no fat is added.*

**1 2¹/₂-pound broiler-fryer chicken
1 cup fat-free chicken broth
¹/₄ teaspoon thyme or sage
¹/₄ teaspoon salt
1 teaspoon chopped parsley
2 tablespoons orange juice
¹/₄ cup dry white wine**

Wash chicken well; remove skin and all visible fat with a sharp
knife and cut into four equal portions. Place chicken in a shallow casserole. Discard the giblets, or give them to someone who
isn't worried about cholesterol.

Mix together remaining ingredients and pour over chicken.
Cover tightly with aluminum foil and bake at 325°F for about 1
hour or until the chicken is tender. Remove from oven and serve
a quarter chicken per serving. (Discard the poaching liquid. It is
too highly spiced to be good for soup and it isn't thick enough or
flavorful enough for a sauce on the chicken.)

Yields 1 chicken—4 servings

Nutritive Values Per Serving

CAL	CARBS (g)	PRO (g)	TOTAL FAT (g)	SAT. FAT (g)	CHOL (mg)	FIBER (g)	NA (mg)
152	trace	23	6	1.5	71	0	133

Food exchanges per serving: 3 lean meat.
Low-sodium diets: Omit salt. Use salt-free chicken broth.
Sugar content per serving: None.

Emperor Chicken Breasts

This recipe comes from the multitalented "Chef Dave."

> ¹/₄ teaspoon Chinese Five Spice seasoning
> (found in the ethnic food section of
> most stores)
> 1 cup soy sauce
> 4 4-ounce boneless, skinless chicken breast
> halves
> 1 tablespoon stick margarine
> ¹/₄ cup cornstarch
> ¹/₄ cup all-purpose flour
> 2¹/₂ cups fat-free chicken broth
> ¹/₄ cup soy sauce
> 2 tablespoons cornstarch
> 2 tablespoons brown sugar
> 3 finely chopped garlic cloves
> 1 tablespoon peanut oil
> 1 teaspoon finely minced fresh ginger
> ¹/₂ cup chopped onions
> ¹/₂ cup chopped fresh green peppers
> ¹/₂ cup chopped celery
> ¹/₂ cup coarsely grated carrots
> 1 8-ounce can sliced bamboo shoots
> 1 cup coarsely chopped Chinese cabbage
> or bok choy

Combine Chinese Five Spice seasoning and 1 cup soy sauce in a shallow baking pan. Wash chicken, drain well, and marinate overnight in soy sauce mixture. Drain well. Use a quarter of the margarine to grease a 9-inch-square nonstick pan. Set aside.

Blend ¹/₄ cup cornstarch and flour in a shallow dish. Dredge chicken in flour mixture. Shake off any excess flour mixture and place chicken in the greased pan. Divide remaining margarine into four equal portions and put one portion on top of each breast half. Bake, uncovered, at 375°F for 30–40 minutes, or until browned.

While chicken is baking, combine chicken broth, ¼ cup soy sauce, 2 tablespoons cornstarch, brown sugar, and garlic. Blend well and set aside.

Preheat a nonstick frying pan, add the peanut oil and the ginger and cook and stir over medium heat until you can smell the ginger. Add onions, green peppers, celery, carrots, bamboo shoots, and Chinese cabbage or bok choy. Cook and stir over medium heat about 5 minutes or until thickened and lightly browned. Mix lightly and pour over browned chicken.

Bake, uncovered, at 325°F for 30 minutes or until chicken is lightly browned. Serve hot, using a half breast topped with a quarter of the chicken broth mixture and a quarter of the vegetable mixture for each serving.

Yields 4 chicken breast halves with sauce—4 servings

Nutritive Values Per Serving

CAL	CARBS (g)	PRO (g)	TOTAL FAT (g)	SAT. FAT (g)	CHOL (mg)	FIBER (g)	NA (mg)
318	29	32	8	1.4	66	3	2,137

Food exchanges per serving: 3 lean meat, 1 starch, 3 vegetable.
Low-sodium diets: Omit salt and use salt-free broth and low-sodium soy sauce.
Sugar content per serving: 1½ teaspoons.

Chicken or Turkey Mushroom Casserole

1 4-ounce can mushroom stems and pieces
1 10¾-ounce can Campbell's Cream of
    Chicken soup
½ cup fat-free chicken broth
1 cup diced cooked chicken or turkey
    without skin or visible fat

½ cup long-grain rice
1 teaspoon chopped parsley

Combine mushrooms, soup, and broth in a small saucepan. Cook and stir over moderate heat until smooth and bubbling.

Add chicken, rice, and parsley to hot soup mixture. Stir to mix well and place in a 1½-quart casserole. Cover tightly and bake at 325°F for 40 minutes or until rice is tender. Serve ¾ cup hot casserole per serving.

Yields 3 cups—4 servings

Nutritive Values Per Serving

CAL	CARBS (g)	PRO (g)	TOTAL FAT (g)	SAT. FAT (g)	CHOL (mg)	FIBER (g)	NA (mg)
240	26	15	8	2.6	37	1	781

Food exchanges per serving: 2 very lean meat, 1 fat, 1 starch, 2 vegetable.
Low-sodium diets: Use low-sodium soup and broth.
Sugar content per serving: None.

Microwave Chicken

This recipe from Dr. Crockett is simple to prepare but it has an intriguing flavor. It can also be baked in a conventional oven, if you prefer.

1 2½-pound broiler-fryer chicken
½ teaspoon salt
¼ teaspoon ground sage
¾ cup orange juice
½ cup dry white wine

Wash chicken well. Remove all skin and visible fat with a sharp knife and cut into pieces. You should have two breast halves, two thighs, two wings, two legs, and the back. Freeze the wings, back, and neck to use later for making broth. Discard the giblets or give them to someone who isn't worried about cholesterol. Place the remaining pieces in an 8- or 9-inch dish suitable for use in the microwave.

Sprinkle salt and sage evenly over the chicken. Pour orange juice and wine over chicken pieces. Cover with plastic wrap or wax paper and cook on high for 5 minutes. Reduce power to low and cook for 15–20 minutes or until tender. Serve hot with a little bit of the juice. Serve one breast half or one leg and one thigh per serving.

Note: If you prefer to use a conventional oven, cover the pan tightly with aluminum foil and bake at 325°F for 45 minutes–1 hour or until the chicken is tender. If you prefer, you can remove the foil the last 15 minutes to allow the chicken to brown a little.

Yields 1 chicken—4 servings

Nutritive Values Per Serving

CAL	CARBS (g)	PRO (g)	TOTAL FAT (g)	SAT. FAT (g)	CHOL (mg)	FIBER (g)	NA (mg)
184	5	25	6	1.7	76	trace	349

Food exchanges per serving: 3 lean meat, 1 vegetable.
Low-sodium diets: Omit salt.
Sugar content per serving: None.

Jambalaya

This is a recipe I developed with help from my friend Della Andreassen for a magazine article.

> 1 tablespoon vegetable oil
> ¹/₂ cup chopped onions
> ¹/₂ cup chopped fresh green peppers
> ¹/₂ cup chopped celery
> 1 16-ounce can tomatoes and juice
> 1 cup fat-free chicken broth
> ¹/₂ cup long-grain rice
> ¹/₂ teaspoon salt
> ¹/₈–¹/₄ teaspoon cayenne pepper, to taste
> 1 tablespoon chopped parsley
> ¹/₂ teaspoon thyme
> 1¹/₂ cups boneless, chopped, cooked
>   chicken with fat and skin removed

**½ cup chopped cooked ham with all
visible fat removed**

Preheat a 2-quart saucepan over medium heat for 1 minute. Swirl oil in bottom of pan. Add onions, green peppers, and celery. Cook, stirring frequently, over medium heat until onions are soft but not browned. Add tomatoes and juice, broth, rice, salt, cayenne pepper, parsley, and thyme. Cook, uncovered, over low heat, stirring frequently, for 20–25 minutes, or until rice is tender. If mixture gets too dry, add hot water, ¼ cup at a time. Add chicken and ham and continue to cook until meat is heated through. Serve hot, using 1 cup per serving.

Yields 5 cups—5 servings

Nutritive Values Per Serving

CAL	CARBS (g)	PRO (g)	TOTAL FAT (g)	SAT. FAT (g)	CHOL (mg)	FIBER (g)	NA (mg)
226	22	18	7	1.5	45	1.5	715

Food exchanges per serving: 2 lean meat, 1 starch, 1 vegetable.
Low-sodium diets: Omit salt. Use low-sodium canned tomatoes and broth. Omit ham and use 2 cups chicken.
Sugar content per serving: None.

Chicken or Turkey à la King

**1 4-ounce can mushroom stems and pieces
2 tablespoons vegetable oil
3 cups fat-free chicken broth
3 tablespoons cornstarch
¼ cup instant nonfat dry milk
⅛ teaspoon white pepper
2 cups cooked diced chicken or turkey
with fat and skin removed
¼ cup chopped drained pimientos**

Drain mushrooms well. Discard juice. Place oil in the bottom of a saucepan. Add the mushrooms and cook and stir over moderate heat until mushrooms are lightly browned.

Mix together broth, cornstarch, dry milk, and pepper until smooth. Add all at once to mushrooms and oil and stir, cooking over moderate heat until thickened. Continue to cook and stir another 2 minutes or until the starchy taste is gone.

Add chicken and pimiento to sauce. Mix lightly. Reheat to serving temperature and serve 1 cup per serving.

Yields 4 cups—4 servings

Nutritive Values Per Serving

CAL	CARBS (g)	PRO (g)	TOTAL FAT (g)	SAT. FAT (g)	CHOL (mg)	FIBER (g)	NA (mg)
280	10	29	13	2.6	77	trace	648

Food exchanges per serving: 3 lean meat, 1 skim milk.
Low-sodium diets: Use low-sodium chicken broth.
Sugar content per serving: None.

Chicken and Broccoli

This recipe is based on one from Judy Ballantine of Madison, Wisconsin.

> 1 tablespoon cornstarch
> 1 tablespoon sherry or fat-free chicken
>   broth
> 2 tablespoons soy sauce
> ½ cup fat-free chicken broth
> ⅛ teaspoon ground ginger
> ⅛ teaspoon garlic powder
> 2 medium-size chicken breast halves
>   without skin or visible fat
> 1 tablespoon vegetable oil
> ½ cup sliced onions
> 2 cups (6 ounces) frozen broccoli cuts
> ½ cup fat-free chicken broth

Combine first six ingredients and mix until smooth to form a marinade. Bone chicken breasts. Freeze bones for later use in broth and cut chicken into bite-size pieces. Place in marinade and refrigerate for 1–4 hours. Drain well, reserving marinade to be used later.

Fry chicken in vegetable oil in heavy frying pan until white and firm. Remove chicken from frying pan with a slotted spoon, leaving as much of the oil as possible still in the frying pan. Add onions and broccoli to the oil in the frying pan. Slice any larger pieces of broccoli to about ½-inch thickness. Cook and stir about 1 minute or until broccoli is thawed.

Add broth to vegetables, mix lightly, cover, and simmer for 5 minutes or until the broccoli is crisp-tender. Add marinade and bring to a boil. Reduce heat to moderate and stir until sauce is thickened and clear. Add chicken and reheat to serving temperature. Serve ⅔ cup per serving over hot rice.

Yields 2 cups—3 servings

Nutritive Values Per Serving (without rice)

CAL	CARBS (g)	PRO (g)	TOTAL FAT (g)	SAT. FAT (g)	CHOL (mg)	FIBER (g)	NA (mg)
179	10	21	6	.9	44	1.4	965

Food exchanges per serving: 2½ very lean meat, 1 vegetable, 1 fat.
Low-sodium diets: Use low-sodium soy sauce and broth.
Sugar content per serving: None.

Italian Chicken over Linguine

This easy-to-make recipe can go from stovetop to table in 15 minutes or less. It is delicious served with a Caesar salad, sliced fresh pears, and an after-dinner mint.

> **1 pound of chicken breast**
> **4 cups yellow and green zucchini squash**
> **(or 8 ounces of your favorite frozen stir-fry vegetable combination)**

1 medium sweet red bell pepper
1 teaspoon olive oil (optional)
Dash salt (optional)
8 ounces (dry) linguine noodles
6 ounces Lite Italian or Lite Zesty Italian
**   Dressing**
3 tablespoons grated Parmesan cheese
Cilantro or parsley to garnish as desired

Cut the chicken breast(s) into 1½-inch strips. Set aside. Wash and slice the zucchini and red peppers. Set aside.

Place a pan of water (8 cups) on the stove to boil. Add 1 teaspoon olive oil and a dash of salt to the water to prevent the noodles from sticking, if so desired. When the water comes to a boil, add the linguine noodles and cook for seven to ten minutes until tender but firm (*al dente*).

While the pasta is cooking, place 2 tablespoons of the Italian dressing in a nonstick frying pan. When the dressing is hot, add the chicken and stir-fry until the chicken is cooked thoroughly and lightly golden brown (about 3 to 5 minutes). Remove the chicken from the pan and add 1 additional tablespoon of dressing; add the vegetables and stir-fry until coated with dressing; add 2 tablespoons of water and continue cooking until tender but crisp (about 3 minutes).

Add the chicken back to the pan. Add ½ cup Italian dressing and cook until heated throughout.

Drain the linguine noodles and place in a pasta bowl. Pour the chicken-vegetable mixture over the linguine and sprinkle with Parmesan cheese. Garnish with fresh parsley or cilantro as desired. Serve immediately while warm. Makes five servings—2 cups each.

Note: If you choose to use frozen vegetables, you will not need to add the 2 tablespoons water when stir-frying. Instead, add the vegetables to the chicken in the pan. Add the ½ cup of Italian dressing and the vegetables and cook until the vegetables are warm throughout.

Yields 10 cups—5 servings

Nutritive Values Per Serving

CAL	CARBS (g)	PRO (g)	TOTAL FAT (g)	SAT. FAT (g)	CHOL (mg)	FIBER (g)	NA (mg)
390	41	28	12	3.5	60	17	880

Food exchanges per serving: 2 starch/bread, 1 vegetable, 2 meat, and 1 fat.
Low-sodium diets: Use a low-sodium Italian dressing or a made-from-scratch Italian dressing with no added salt.
Sugar content per serving: 1 1/4 teaspoon.

Tomato Chicken Sauce for Spaghetti

6 ounces raw boneless chicken without skin or visible fat
2 tablespoons vegetable oil
1/2 cup chopped onions
1/2 cup chopped fresh green peppers
1/2 cup chopped celery
2 cups canned tomato sauce
1/4 teaspoon Italian seasoning
1/4 teaspoon salt
1/4 teaspoon leaf oregano
1/4 teaspoon basil
1/2 teaspoon paprika
Whisper of white pepper

Cut chicken into 1/2-inch cubes and set aside for later use.

Place oil in the bottom of a saucepan. Heat over moderate heat for 1 minute. Add onions, peppers, celery, and chicken and cook and stir about 5 minutes or until chicken is white and firm, and vegetables are softened but not browned.

Add remaining ingredients to vegetables and chicken and cook, stirring almost constantly, for 5 minutes. Serve hot, 1/2 cup per serving, over hot spaghetti or hot, thin, homemade noodles.

servings

Nutritive Values Per Serving

	TOTAL FAT (g)	SAT. FAT (g)	CHOL (mg)	FIBER (g)	NA (mg)
	6	.8	20	1.7	614

Food exchanges per serving: 1 lean meat, 1½ vegetable, 1 fat.
Low-sodium diets: Omit salt. Use low-sodium tomato sauce.
Sugar content per serving: None.

Chicken and Bean Sprouts with Mushrooms

1 4-ounce can mushroom pieces
Fat-free chicken broth as necessary
3 tablespoons soy sauce
1 teaspoon sugar
1½ tablespoons cornstarch
1 tablespoon sherry
2 large chicken breast halves without skin
    or visible fat
2 tablespoons vegetable oil
1 16-ounce can bean sprouts

Drain mushrooms, reserving the liquid. Set drained mushrooms aside. Place the mushroom juice in a 1 cup measure and add enough broth to total 1 cup liquid. Set aside.

Mix together soy sauce, sugar, cornstarch, sherry, and 2 tablespoons of broth mixture in a small bowl until smooth, and set aside. Bone chicken breasts. You should have about 8 ounces chicken. Discard bones and cut chicken into ¾-inch cubes. Place chicken into the soy sauce mixture and let marinate for 10 minutes. Drain well, reserving the marinade for later.

Place oil in a heavy frying pan and heat over moderate heat until oil has a haze over it. Add the chicken to the hot oil and fry over moderate heat until chicken is firm and white, stirring frequently. Push chicken to the side of the frying pan. Add mushrooms and cook and stir until mushrooms are hot but not browned. Mix lightly with chicken. Add remainder of marinade and chicken broth mixture and bring to a boil, then cook and stir over moderate heat until the sauce is thickened and clear.

Drain bean sprouts well and stir into chicken and sauce. Cook and stir until hot and the sprouts are covered with sauce. Serve hot over rice, using ¾ cup per serving.

Yields 3 cups—4 servings

Nutritive Values Per Serving (without rice)

CAL	CARBS (g)	PRO (g)	TOTAL FAT (g)	SAT. FAT (g)	CHOL (mg)	FIBER (g)	NA (mg)
197	8	22	8	1	49	1	1,090

Food exchanges per serving: 3 lean meat, 1 vegetable.
Low-sodium diets: Use low-sodium soy sauce and broth.
Sugar content per serving: .3 teaspoon.

Chicken or Turkey Sandwich Spread

This is a favorite of my friend Jan Franks. Beef may be substituted for the chicken with no change in the food exchanges. This spread is also good for appetizers, and 1 tablespoon (about three appetizers) may be eaten without counting the spread.

> 1 cup diced, cooked chicken or turkey
> without skin or visible fat
> 3 tablespoons Kay's Cooked Dressing (see
> Index)
> 2 tablespoons Mrs. Riley's Pickles, finely
> chopped (see Index)

Chop chicken rather fine in a food processor or grind in a food grinder, using the coarse blade.

Add dressing and pickles to chicken and mix well. Refrigerate until served using ¼ cup per serving for a sandwich.

Yields 1 cup—4 servings

Nutritive Values Per Serving

CAL	CARBS (g)	PRO (g)	TOTAL FAT (g)	SAT. FAT (g)	CHOL (mg)	FIBER (g)	NA (mg)
121	1	17	5	1.3	50	trace	222

Food exchanges per serving: 2 lean meat.
Low-sodium diets: Use low-sodium variation of the dressing.
Sugar content per serving: None.

Chicken or Turkey Loaf

This makes excellent sandwiches, hot or cold.

> **2 pounds ground raw chicken or turkey**
> **1 cup dry bread crumbs**
> **2 large egg whites**
> **2 chicken bouillon cubes dissolved in**
> **½ cup water**
> **1 tablespoon Worcestershire sauce or**
> **½ teaspoon rubbed sage or thyme**
> **1 tablespoon chopped parsley**
> **Dash of white pepper**
> **½ cup finely chopped onions**

It is best to grind the meat yourself since the ground chicken and turkey you buy generally has the skin and some fat in it. If your market will grind it for you without skin or fat you are in luck; but if not, figure that you will need about 3 pounds raw chicken or turkey for each pound of ground meat. Remove all skin and visible fat with a sharp knife. Bone the chicken or turkey, and then grind it in a meat grinder or chop it in a food processor. (Freeze the bones, wings, and neck to use to make broth later.) Refrigerate until needed. The ground poultry can also be used to make chicken or turkey patties.

Place remaining ingredients in mixing bowl. Mix well. Add chicken and mix lightly but thoroughly. Form into a loaf and place in a 9" × 5" × 3" loaf pan that has been greased with margarine. Bake at 325°F about 1½ hours or until firm and lightly browned. Remove from oven and let set for 15 minutes. Slice into 12 equal slices and serve one slice per serving.

Yields 1 loaf—12 servings

Nutritive Values Per Serving

CAL	CARBS (g)	PRO (g)	TOTAL FAT (g)	SAT. FAT (g)	CHOL (mg)	FIBER (g)	NA (mg)
136	8	18	3	.8	53	trace	323

Food exchanges per serving: 2 lean meat, ½ starch.
Low-sodium diets: Use ½ cup strong low-sodium, fat-free chicken broth instead of the bouillon cubes and water. Use sage or thyme instead of Worcestershire sauce.
Sugar content per serving: None.

Chicken or Turkey Gravy

2¼ cups fat-free chicken or turkey
   drippings or broth
2 tablespoons cornstarch
⅛ teaspoon rubbed sage or thyme
1½ teaspoons margarine
Whisper of white pepper

Combine all ingredients in a small saucepan and cook over moderate heat, stirring constantly, until thickened and smooth. Continue to cook and stir for another 2 minutes over low heat until the starchy taste is gone. Serve hot using ¼ cup gravy per serving. (The flavor of the gravy will depend upon the flavor of the drippings or broth, so it is a good idea to use the most flavorful drippings or broth possible.)

Yields 2 cups—8 servings

Nutritive Values Per Serving

CAL	CARBS (g)	PRO (g)	TOTAL FAT (g)	SAT. FAT (g)	CHOL (mg)	FIBER (g)	NA (mg)
19	2	1	1	trace	0	trace	190

Food exchanges per serving: 1 serving may be considered free. ¹/₂ cup is 1
   vegetable exchange.
Low-sodium diets: Use low-sodium drippings or broth.
Sugar content per serving: None.

Bread Dressing

*This costs a lot in bread exchanges but I included it because it
illustrates how to adapt bread dressing to a low-cholesterol diet.
I like it well enough to consider it worth the bread exchanges it
costs me.*

> **2 tablespoons vegetable oil**
> **³/₄ cup finely chopped celery**
> **¹/₂ cup finely chopped onions**
> **2 cups fat-free chicken or beef broth**
> **³/₄ teaspoon ground sage or thyme**
> **Whisper of black pepper**
> **12 slices day-old white bread**
> **2 egg whites**

Place oil in the bottom of a saucepan. Add celery and onions and
cook over moderate heat for 5 minutes, stirring frequently.
Remove from heat. Add broth and seasonings to vegetables. Mix
well and cool to lukewarm, if necessary.

Cut bread into cubes. It is a good idea to leave the bread
spread out on a tray overnight before it is used—the bread won't
absorb enough liquid to give it a good flavor if it isn't somewhat
dry. Place cubes in a large mixing bowl.

Add egg whites to lukewarm vegetables and broth. Mix well
and pour over bread cubes. Toss lightly but thoroughly. Spread

evenly in an 8-inch square cake pan or 1-quart shallow casserole that has been well greased with margarine. Bake at 375°F for 45 minutes. Cut 3 × 4 into 12 equal servings, allowing one square per serving.

Yields 8-inch square pan—12 servings

Nutritive Values Per Serving

CAL	CARBS (g)	PRO (g)	TOTAL FAT (g)	SAT. FAT (g)	CHOL (mg)	FIBER (g)	NA (mg)
105	15	4	3	.5	trace	.9	276

Food exchanges per serving: 1 starch.
Low-sodium diets: Use low-sodium broth.
Sugar content per serving: None.

12

Meats

Planning and preparing meat dishes is probably the hardest part of the low-cholesterol diabetic diet. Most of us are used to using a lot of plain roast meat, and this is still a good idea as long as we pick the leanest cuts and prepare them so that we remove as much of the remaining fat as possible.

Specific cuts with a lower fat content that are good for the low-cholesterol diabetic diet include the following:

- *Beef*—round, rump, sirloin, tenderloin, and dried beef
- *Pork*—loin, center cut roasts or chops, tenderloin, lean ham, center cut ham, and Canadian bacon
- *Veal*—round, rump, leg, sirloin, cutlets, and loin chops
- *Lamb*—sirloin, leg, cutlets, and sirloin chops

Baking, boiling, broiling, and roasting are all good methods for preparing meat because they help remove any remaining fat after all of the visible fat has been removed with a sharp knife. Baked or roasted meats should be placed on a rack so that the liquids will drip down in the bottom of the pan and the meat won't be cooking in its own fat. If necessary, the meat can be basted with broth or a marinade. Drippings in the bottom can be chilled and used for gravy or soups after the fat is removed.

Meats can be pan-broiled if salt or only a small amount of fat used in the bottom of the frying pan—and you will be surprised how little fat is really needed for pan-broiling. Sprinkle the pan first with salt; but if you can't do that, you can use just a tablespoon of oil in the bottom of the frying pan with excellent results. Oil is better than margarine for pan-frying because it doesn't get brown and burn as easily as margarine does.

Roasts should be cooked at about 325°F. There is a classic example I use when teaching meat cookery to illustrate the advantages of using the lower temperature: we take two identical roasts, roasting one at 325°F and the other at 400°F—the one cooked at 400°F is always obviously shrunken and less tender. All roasting time is approximate because of the variability of the tenderness of the meat, thickness, and whether the roast has been in the refrigerator or is at room temperature. A meat thermometer should be used for accuracy. It should be inserted in the thickest part of the roast without touching any fat or bone. Rare meat is more tender than well done.

Round of beef has the lowest fat content, so you don't have to worry about the amount of fat left in the cooked roast. Round of beef is found in many different forms in your supermarket. You can get a boneless top round roast, eye of round roast, and the less tender bottom round pot roast. You can find thick round steaks for broiling and thinner round steaks for grilling or pan-frying. There are thinly sliced minute steaks for sandwiches, and top round can be found that has been cut into cubes for stews or broiling on skewers. The less tender bottom round can be cut into cubes or ground for use in spaghetti sauce, stew, or chili. Bottom round is also the top choice ground for hamburgers.

Roast round of beef requires a little extra care to make it tender. Top round or eye of round are best for roasting. Roast it, uncovered, at 300°F to about 130–140°F internally for rare or medium rare. Don't overcook it. Well done round of beef will be tough unless you pot-roast it until it is falling apart. It is better if it is soaked in a marinade for several hours or overnight in the refrigerator—or a commercial tenderizer can be used according to the directions on the package. (Never use tenderizer on hamburger; it makes it mushy.) Don't bother to include oil in your marinade. It doesn't help tenderize the meat and adds calories and fat exchanges. Wine, vinegar, and tomato juice contain natural acids that tenderize meat without adding many calories.

Flank steak, rump, round, or sirloin tip are best used for stews and casseroles. If you must use stew meat, remove all visible fat before it is cooked. All stew meat should be browned first in as little fat as possible, covered with liquid, and simmered until tender. It can then be drained and the broth refrigerated until it is cool and the fat has risen to the top. You will be surprised at the amount of fat you will be able to skim off the broth before it is recombined with the meat and the stew or casserole finished. This is a time-consuming task, so I generally do several pounds of meat at once and then freeze what I'm not going to use that day in portions for future use.

Recipes including ground beef should be prepared so that you get as much of the fat as possible out of the meat. Buy lean ground beef, ground round of beef or veal, or ground leg of lamb. You should try to use recipes that allow the meat to be browned, drained, and rinsed with hot water before it is combined with other ingredients. Meat loaves aren't all that good for you if they contain much filler such as bread crumbs or oatmeal, because the fillers absorb the saturated fat from the meat while the loaf is cooking. This is too bad because meat loaves are handy to have for sandwiches. Because meat loaves tend to hold fat, it is a good idea to use only the leanest meat in them, or chicken or turkey, which also make a good meat loaf (see Index). The best way to do it when you want to make a beef meat loaf is to buy round steak, have the butcher remove any visible fat, and then grind the meat for you. If you don't have a butcher who will do it for you, a food processor will do a good job. Most heavy-duty mixers have good grinders, or you can buy an electric or hand grinder to use. If you grind the meat yourself you can be sure that you have removed all possible visible fat before grinding.

Hamburgers are good and we all love them, but it isn't a good idea to buy them at a restaurant because the fat content is generally very high. If you do buy them at a restaurant, take a paper napkin and blot the fat off both sides of the hamburger before you eat it. When you cook hamburgers at home be sure to use lean ground meat and the seasonings you like; however, it is best not to add bread crumbs or other fillers to the meat because they trap the fat that you are trying to get rid of. It will taste good but it will have more saturated fat than you really should be using. Hamburgers can be prepared according to one of the following methods:

- *Grilled.* Rub a grill lightly with oil or sprinkle with salt (if permissible), heat until it is sizzling hot, and brown the burgers on both sides. Cook them 2–8 minutes on each side depending upon whether you like them rare or well done.
- *Pan-fried.* Heat a heavy frying pan until sizzling hot, rub lightly with oil or sprinkle with salt (if permissible), and brown the burgers on both sides. Reduce the heat and cook them over medium heat 2–8 minutes on each side depending upon whether you like them rare or well done.
- *Broiled.* Arrange hamburger patties on a cold broiler rack. Broil 3–4 inches from the heat, turning once, for about 4–6 minutes on each side depending upon how thick they are and how well done you like them to be.

It is a good idea to stick to the *good* grade of beef. *Choice* beef may be a little more tender, but that is because it has more marbling of fat and this is what you want to avoid. Check the grade of beef before you buy it, and if you are in doubt always check with the butcher or salesperson behind the counter. If it is practical for you, it is a good idea to buy your meat at a store where you can be sure you are getting the *good* grade of beef, and then instruct them to remove every bit of fat possible before the meat is ground.

Swine breeders have developed much leaner hogs in the last few years, so that pork is no longer as fat as it used to be and may be used occasionally on a low-cholesterol diabetic diet. However, it is still wise to use the leanest cuts, avoiding spareribs, pork sausage, and other cuts, such as the shoulder, with a higher fat content. The tenderloin is particularly good and is luscious when cut thick and broiled. Fresh ham and center cut loin are also good for roasting after all the visible fat has been removed. Pork chops should be center cut and have all visible fat removed before cooking, and they should not be cooked with dressing or stuffing because the dressing or stuffing picks up too much fat from the pork chops while they are baking.

Ham can be very lean, and if you don't have to worry about salt restrictions can be a very good buy, particularly some of the low-fat hams. Most hams available are precooked so you only need to reheat them to an interior temperature of 130°F. This should take about 15–20 minutes per pound at 325°F or you can do it in the microwave, according to directions that come with your microwave. The center cut of smoked ham is generally acceptable also if all of the visible fat is removed. It may be broiled or pan-broiled.

- *Broiled.* Remove all visible fat from a center cut of ham about 1 inch thick. Broil about 15 minutes for precooked ham and about 25 minutes for uncooked ham, turning it once while it is broiling.
- *Pan-broiled.* Remove all visible fat from a center cut of ham about ¼–½ inch thick. Rub a frying pan with a little oil and cook over medium heat, turning at least once while it is frying. Cook about 6–8 minutes for precooked ham and about 12–16 minutes for uncooked ham.

Here in Iowa we have what they call Iowa Pork Chops. These are lean chops that weigh about 8–9 ounces each. One chop is far too much for our meat allowance, but I like to brown them, put them in a small roaster with a rack, and continue cooking them, covered, in the oven at 325°F for about an hour or until they are tender. I cut off the amount of meat that I am allowed for that meal and save the rest for another meal. It tastes like luscious roast pork and is really very good. If they aren't available in your area, I'm sure your butcher would be happy to cut some for you from the center loin. Of course, I cut off all visible fat before preparing them, and they are really very lean when prepared that way.

Properly cooked lamb has a delicious, mild flavor and an appetizing aroma. It should be served hot or cold—never lukewarm. In the past, recipes generally specified well-done lamb; however, today the accepted procedure is to cook it to 165°F, which is slightly rare. This gives you a more flavorful and juicy roast. Lamb is good for a low-cholesterol diet because it is lower in fat than many of the beef cuts. The leg is the leanest part of the lamb and it can be cut into a leg of lamb roast or a sirloin roast. The sirloin may also be cut into chops or ground. Lamb patties, which are traditionally lean, are often wrapped in bacon. We can't do this but I find that if I add a little seasoning and broil the patty until it is medium well done, it will be moist and juicy. If you buy the whole leg of lamb you will find it is covered with a whitish, brittle fat that is called the fell. This should be removed before the roast is cooked because it tends to make the flavor of the meat strong, as well as adding additional fat that you don't need.

Veal has a delicate flavor when it is cooked properly. Good veal is light pink in color rather than red and has a small amount of very white fat. It is not suited for broiling because of the small amount of fat, but that small amount of fat makes it an excellent choice for a low-cholesterol diabetic diet. Veal cutlets are very lean and may be pan-broiled. They are often dipped in egg white and then cracker crumbs and deep fat fried. This method would be satisfactory except that it does add more fat exchanges. The veal cutlets may also be dipped in egg white and then crumbs and pan-broiled using very little oil, which uses fewer fat exchanges and still tastes like a good veal cutlet. Veal is a good choice for stews and casseroles because of its low fat content—and roast leg of veal is an excellent entrée for a dinner or special occasion.

If you have a favorite meat recipe that isn't included in this book, you can calculate the nutritive values for it using the information in Chapter 3. Roast meats are calculated using nutritive values of one meat exchange per 1 ounce serving of meat. If gravy is used it will have to be figured separately. I have tried to illustrate different methods of preparation hoping that you could use them as a basis for your own recipes—but remember, if you add or subtract something, unless it is very, very low in food value like celery or mushrooms, you must recalculate the recipe to arrive at the correct exchanges for your diet pattern.

Broiled Round Steak

Who says we can't have steak on a low-cholesterol diet? I think you will be surprised when you taste this broiled steak.

It is really a method more than an exact recipe. You can vary the marinade to suit yourself, which will change the flavor a little bit. The steak will be more tender if it is rare or, at the least, medium done. This method also will work for a round bone pot roast, although the round is better for a low-cholesterol diet.

> **2 pounds round of beef, 2 inches thick,**
>   **with all visible fat removed**
> **¼ cup vegetable oil**
> **¼ cup red wine vinegar**
> **¼ cup red wine**
> **¼–½ teaspoon garlic powder**
> **1 teaspoon leaf thyme**
> **1 teaspoon leaf oregano**
> **3 tablespoons chopped parsley**
> **Salt and pepper to taste**

Place steak in a shallow dish. Mix together all remaining ingredients except salt and pepper and pour over the round steak. Cover tightly and let it marinate at room temperature for about 2 hours, or overnight in the refrigerator. Remove meat from the marinade. Pat it dry with a paper towel and discard the marinade. Broil 3–4 minutes on each side about 4 inches from the heat for rare, or more as desired.

Season meat with salt and pepper and serve hot. It can be carved in thin slices across the grain or served in large pieces for each person to cut his or her own. Food exchanges will depend upon the serving size, with 1 ounce cooked meat counted as one lean meat exchange. Low-sodium diets should omit salt.

Yields 21 to 24 ounces

Nutritive Values Per 3-Ounce Serving

CAL	CARBS (g)	PRO (g)	TOTAL FAT (g)	SAT. FAT (g)	CHOL (mg)	FIBER (g)	NA (mg)
180	trace	25	8	2.4	66	0	55

Food exchanges per 3-ounce serving: 3 lean meat.
Low-sodium diets: Omit salt.
Sugar content per serving: None.

Beef with Green Beans

I find this easier to prepare in an electric frying pan.

> **8 ounces round of beef with all visible fat
>   removed before it is weighed**
> **2 tablespoons soy sauce**
> **1 tablespoon cornstarch**
> **½ teaspoon salt**
> **1 tablespoon sherry or beef broth**
> **1 tablespoon vegetable oil**
> **¼ cup water**
> **1 pound frozen green beans cut into 1-inch
>   lengths**

Cut beef into pieces about ⅛–¼ inch thick and about 1 inch long. (This is easier if the meat is slightly frozen.) Refrigerate until needed.

Mix soy sauce, cornstarch, salt, and sherry well. Pour over the meat. Mix lightly and let stand at room temperature for about ½ hour, or refrigerate for several hours or overnight. Drain well, reserving the marinade.

Spread oil over the bottom of a frying pan. Heat to a frying temperature. Fry, stirring frequently, until the meat is no longer pink. Add ¼ cup water to the meat along with the reserved marinade. Stir lightly over medium heat.

Add green beans to meat mixture. Cook and stir until beans and meat are both well coated with the sauce. Cover and cook, stirring occasionally, until beans are crisp-tender. Serve about ¾ cup per serving over rice or noodles.

Yields 3 cups—4 servings

Nutritive Values Per Serving (without rice or noodles)

CAL	CARBS (g)	PRO (g)	TOTAL FAT (g)	SAT. FAT (g)	CHOL (mg)	FIBER (g)	NA (mg)
164	12	15	6	1.4	33	2	824

Food exchanges per serving: 2 lean meat, 1 other carbohydrate.
Low-sodium diets: Omit salt and use low-sodium soy sauce.
Sugar content per serving: None.

Texas Round Steak

½ cup all-purpose flour
1 teaspoon salt
1½ teaspoons chili powder
1 pound 2 ounces round of beef about ½
    inch thick (weighed after fat and bone
    are removed), cut into 6 3-ounce steaks
2 tablespoons vegetable oil
½ cup chopped fresh green peppers
½ cup chopped onions
1 cup fat-free beef broth
½ cup tomato sauce
½ cup tomato juice
1 teaspoon chili powder
¼ teaspoon garlic powder
¼ teaspoon ground cumin

Blend flour, salt, and 1½ teaspoons chili powder well and place in a pie pan. Dredge meat in the flour mixture. You should use about half of the mixture. (You can discard the rest; however, it is necessary to have this amount to make dredging practical.)

Place oil in a heavy frying pan and heat to frying temperature over moderate heat. Add meat and brown on both sides. Transfer steaks to a 1½-quart casserole.

Fry peppers and onions over moderate heat in the pan in which the meat was browned, stirring frequently. Remove vegetables with a slotted spoon and spread over the meat. Pour out any remaining fat. Add beef broth to frying pan and cook and stir over moderate heat to absorb any brown particles remaining in the pan.

Add remaining ingredients to broth. Mix well and pour over meat. Stir the meat and vegetables lightly with a fork to distribute the broth and vegetables. Cover tightly and bake at 325°F for about 1–1½ hours or until the meat is tender. Serve one piece of steak with some of the sauce per serving.

Yields 6 steaks—6 servings

Nutritive Values Per Serving

CAL	CARBS (g)	PRO (g)	TOTAL FAT (g)	SAT. FAT (g)	CHOL (mg)	FIBER (g)	NA (mg)
220	13	21	9	2	50	1.4	728

Food exchanges per serving: 3 lean meat, 1 other carbohydrate.
Low-sodium diets: Omit salt. Use low-sodium broth, tomato sauce, and tomato juice.
Sugar content per serving: None.

Beef Mushroom Spaghetti Sauce

12 ounces round of beef weighed and
  ground after fat is removed
1 tablespoon vegetable oil
½ cup finely chopped onions
2 4-ounce cans mushroom stems and
  pieces
3½ cups (29-ounce can) tomato purée
2 cups tomato juice
2 tablespoons chopped parsley
1 teaspoon salt
½ teaspoon dehydrated garlic
½ teaspoon basil
½ teaspoon leaf oregano
1 teaspoon Italian seasoning

Place beef in a 5- or 6-quart Dutch oven or heavy pot. Cook and stir over moderate heat until it is separated and lightly browned. Place in a strainer and strain off any fat. Set aside to drain. Rinse out the pan with hot water and return it to the heat.

Place oil in Dutch oven. Add onions. Drain mushrooms well. Discard juice and add mushrooms to onions. Cook and stir over moderate heat until onions are soft.

Add remaining ingredients along with meat to onions and mushrooms. Cook over low heat for 30 minutes, stirring frequently. Serve hot over cooked, well-drained spaghetti, ½ cup sauce per serving.

Yields 7 cups—14 servings

Nutritive Values Per Serving (without spaghetti)

CAL	CARBS (g)	PRO (g)	TOTAL FAT (g)	SAT. FAT (g)	CHOL (mg)	FIBER (g)	NA (mg)
78	9	7	2	.5	14	1.7	570

Food exchanges per serving: 1 lean meat, 2 vegetable.
Low-sodium diets: Omit salt. Use low-sodium tomato purée and tomato juice.
Sugar content per serving: None.

Vegetable-Beef Stew

1 pound round of beef or veal weighed
   after fat and bone are removed
1 tablespoon vegetable oil
3 cups hot fat-free beef broth
¼ teaspoon thyme
⅛ teaspoon pepper
¼ teaspoon garlic powder
1 teaspoon salt
1 cup carrots cut into 1-inch pieces
4 large stalks celery cut into 1-inch lengths
½ cup coarsely chopped onions
¼ cup chopped fresh green peppers
10-ounce package frozen Brussels sprouts

2 tablespoons cornstarch
¼ cup water

Cut meat into ¾-inch cubes. (This is easier if the meat is slightly frozen.) Place oil on the bottom of a heavy pot. (I use a deep iron frying pan with a glass cover.) Bring to a frying temperature. Add meat and cook, stirring occasionally, until meat is browned.

Add broth and seasonings to meat. Cover and simmer 45 minutes to 1 hour or until meat is tender.

Add carrots, celery, onions, and peppers to meat. Cover and simmer 10 minutes. Add Brussels sprouts to stew. Cover and simmer another 12 minutes.

Mix cornstarch and water until smooth. Add to stew and cook and stir until thickened. Continue to simmer for another 2 to 3 minutes or until starchy taste is gone. Serve hot, 1 cup stew with gravy per serving.

Yields 6 cups—6 servings

Nutritive Values Per Serving

CAL	CARBS (g)	PRO (g)	TOTAL FAT (g)	SAT. FAT (g)	CHOL (mg)	FIBER (g)	NA (mg)
181	11	21	6	1.6	44	2.3	767

Food exchanges per serving: 2 lean meat, 2 vegetable.
Low-sodium diets: Omit salt. Use low-sodium broth.
Sugar content per serving: None.

Stir-Fry Beef and Vegetables

This stir-fry recipe is an adaptation of a Chinese recipe.

8 ounces beef sirloin with fat and gristle
removed
¼ cup dry red wine or fat-free beef broth
3 tablespoons soy sauce
1 teaspoon sugar
1½ tablespoons cornstarch

Water
1 tablespoon vegetable oil
2 cups coarsely chopped onions
½ cup thinly sliced celery
½ cup coarsely chopped fresh green
   peppers
2 tablespoons chopped roasted cashews

Place meat in freezer until it is firm but not frozen. Cut across the grain into bite-size pieces and set aside. Place wine or broth, soy sauce, sugar, and cornstarch in a 2-cup measure. Add enough water to total 1 cup. Stir until smooth and set aside.

Preheat a 10-inch, nonstick-surfaced frying pan. (I use a wok frying pan with a T-Fal lining.) Swirl oil around bottom of frying pan, add onions, celery, and green peppers, and cook, stirring frequently, over medium heat until onions are soft but not browned.

Push vegetables to one side of pan, add meat, and cook, stirring the meat frequently, until the meat is rare to well done, as you prefer. Pour wine sauce over meat and vegetables and cook and stir until sauce is clear and thickened. Serve hot over rice or noodles using 1 cup per serving. Garnish each serving with 2 teaspoons of cashews.

Yields 3 cups—3 servings

Nutritive Values Per Serving (without rice or noodles)

CAL	CARBS (g)	PRO (g)	TOTAL FAT (g)	SAT. FAT (g)	CHOL (mg)	FIBER (g)	NA (mg)
264	20	19	11	2.3	46	2.5	1,096

Food exchanges per serving: 2 medium-fat meat, 1 vegetable, 1 other
   carbohydrate.
Low-sodium diets: Use low-sodium soy sauce.
Sugar content per serving: .3 teaspoon.

Mary's Meatballs

This recipe is based on one from Mary Hinkle here in Wadena, Iowa.

¼ cup ketchup
¼ cup tomato juice
1 tablespoon liquid smoke
½ teaspoon Durkee's barbecue seasoning
1 teaspoon sugar
½ cup oatmeal
¼ cup dry bread crumbs
3 tablespoons grated onions
½ teaspoon salt
¼ teaspoon black pepper
1 cup skim milk
1½ pounds round of beef weighed and
    ground after fat is removed

Blend first five ingredients together well to form a barbecue sauce and set aside at room temperature for later use.

Place oatmeal, crumbs, onions, salt, pepper, and milk in a mixer bowl and mix together at low speed to mix well. Add beef to milk mixture and mix at low speed until blended. Do not over-mix. Shape into balls using 2 tablespoons of the mixture for each meatball. Place on a cookie sheet and broil 2–4 minutes. Remove from cookie sheet and place in a casserole, brushing the meatballs with the barbecue sauce as you put them in the casserole. Pour any remaining sauce over the meatballs, cover, and bake at 325°F for about 45 minutes or until done. Serve hot, two meatballs per serving.

Yields 28 meatballs—14 servings

Nutritive Values Per Serving

CAL	CARBS (g)	PRO (g)	TOTAL FAT (g)	SAT. FAT (g)	CHOL (mg)	FIBER (g)	NA (mg)
99	6	12	3	.9	29	.5	208

Food exchanges per serving: 1¼ lean meat, 1 vegetable.
Low-sodium diets: Omit salt. Use low-sodium ketchup.
Sugar content per serving: Trace.

Norwegian Meatballs

This recipe is based on one from Doris Walker of Grinnell, Iowa.

2 tablespoons cornstarch
³/₄ teaspoon salt
¹/₂ teaspoon nutmeg
2 large egg whites
³/₄ cup skim milk
1 pound ground round of beef weighed
**   and ground after fat is removed**
²/₃ cup Campbell's Cream of Mushroom
**   soup**

Place first four ingredients and ¼ cup of the milk in mixer bowl and mix at low speed to blend well. Add beef to mixer bowl and mix at low speed to blend well. Shape 18 meatballs using about 1½ tablespoons mix per meatball. (The mixture will be soft.) Place in a 9″ × 13″ cake pan that has been lined with aluminum foil or sprayed with cooking spray. Bake 30 minutes at 375°F. Remove from pan while still hot and place in a 1½-quart casserole.

Mix soup and remaining ½ cup milk well and pour over meatballs. Cover and bake at 350°F for 30 minutes. Serve three meatballs per serving with a sixth of the sauce.

Yields 18 meatballs—6 servings

Nutritive Values Per Serving

CAL	CARBS (g)	PRO (g)	TOTAL FAT (g)	SAT. FAT (g)	CHOL (mg)	FIBER (g)	NA (mg)
156	6	19	5	1.9	45	trace	546

Food exchanges per serving: 3 lean meat, 1 vegetable.
Low-sodium diets: Omit salt. Use low-sodium soup.
Sugar content per serving: None.

Chicago Chili

This is the recipe Chuck developed when he owned a restaurant in Chicago. He always served it in a bowl with the beans on the side. If you add canned beans to your chili, add one bread exchange for each 1/3 cup hot, cooked, drained kidney or pinto beans that you stir into a bowl of chili.

1 tablespoon vegetable oil
1 cup chopped onions
1 pound ground round of beef weighed
    and ground after bone and fat are
    removed
2 cups chopped solid-pack canned
    tomatoes with juice
1 cup tomato purée
1 cup tomato juice
3 cups fat-free chicken broth
1 teaspoon sugar
1½ teaspoons salt
¼ teaspoon pepper
½ teaspoon garlic powder
¼ teaspoon ground cumin
½ teaspoon ground oregano
1 teaspoon chili powder

Pour the oil into a heavy pot. Bring to frying temperature over moderate heat. Add the onions and cook and stir over moderate heat until onions are soft but not golden.

Add beef to onions. Cook and stir over moderate heat until meat is well browned and broken into small pieces. Pour meat and onions into a colander and drain off any fat and liquid. Discard fat and liquid, rinse the pot out with hot water, and then return the meat and onions to the pot.

Add remaining ingredients to meat mixture. Bring to a boil, reduce heat, and simmer, uncovered, for 1¼ hours, stirring occasionally. Serve hot using 1 cup chili per serving.

Yields 6 cups—6 servings

Nutritive Values Per Serving

CAL	CARBS (g)	PRO (g)	TOTAL FAT (g)	SAT. FAT (g)	CHOL (mg)	FIBER (g)	NA (mg)
189	13	21	6	1.6	44	2.4	1,363

Food exchanges per serving: 2 lean meat, 2 vegetable.

Low-sodium diets: Omit salt. Use low-sodium tomatoes, tomato purée, tomato juice, and broth.

Sugar content per serving: .2 teaspoon.

Barbecue Meat Loaf

¼ cup finely chopped onions
¼ cup finely chopped celery
¼ cup ketchup
2 large egg whites
¼ cup dry bread crumbs
1 teaspoon liquid smoke
1 teaspoon salt
Whisper of black pepper
1 pound round of beef weighed and
  ground after fat is removed

Place all ingredients except beef in mixer bowl and mix at low speed to blend well.

Add beef to ketchup mixture and mix at low speed until blended. Do not overmix. Shape into a loaf about 3½" × 7". Place in a pan that has been sprayed with cooking spray or lined with aluminum foil. Bake at 325°F about 1 hour or until browned and firm. Pour off any fat and drippings and let stand for 10 minutes before cutting into six equal slices. Serve one slice per serving.

Yields 1 loaf—6 servings

Nutritive Values Per Serving

CAL	CARBS (g)	PRO (g)	TOTAL FAT (g)	SAT. FAT (g)	CHOL (mg)	FIBER (g)	NA (mg)
143	7	19	4	1.3	44	.5	591

Food exchanges per serving: 2 very lean meat, 1 fat, 1 vegetable.

Low-sodium diets: Omit salt. Use low-sodium ketchup.

Sugar content per serving: None.

Meat Loaf with Fiber

---

1 cup All-Bran, Bran Buds, or 100% Bran
¼ cup finely chopped onions
3 large egg whites
1 cup tomato sauce
1 teaspoon Worcestershire sauce
1 teaspoon dry mustard
½ teaspoon salt
¹⁄₁₆ teaspoon pepper
1 pound 4 ounces round of beef weighed
    and ground after fat is removed

Place all ingredients except beef in mixer bowl and mix at low speed to blend.

Add beef to bran mixture and blend at low speed. Do not overmix. Shape into a loaf and place in a pan that has been sprayed with cooking spray or lined with aluminum foil. Bake at 325°F about 1¼ hours or until browned and firm. Pour off any fat and drippings and let stand for 10 minutes. Cut into eight equal slices. Serve one slice per serving.

Yields 1 loaf—8 servings

Nutritive Values Per Serving

CAL	CARBS (g)	PRO (g)	TOTAL FAT (g)	SAT. FAT (g)	CHOL (mg)	FIBER (g)	NA (mg)
137	8	18	4	1.2	41	3	459

Food exchanges per serving: 2 very lean meat, 1 fat, 1 vegetable.
Low-sodium diets: Omit salt. Use low-sodium tomato sauce.
Sugar content per serving: None.

Baked Pork and Rice

**12-ounces pork tenderloin weighed after
visible fat is removed**
1 cup thinly sliced celery
½ cup chopped onions
1½ cups fat-free chicken broth
½ cup long-grain rice
2 tablespoons soy sauce
Whisper of black pepper
3 tablespoons chopped pimientos

Cut pork into ½-inch cubes. Place in a shallow pan and bake at 350°F about 30 minutes or until browned. Remove from pan with a slotted spoon and place in a 1½-quart casserole.

Place celery, onions, and broth in a small saucepan. Bring to a boil, reduce heat, cover, and simmer for 10 minutes. Add rice, soy sauce, and pepper to hot broth. Mix lightly and add to meat in casserole. Mix lightly. Cover tightly and bake at 350°F about 40 minutes or until rice is tender. Remove from oven.

Stir pimientos into hot pork and rice. Serve hot, using a quarter of the total (about ¾ cup) per serving.

Yields about 3 cups—4 servings

Nutritive Values Per Serving

CAL	CARBS (g)	PRO (g)	TOTAL FAT (g)	SAT. FAT (g)	CHOL (mg)	FIBER (g)	NA (mg)
212	23	22	3	1	55	1	828

Food exchanges per serving: 2½ very lean meat, 1 starch, 1 vegetable.
Low-sodium diets: Use low-sodium soy sauce and broth.
Sugar content per serving: None.

Sweet and Sour Pork

**1 pound lean pork from fresh ham or
  tenderloin weighed after bone and fat
  are removed**
1 tablespoon vegetable oil
2 cups fat-free chicken broth
1½ cups thinly sliced celery
½ cup coarsely chopped onions
¼ cup soy sauce
2 tablespoons cornstarch
⅓ cup vinegar
**¼–⅓ cup Sugar Twin Brown Sugar
  Replacement**
1 large tomato cut into wedges
**1 cup drained, canned unsweetened
  pineapple tidbits**

Cut pork into small pieces about 1″ × ¼″. (It is easier to cut the pork this thin if it is slightly frozen.) Place oil in the bottom of a heavy frying pan or saucepan. Bring to frying temperature. Add pork and cook and stir over moderate heat until pork is browned and cooked through. Remove pork with slotted spoon and set aside for later use. Pour off as much of the fat as possible from the pan and then blot up any remaining fat with a paper towel.

Add broth to frying pan. Cook and stir over low heat to incorporate the browned bits in the bottom of the pan. Add celery and onions to hot chicken broth. Cover and simmer 10 minutes.

Mix soy sauce, cornstarch, and vinegar until smooth. Add to vegetables and cook and stir over moderate heat until thickened. Add sweetener to vegetables to taste and mix lightly.

Add tomatoes and pineapple to vegetables along with the pork. Cook over low heat until serving temperature, stirring occasionally. Do not allow to boil. The tomato wedges should be hot but not cooked. Serve hot over cooked rice, using 1 cup as a standard serving.

Yields 5 cups—5 servings

Nutritive Values Per Serving (without rice)

CAL	CARBS (g)	PRO (g)	TOTAL FAT (g)	SAT. FAT (g)	CHOL (mg)	FIBER (g)	NA (mg)
228	18	22	8	2	62	1.6	1,166

Food exchanges per serving: 2¹/₂ lean meat, 2 vegetable, ¹/₂ fruit.
Low-sodium diets: Use low-sodium broth and soy sauce.
Sugar content per serving: None.

Brown Gravy

The flavor of this gravy depends upon the flavor of the drippings or broth that you use as a base. It can be luscious or it can be bland. I prefer to use drippings from roasts. I chill them and remove the fat and the murky stuff at the bottom and then save them for gravy.

> **2¹/₄ cups cold fat-free drippings or broth**
> **2 tablespoons cornstarch**
> **Whisper of pepper**
> **¹/₂ teaspoon Kitchen Bouquet**
> **Salt to taste**

Place drippings, cornstarch, and pepper in a small saucepan and mix together until smooth. Place over moderate heat and cook and stir until smooth and thickened, using a wire whisk. Taste for flavoring and add salt and Kitchen Bouquet if necessary. Serve hot, using ¹/₄ cup per serving.

Yields 2 cups—8 servings

Nutritive Values Per Serving

CAL	CARBS (g)	PRO (g)	TOTAL FAT (g)	SAT. FAT (g)	CHOL (mg)	FIBER (g)	NA (mg)
13	2	1	0	0	0	0	178

Food exchanges per serving: ¹/₄ cup may be considered free.
Low-sodium diets: Omit salt. Use salt-free broth or drippings.
Sugar content per serving: None.

Pan Gravy

This gravy is a great favorite in the Midwest. It is served often and in large quantities.

> **1 tablespoon vegetable oil**
> **¼ cup all-purpose flour**
> **2½ cups cold water**
> **½ teaspoon salt**
> **Whisper of pepper**

Pour all of the fat out of a pan in which you have pan-fried steak, chicken, pork chops, or other meats. Blot out remaining fat with a paper towel. Add the oil to the pan and bring the pan to a frying temperature. Add flour to oil and cook and stir until browned and smooth.

Add the water to the flour mixture; cook and stir over moderate heat until thickened and you have scraped all of the brown bits from the pan. Add salt and pepper to the gravy. Mix lightly and serve hot, using ¼ cup gravy per serving.

Yields 2 cups—8 servings

Nutritive Values Per Serving

CAL	CARBS (g)	PRO (g)	TOTAL FAT (g)	SAT. FAT (g)	CHOL (mg)	FIBER (g)	NA (mg)
29	3	trace	2	trace	0	trace	137

Food exchanges per serving: ½ vegetable.
Low-sodium diets: Omit salt.
Sugar content per serving: None.

Brown Rice Dressing

1 cup raw brown rice
2½ cups fat-free chicken broth
1 tablespoon vegetable oil
2 cups thinly sliced celery
1 cup chopped onions
1 4-ounce can drained mushroom stems
  and pieces
1 8-ounce can water chestnuts
½ teaspoon leaf thyme
½ teaspoon rosemary
¹⁄₁₆ teaspoon black pepper
¼ teaspoon salt
½ teaspoon sage

Combine rice and broth in a saucepan. Heat to boiling. Stir, cover, and reduce heat. Simmer 45–50 minutes or until tender.

Place oil in saucepan. Bring to frying temperature. Add celery, onions, and mushrooms to hot oil. Cook, stirring frequently, over moderate heat, until onions are just tender. Drain chestnuts well. Slice into thin slices and add to hot vegetables.

Add remaining seasonings to vegetables and cook over low heat for 4 minutes, stirring frequently. Add rice and toss lightly. Reheat, if necessary, stirring gently over low heat. Serve hot using ½ cup per serving.

Yields 6 cups—12 servings

Nutritive Values Per Serving

CAL	CARBS (g)	PRO (g)	TOTAL FAT (g)	SAT. FAT (g)	CHOL (mg)	FIBER (g)	NA (mg)
87	16	2	2	trace	0	1.4	221

Food exchanges per serving: 1 starch.
Low-sodium diets: Omit salt. Use low-sodium broth.
Sugar content per serving: None.

13

Vegetables, Etc.

There is such an abundance of interesting fresh, frozen, dried, and canned vegetables available these days that we shouldn't ever complain that we don't know what vegetable to have for dinner. They can be prepared very simply or they can be the star of the menu—and you can eat your fill of vegetables without adding all that much carbohydrate to the meal. Vegetables don't contain any cholesterol so we should really appreciate them from both the low-cholesterol and the low-calorie viewpoints.

Vegetables contain a great deal of fiber, vitamins, and minerals; they even have a little protein, although only a trace of fat. They also taste delicious, which is a definite plus.

Vegetables fresh from the garden are wonderful in the summer. If you can't get vegetables fresh from the garden, frozen ones are next best. Sometimes frozen vegetables can be even better than fresh because they are picked and frozen at the peak of their perfection (and haven't stayed in the refrigerator until you get around to using them).

It is best to use fresh or frozen vegetables on a low-sodium diet because most canned vegetables have salt added to them when they are processed. If you can't get either fresh or frozen vegetables for your low-sodium diet, drain the liquid off the vegetables (except for tomatoes or some other vegetable where the liquid is important) and replace it with water. This will lower the sodium content somewhat. There are also vegetables available now that are canned without added salt, and they are a good buy on a low-sodium diet—or you can can your own vegetables (see Chapter 21) without adding any salt when you process them.

If you aren't on a low-sodium diet, canned vegetables are an excellent source of fiber, vitamins, and minerals. There is such a variety of them and they are always available. If you do keep some canned vegetables on hand, they should be kept in a cool place (around 70°F or lower), out of direct light, and should be rotated. Use the oldest cans first.

If the cans show any signs of spoilage they should be discarded. If they are bulging or leaking or have a bad smell when you open them, discard them immediately. Don't ever taste them to see if they are good. Just tasting them, if there is botulism in the cans, can cause death. Very few cases of botulism have been reported in this country in recent years, but it still pays to be cautious.

Although many vegetables are very low in carbohydrate, some vegetables are higher in carbohydrate and need to be included under the bread exchanges on a diabetic diet. I would have liked to have included more beans, brown rice, peas, and other starchy vegetables in this chapter because of their good fiber content; however, we will get sufficient fiber in our diet if we eat a good supply of the other vegetables. Most dietitians will tell you that if you eat whole wheat bread, an occasional special bran bread or muffin, and five or more servings of fruits and vegetables daily, you will get enough fiber.

I usually consider beans a special treat that I can have when the carbohydrate content of my meal is very low—or I use a couple of tablespoons of them in a lettuce salad to add interest to the salad (2 tablespoons of baked beans is one vegetable exchange). If you have a liberal diabetic diet and can afford it, I highly recommend that you use a good quantity of beans and other starchy vegetables because of their taste and good fiber content.

All of our diabetic lists include the values for vegetables, so I haven't included many plain vegetables in this chapter. I have tried to show you how to add a little zing to a few of them. I hope you'll try them, and perhaps adapt some of your own vegetable recipes using the information in Chapter 3, "Calculating Food Exchanges," and also develop some of your own special recipes.

Green Bean and Mushroom Casserole

This recipe was given to me by M. J. Smith, a registered dietitian from Guttenberg, Iowa. She is an innovative dietitian who has written several cookbooks for people on low-fat diets.

> 1 10-ounce package frozen French-cut
>   green beans
> 1 teaspoon liquid margarine
> 8 ounces fresh mushrooms, sliced
> ½ cup plain low-fat yogurt
> 1 tablespoon all-purpose flour
> 1 tablespoon dry sherry
> 2 teaspoons Worcestershire sauce

Thaw the green beans. Preheat a small (8-inch) nonstick-surfaced frying pan over medium heat for 1 minute. Swirl margarine in it, add mushrooms, and cook and stir over medium heat until mushrooms are tender.

Combine yogurt, flour, sherry, and Worcestershire sauce in a 1½-quart casserole and stir until smooth. Fold mushrooms and beans into sauce and bake at 350°F for 35–40 minutes. Serve hot, using 1 cup per serving.

Yields 4 cups—4 servings

Nutritive Values Per Serving

CAL	CARBS (g)	PRO (g)	TOTAL FAT (g)	SAT. FAT (g)	CHOL (mg)	FIBER (g)	NA (mg)
76	12	4	2	.5	2	2	62

Food exchanges per serving: 2 vegetable.
Low-sodium diets: May be used as written.
Sugar content per serving: None.

Creole Green Beans

1 tablespoon vegetable oil
¼ cup chopped onions
¼ cup thinly sliced celery
1 tablespoon flour
1 cup tomato juice
¼ teaspoon salt
Whisper of pepper
2 16-ounce cans green string beans

Place oil in a saucepan and heat to frying temperature over moderate heat. Add onions and celery to oil and cook and stir over moderate heat until the onions are soft but not browned. Add flour to vegetables and cook and stir until the flour is absorbed by the vegetables. Add tomato juice, salt, and pepper to the vegetables and cook and stir over moderate heat until slightly thickened and smooth.

Drain beans well. Add to hot sauce and simmer 2 minutes over moderate heat. Serve hot, using ½ cup per serving.

Yields 4 cups—8 servings

Nutritive Values Per Serving

CAL	CARBS (g)	PRO (g)	TOTAL FAT (g)	SAT. FAT (g)	CHOL (mg)	FIBER (g)	NA (mg)
40	6	1	2	trace	0	1.2	352

Food exchanges per serving: 1 vegetable.
Low-sodium diets: Omit salt. Drain green beans and wash them well before using them.
Sugar content per serving: None.

Broccoli Rice Casserole

1 tablespoon vegetable oil
1 cup chopped onions
1 pound fresh or frozen broccoli pieces
1 can cream of mushroom soup
¼ cup skim milk
1 cup cooked rice
2 tablespoons grated Parmesan cheese

Place oil in a saucepan and bring to a frying temperature. Add onions to oil and cook and stir over moderate heat until soft but not browned. Add broccoli to onions and cook and stir over moderate heat until hot but not cooked. Mix soup and milk together to blend and add to broccoli mixture.

Add rice to vegetables. Cook and stir over low heat until hot and mixed. Place in a 1½- or 2-quart casserole that has been greased with margarine.

Sprinkle Parmesan evenly over the top of the broccoli mixture. Bake, uncovered, at 350°F for 35–40 minutes or until the casserole is bubbly and the broccoli is cooked. Serve hot using ½ cup per serving.

Yields 5 cups—10 servings

Nutritive Values Per Serving

CAL	CARBS (g)	PRO (g)	TOTAL FAT (g)	SAT. FAT (g)	CHOL (mg)	FIBER (g)	NA (mg)
96	12	3	4	1	2	1.6	276

Food exchanges per serving: 2 vegetable, 1 fat.
Low-sodium diets: Cook rice without salt and use low-sodium soup.
Sugar content per serving: None.

Chinese Vegetables

1 tablespoon vegetable oil
½ cup coarsely chopped onions
1 cup thinly sliced celery
1 4-ounce can of well-drained mushrooms
1 cup water
1½ tablespoons cornstarch
¼ cup soy sauce
1 14-ounce can of well-drained bean
   sprouts
2 tablespoons chopped cashew nuts
   roasted in oil

Place oil in a saucepan and bring to a frying temperature. Add onions, celery, and mushrooms to hot oil. Cook and stir over moderate heat for 2–3 minutes or until onions are softened. Add ¼ cup water to vegetables. Cover and cook over low heat about 8 minutes or until vegetables are tender.

Mix together ¾ cup water, cornstarch, and soy sauce until smooth. Add to vegetables and cook and stir over moderate heat until thickened and clear. Add sprouts and nuts to vegetables and heat to serving temperature. Serve hot using ½ cup per serving.

Yields 3 cups—6 servings

Nutritive Values Per Serving

CAL	CARBS (g)	PRO (g)	TOTAL FAT (g)	SAT. FAT (g)	CHOL (mg)	FIBER (g)	NA (mg)
65	7	2	4	.5	0	1	781

Food exchanges per serving: 1 vegetable, 1 fat.
Low-sodium diets: Use low-sodium soy sauce.
Sugar content per serving: None.

Shredded Cabbage

1 pound white cabbage
¼ cup water
½ teaspoon salt
1 tablespoon margarine
Whisper of pepper

Trim and wash cabbage. Shred coarsely or cut into slices about ⅛ inch wide. Place water and salt in a saucepan and bring to a boil. Add cabbage. Mix lightly and cover tightly. Simmer over low heat for 12 minutes, stirring once during the cooking period. Drain well. Add margarine and pepper to cabbage. Toss lightly and serve hot, using ½ cup cabbage per serving.

Yields 2 cups—4 servings

Nutritive Values Per Serving

CAL	CARBS (g)	PRO (g)	TOTAL FAT (g)	SAT. FAT (g)	CHOL (mg)	FIBER (g)	NA (mg)
50	6	1	3	.5	0	2.5	187

Food exchanges per serving: 1 vegetable, ½ fat.
Low-sodium diets: Omit salt. Use salt-free margarine.
Sugar content per serving: None.

Cauliflower Parmesan

Chuck's cousin Dave Cavaiani's wife Etta cooked this for us when we visited them in Iron Mountain and we really liked it. The cheese adds to the flavor of the cauliflower in a most attractive way.

1 pound frozen cauliflower
2 cups boiling water
1 teaspoon salt

1 tablespoon margarine
2 tablespoons grated Parmesan cheese

Place cauliflower, water, and salt in a saucepan, cover, and simmer about 8 minutes or until the cauliflower is tender; or cook in the microwave oven according to directions on the package. Drain well.

Sprinkle margarine and cheese over the cauliflower. Toss lightly to coat the cauliflower and serve hot, using a quarter of the cauliflower (about ½ cup) per serving.

Yields about 2 cups—4 servings

Nutritive Values Per Serving

CAL	CARBS (g)	PRO (g)	TOTAL FAT (g)	SAT. FAT (g)	CHOL (mg)	FIBER (g)	NA (mg)
64	5	3	4	1	2	3	381

Food exchanges per serving: 1 vegetable, 1 fat.
Low-sodium diets: Omit salt. Use salt-free margarine.
Sugar content per serving: None.

Eggplant and Tomatoes

1 1-pound eggplant
¼ cup vegetable oil
½ cup coarsely chopped onions
½ cup coarsely chopped fresh green peppers
1 finely minced garlic clove
2 cups (1-pound can) Italian plum tomatoes
¼ cup chopped fresh parsley
⅛ teaspoon pepper
1 teaspoon salt
1 teaspoon sugar

Wash eggplant and remove ends. Cut into ½-inch cubes without removing the skin. Place oil in the bottom of a heavy pot or frying pan. Add eggplant along with onions, peppers, and garlic and fry over moderate heat, stirring occasionally, until eggplant is transparent and tender.

Add remaining ingredients to eggplant mixture and cook, stirring frequently, over moderate heat for about 5 minutes. Serve hot or at room temperature, using ½ cup per serving.

Yields 6 cups—12 servings

Nutritive Values Per Serving

CAL	CARBS (g)	PRO (g)	TOTAL FAT (g)	SAT. FAT (g)	CHOL (mg)	FIBER (g)	NA (mg)
64	5	1	5	.6	0	1	251

Food exchanges per serving: 1 vegetable, 1 fat.
Low-sodium diets: Omit salt. Use low-sodium canned or fresh tomatoes.
Sugar content per serving: Trace.

Sauerkraut with Tomatoes

Many thanks to Dave Christen, who gave me this recipe.

> **1 29-ounce can sauerkraut**
> **1 16-ounce can whole tomatoes with juice**
> **½ cup cooked, diced, very lean ham with**
>   **all visible fat removed**
> **½ cup chopped onions**
> **2 tablespoons packed brown sugar**
> **½ teaspoon Sugar Twin Brown Sugar**
>   **Replacement**

Place sauerkraut in a colander, rinse with 2 quarts cold water, and drain well. Place sauerkraut in a large bowl, add tomatoes and juice, ham, onions, and brown sugar, and mix well. Place in a 2-quart casserole. Cover and bake at 325°F for 1 hour.

Remove cover, stir lightly, and bake 1 more hour. (Dave says he sometimes does this in a Crock-Pot for picnics.) Stir sugar substitute into sauerkraut mixture and serve hot, using ½ cup per serving.

Yields 1 quart—8 servings

Nutritive Values Per Serving

CAL	CARBS (g)	PRO (g)	TOTAL FAT (g)	SAT. FAT (g)	CHOL (mg)	FIBER (g)	NA (mg)
52	9	3	1	trace	5	1.9	431

Food exchanges per serving: ¼ lean meat, 1½ vegetable.
Low-sodium diets: Use low-sodium canned or fresh tomatoes and rinse and drain sauerkraut very well.
Sugar content per serving: .8 teaspoon.

Southern-Style Greens

1 pound frozen mustard or turnip greens
4 ounces chopped center-cut ham with fat,
   bone, and skin removed
Whisper of black pepper
1½ cups boiling water

Greens should be almost completely thawed before cooking. Place greens in a saucepan. Add ham, pepper, and water to greens. Bring to a boil, reduce heat, and simmer uncovered for 30 minutes or until tender, adding more hot water if necessary. Cut through the greens several times with a sharp knife. Serve hot with some of the juice using ½ cup greens per serving.

Yields about 2 cups—4 servings

Nutritive Values Per Serving

CAL	CARBS (g)	PRO (g)	TOTAL FAT (g)	SAT. FAT (g)	CHOL (mg)	FIBER (g)	NA (mg)
60	4	8	2	.5	13	3	438

Food exchanges per serving: 1 very lean meat, 1 vegetable.
Low-sodium diets: May be used as written.
Sugar content per serving: None.

Pickled Vegetables

These vegetables can be canned but I never bother to do so. I pre-pare them one recipe at a time and keep them in the refrigerator where they keep well for several weeks.

> **3 cups vinegar**
> **3 cups water**
> **3 tablespoons pickling spices**
> **1 pound fresh carrots**
> **1 10-ounce package frozen Brussels sprouts**
> **2 cups celery cut into thin slices**
> **2 cups (1-pound can) drained canned green beans**
> **2 cups (1-pound can) drained canned yellow wax beans**
> **2 cups julienne-cut fresh green peppers**
> **2 cups coarsely chopped onions**
> **Sugar substitute equal to 2 cups sugar**

Combine vinegar, water, and pickling spices in a saucepan. Bring to a boil and simmer, covered, for 3 minutes. Remove from heat, cover, and let stand at room temperature for about a week or until the vinegar mixture tastes spicy according to your taste. Discard spices.

Clean carrots and cut into julienne pieces. Combine carrots, Brussels sprouts, and celery. Cover with boiling water and cook 3 minutes. Remove from heat; drain. Cover with cold water and drain again. Place in a large kettle with the vinegar mixture. Drain beans well and add to carrot and vinegar mixture.

Add peppers and onions to vegetables. Bring to a boil but remove immediately from heat. The vegetables should not be allowed to boil. Add sweetener to vegetable mixture. Mix lightly. Cover and allow to come to room temperature. Refrigerate at least 3 days before serving (½ cup per serving).

Yields about 1 gallon—32 servings

Nutritive Values Per Serving

CAL	CARBS (g)	PRO (g)	TOTAL FAT (g)	SAT. FAT (g)	CHOL (mg)	FIBER (g)	NA (mg)
23	6	1	trace	0	0	1.2	56

Food exchanges per serving: 1 vegetable.
Low-sodium diets: Rinse canned vegetables thoroughly.
Sugar content per serving: None.

Sautéed Vegetables

2 teaspoons vegetable oil
2 cups coarsely shredded cabbage
1 cup coarsely shredded carrots
1½ cups thinly sliced celery
¼ cup chopped fresh green peppers
½ cup coarsely chopped onions
½ teaspoon salt
¼ cup water
Soy sauce as desired

Place oil in the bottom of a heavy saucepan and heat to frying temperature. Add vegetables and salt to oil. Cook over medium heat for 5 minutes, stirring frequently.

Add ¼ cup water to vegetables, cover, and cook over low heat for 5–7 minutes or until vegetables have reached the desired tenderness. Serve vegetables hot, using ½ cup per serving with soy sauce to be added as desired.

Yields 3 cups—6 servings

Nutritive Values Per Serving (without soy sauce)

CAL	CARBS (g)	PRO (g)	TOTAL FAT (g)	SAT. FAT (g)	CHOL (mg)	FIBER (g)	NA (mg)
38	6	1	2	trace	0	1.9	219

Food exchanges per serving: 1 vegetable.
Low-sodium diets: Omit salt. Use low-sodium soy sauce.
Sugar content per serving: None.

Spinach Frittata

I'm very fond of frittatas and make them frequently. I use a variety of vegetables, and sometimes I use ¼ cup cooked rice instead of bread.

2½ ounces frozen chopped spinach
¼ cup finely chopped onions
1 tablespoon imitation bacon bits
⅛ teaspoon salt
Whisper of pepper
Whites from 2 large or 3 medium eggs
½ slice whole wheat bread cut into cubes
½ teaspoon margarine

Cut a 10-ounce package of frozen chopped spinach into quarters. Defrost one quarter and return the rest to the freezer. Press any liquid out of spinach. Put spinach into a small bowl with onions, bacon bits, salt, pepper, and egg whites. Mix well with a fork. Add bread cubes and mix lightly, until they are covered with egg mixture but not soaked.

Preheat a small (8-inch) nonstick-surfaced frying pan over medium heat for 1 minute. Swirl margarine around bottom of pan. Add spinach mixture and fry over medium heat until bottom is lightly browned. Turn frittata over and cook until firm and bottom is lightly browned. Serve hot, using one frittata per serving. *Note:* If you want to make several frittatas, it is best to make them individually.

Yields 1 frittata—1 serving

Nutritive Values Per Serving

CAL	CARBS (g)	PRO (g)	TOTAL FAT (g)	SAT. FAT (g)	CHOL (mg)	FIBER (g)	NA (mg)
143	16	14	4	.5	0	3.6	717

Food exchanges per serving: 2 very lean meat, 1 starch.
Low-sodium diets: Omit salt. Use salt-free margarine.
Sugar content per serving: None.

Creamed Spinach with Peanuts

My husband Chuck developed this recipe when we lived in Chicago to persuade a friend who insisted he didn't like spinach that it could be very good.

> 1 10-ounce package frozen chopped
>   spinach
> 1 quart boiling water
> 1½ cups fat-free chicken broth
> 2 tablespoons instant nonfat dry milk
> 3 tablespoons all-purpose flour
> ¼ teaspoon salt
> ⅛ teaspoon nutmeg
> Whisper of white pepper
> 2 tablespoons chopped salted peanuts

Defrost spinach, break it up with a fork, and place it in a bowl. Add boiling water and let it sit for 5 minutes. Drain well and set aside.

Place broth, dry milk, flour, salt, nutmeg, and pepper in a small saucepan. Stir until smooth and then cook, stirring over medium heat until smooth and thickened. Add spinach and peanuts to the sauce. Stir lightly and serve hot, using ½ cup per serving.

Yields 2½ cups—5 servings

Nutritive Values Per Serving

CAL	CARBS (g)	PRO (g)	TOTAL FAT (g)	SAT. FAT (g)	CHOL (mg)	FIBER (g)	NA (mg)
63	8	5	2	.3	trace	1.6	368

Food exchanges per serving: 1 vegetable.
Low-sodium diets: Omit salt. Use low-sodium broth and unsalted peanuts.
Sugar content per serving: None.

Summer Squash with Ginger

I've never cared much for summer squash but when Chef Dave Hutchins served this to us at a luncheon, I knew I had finally found a recipe for summer squash I could enjoy.

> **1 tablespoon vegetable oil**
> **3 cups ¼-inch slices of summer squash**
>   **(about 6 small)**
> **1½ teaspoons finely chopped fresh ginger**
> **4 crushed garlic cloves**
> **1 cup peeled, seeded, and chopped fresh**
>   **tomatoes**
> **1 teaspoon grated Parmesan cheese**
> **½ teaspoon salt**
> **Whisper of pepper**

Preheat a large (12-inch) nonstick-surfaced frying pan. Swirl oil around pan, add squash, ginger, and garlic, and cook, stirring frequently, until squash is soft but not transparent. Add tomato to the sauce and continue to cook over medium heat, stirring frequently, until squash is transparent. Stir in Parmesan, salt, and pepper. Serve hot, using ½ cup per serving.

Yields 3 cups—6 servings

Nutritive Values Per Serving

CAL	CARBS (g)	PRO (g)	TOTAL FAT (g)	SAT. FAT (g)	CHOL (mg)	FIBER (g)	NA (mg)
40	4	1	3	trace	trace	.8	193

Food exchanges per serving: 1 vegetable, ½ fat.
Low-sodium diets: Omit salt.
Sugar content per serving: None.

Fran's Butternut Squash Casserole

This recipe was a favorite of my friend Frances Nielsen. She always fixed it for us when she came to visit every fall. You can use 1 cup canned tomatoes and juice instead of the fresh tomatoes, but the fresh tomatoes are the best.

2 pounds butternut squash
2 medium-size fresh tomatoes
1 cup coarsely chopped onions
1 cup coarsely chopped fresh green
  peppers
1 teaspoon Italian seasoning
¾ teaspoon salt
2 tablespoons (¼ stick) margarine

Peel squash, remove seeds and fiber, and cut into slices about ½ inch thick. Wash and peel tomatoes and slice. Layer vegetables in a casserole dish with the squash on the bottom, then tomatoes, onions, and peppers. Add seasoning and dot with margarine. Cover and bake at 350°F for 1½ hours. Remove the cover, stir lightly, and continue to bake about another ½ hour or until lightly browned and almost dry. Stir lightly and serve hot using ½ cup per serving.

Yields 3 cups—6 servings

Nutritive Values Per Serving

CAL	CARBS (g)	PRO (g)	TOTAL FAT (g)	SAT. FAT (g)	CHOL (mg)	FIBER (g)	NA (mg)
115	20	2	4	.7	0	3.5	332

Food exchanges per serving: 1 starch, 1 fat, 1 vegetable.
Low-sodium diets: Omit salt. Use fresh tomatoes or low-sodium canned
   tomatoes and salt-free margarine.
Sugar content per serving: None.

Monk's Rice

Margaret "Monk" Sellers prepared this rice when we both visited her sister and brother-in-law, Frances and Bud Gunsallus, in Miami. Monk said that she likes this version because the rice and vegetables aren't soupy or gummy as they are when you cook them all in the same pot. She prepared a big roaster full of it for the family party that night and we ate every bite of it.

> ½ cup long-grain rice
> 1 cup chicken broth
> 1 tablespoon vegetable oil
> 2 cups broccoli ends and pieces
> 1 cup coarsely chopped onions
> 1 cup coarsely grated carrots
> ½ cup chopped fresh green peppers
> ½ cup thinly sliced celery
> 1 4-ounce can well-drained mushroom
>   stems and pieces
> ¼ teaspoon salt

Combine rice and broth and bring to a boil. Pour in a small casserole, cover tightly, and bake at 350°F for 30 minutes. Remove cover and set aside for later use.

Spread oil in a heavy 9- or 10-inch frying pan. Bring to a cooking temperature over moderate heat. Add vegetables and salt to hot oil in frying pan. Cook, stirring frequently, over moderate heat 10 to 15 minutes or until vegetables are crisp-tender (or soft if you prefer them that way). Add rice and mix lightly. Serve ½ cup per serving.

Yields 5 cups—10 servings

Nutritive Values Per Serving							
CAL	CARBS (g)	PRO (g)	TOTAL FAT (g)	SAT. FAT (g)	CHOL (mg)	FIBER (g)	NA (mg)
67	12	2	2	trace	0	1.4	160

Food exchanges per serving: ½ starch, 1 vegetable.
Low-sodium diets: Omit salt. Use low-sodium broth.
Sugar content per serving: None.

Baked Tomato Halves

Frances Nielsen taught me to make these when she lived here in Wadena. The tomatoes are best right out of the garden. They should be fully ripe but still firm. The seasoning can be varied using basil, oregano, or any other favorite seasoning instead of the garlic.

4 fresh, ripe, medium-size tomatoes
2 tablespoons melted margarine
1 teaspoon garlic salt
¹/₁₆ teaspoon pepper
4 teaspoons grated Parmesan cheese
2 teaspoons dried parsley flakes

Wash tomatoes and remove the stems. Cut the tomatoes in half crosswise and place the halves on a rimmed cookie sheet that has been greased with margarine or sprayed with cooking spray. Brush the tomato halves with margarine using a pastry brush.

Sprinkle the garlic salt and pepper on the tops of the tomato halves and then sprinkle the halves with the Parmesan cheese and parsley flakes, using ½ teaspoon of cheese for each tomato half. Bake at 350°F for 35–45 minutes or until tender and lightly browned. Serve hot using two halves per serving.

Yields 8 halves—4 servings

Nutritive Values Per Serving

CAL	CARBS (g)	PRO (g)	TOTAL FAT (g)	SAT. FAT (g)	CHOL (mg)	FIBER (g)	NA (mg)
85	6	2	7	1.3	1	1.6	470

Food exchanges per serving: 1 vegetable, 1 fat.
Low-sodium diets: Omit garlic salt. Sprinkle with garlic powder.
Sugar content per serving: None.

Stir-Fry Tomatoes

1 tablespoon vegetable oil
1 cup thinly sliced celery
1 cup julienne-cut fresh green peppers
1 6- to 8-inch zucchini cut into ¼-inch
  slices
4 medium-size tomatoes at room
  temperature
1 cup fat-free chicken broth
1 tablespoon cornstarch
¼ teaspoon salt
½ teaspoon ground ginger
¼ teaspoon pepper

Place oil in heavy saucepan or deep, heavy frying pan and bring to frying temperature. Add celery, peppers, and zucchini to frying pan. Cook and stir over moderate heat about 5 minutes, or until crisp-tender. Wash tomatoes and remove stems. Cut into wedges and add to vegetable mixture. Cook and stir until tomatoes are hot.

Stir together broth, cornstarch, and seasonings until smooth. Add to vegetables and cook and stir about 2 minutes or until thickened. Serve hot using about ¾ cup per serving.

Yields about 6 cups—8 servings

Nutritive Values Per Serving

CAL	CARBS (g)	PRO (g)	TOTAL FAT (g)	SAT. FAT (g)	CHOL (mg)	FIBER (g)	NA (mg)
45	6	2	2	trace	0	1.4	168

Food exchanges per serving: 1 vegetable.
Low-sodium diets: Omit salt. Use low-sodium broth.
Sugar content per serving: None.

Zucchini Scramble

My sister-in-law, Josephine Serevino of Chicago, said this was one of her favorite summer vegetable combinations.

> **1 tablespoon vegetable oil**
> **1 6- to 8-inch zucchini cut into ¼-inch slices**
> **1 cup julienne-cut fresh green peppers**
> **½ cup diced fresh potatoes**
> **½ cup coarsely chopped onions**
> **1 large fresh tomato cut into wedges**
> **¼ teaspoon garlic powder**
> **½ teaspoon salt**
> **1 bay leaf**

Place oil in a heavy saucepan or deep, heavy frying pan and bring to frying temperature.

Add vegetables and seasonings to hot oil. Cook and stir over moderate heat for about 3 minutes. Reduce heat to low, cover, and cook, stirring occasionally, about 20 minutes or until vegetables are tender. Remove bay leaf and serve hot, using about ½ cup per portion.

Yields about 4 cups—8 servings

Nutritive Values Per Serving

CAL	CARBS (g)	PRO (g)	TOTAL FAT (g)	SAT. FAT (g)	CHOL (mg)	FIBER (g)	NA (mg)
38	5	1	2	trace	0	.9	140

Food exchanges per serving: 1 vegetable.
Low-sodium diets: Omit salt.
Sugar content per serving: None.

Pandy's Zucchini and Corn

This recipe came from my friend Pandy Williams of Ajo, Arizona. She isn't on a low-cholesterol diet, so she sprinkles it with 8 ounces grated longhorn or Monterey Jack cheese just before she serves it. The cheese melts and it is absolutely luscious. Since she is diabetic she counts the 8 ounces of cheese as one meat exchange per serving.

> **1 pound fresh 6- to 8-inch zucchini**
> **1 tablespoon vegetable oil**
> **1 cup coarsely chopped onions**
> **1 cup coarsely chopped fresh green peppers or 4-ounce can diced green chilies**
> **2 cups fresh or canned chopped tomatoes and juice**
> **1 cup canned or fresh whole kernel corn**
> **1 teaspoon garlic salt**
> **Whisper of pepper**

Wash and trim the ends from the zucchini. Cut crosswise into 1-inch slices and set aside.

Heat oil in a nonstick-surfaced frying pan, add onions and peppers, and stir over medium heat until the onions begin to soften. Add tomatoes and cook 2 minutes. Add zucchini and cook, stirring occasionally, for 10 minutes. Add corn, salt, and pepper, cover, and cook, stirring occasionally, 10 to 12 minutes or until the zucchini is transparent. Serve hot, using ½ cup per serving.

Yields 4 cups—8 servings

Nutritive Values Per Serving

CAL	CARBS (g)	PRO (g)	TOTAL FAT (g)	SAT. FAT (g)	CHOL (mg)	FIBER (g)	NA (mg)
64	11	2	2	trace	0	1.7	258

Food exchanges per serving: 2 vegetable.
Low-sodium diets: Use fresh tomatoes, fresh or frozen peppers and corn, and ¼ teaspoon garlic powder instead of salt.
Sugar content per serving: None.

Vegetable Purées

This is a method, not a recipe, but I urge you to try it. The vegetable purées are very flavorful and attractive—a whole new taste sensation. Since they are more concentrated than the regular vegetables, ⅓ of a cup of puréed vegetable is equal to ½ cup of the same vegetable—but it is worth it. Add margarine and other seasonings after the vegetables are puréed, except for the salt that you should add when cooking the vegetable. If you add 1 tablespoon of margarine per cup of cooked puréed vegetables, you will have 1 vegetable exchange and 1 fat exchange per ⅓ cup of puréed vegetable.

Start with good fresh vegetables. Wash them, and peel them if necessary. Cook them until tender but not mushy. If you have cooked them in water, drain them well and shake the pan over low heat for a few seconds to get rid of as much moisture as possible. If you have cooked them in the microwave, drain them well and cover them with a clean napkin or dish towel for a few minutes to absorb as much of the steam as possible.

Vegetables can be sieved or put into the food processor. I don't recommend the blender because you have to add a little water and the results aren't firm enough. Remove any seeds or skin you don't want to be in the purée before you put the food in the food processor because it will process everything together.

The vegetable purée will probably be cold after it is processed. Add seasonings then along with the margarine. The purée can be reheated by placing it in the microwave, or it can be stirred over low heat in a saucepan until it is at serving temperature. You can also freeze the purées in ⅓ cup portions to use in the future. If you do this, it is better not to add the margarine until you are ready to defrost and reheat the vegetables.

Potatoes should not be prepared in the food processor because the action of the food processor will make the potatoes gummy. However, winter squash and carrots both react well in the food processor. I also like to combine vegetables, puréeing them separately or together, such as adding onions to winter squash or broccoli, or a little green pepper to carrots. One of my favorites is to add some dill seed to puréed winter squash. There are so many good combinations to explore that your vegetable exchanges should never be dull.

Baked Beans

These are my sister Shirley's favorite. I wish I could use more of them in my diet because they are a good source of fiber, but they are so high in carbohydrate that I don't use them too often. Sometimes I add a couple of tablespoons of them to a big lettuce salad—which is very good and only costs me a vegetable exchange.

> **1 pound dry great northern beans**
> **Cold water as necessary**
> **4 ounces chopped center-cut ham with fat,**
> **bone, and skin removed**
> **1 cup chopped onions**
> **6 ounces tomato paste**
> **1½ teaspoons salt**
> **2 tablespoons salad mustard**
> **¾ cup Sugar Twin Brown Sugar**
> **Replacement**

Wash beans and discard any imperfect ones. Add cold water to cover and bring to a boil. Simmer for 5 minutes. Remove from heat and let stand for 2–3 hours. Drain well. Cover again with cold water to about ½ inch over the top of the beans. Bring to a boil, reduce heat, cover, and let simmer for about 2½ hours or until the beans are soft.

Thoroughly mix beans with remaining ingredients. Place in a shallow baking dish and bake, uncovered, at 325°F for 2 to 3 hours or until the beans are rather dry, stirring every hour. Serve hot or cold, using ⅓ cup beans per serving.

Yields 6 cups—18 servings

Nutritive Values Per Serving

CAL	CARBS (g)	PRO (g)	TOTAL FAT (g)	SAT. FAT (g)	CHOL (mg)	FIBER (g)	NA (mg)
109	19	7	1	trace	3	10.6	373

Food exchanges per serving: 1 starch, 1 very lean meat.
Low-sodium diets: Omit salt. Use low-sodium tomato paste.
Sugar content per serving: None.

Red Beans and Rice

Judy Ballantine from Madison, Wisconsin, loves this combination.

> 1 pound dry kidney beans
> Water as necessary
> 1 cup chopped onions
> ³/₄ cup chopped fresh green peppers
> 1 cup finely chopped celery
> 4 ounces chopped center-cut ham with fat,
>   skin, and bone removed
> 2 teaspoons salt
> ¹/₂ teaspoon cayenne pepper
> ¹/₄ teaspoon black pepper
> 3 tablespoons thinly sliced green onion
>   tops
> 1¹/₂ tablespoons parsley flakes
> 6 cups hot fluffy cooked rice
> Fresh onion slices

Wash and sort beans. Add 2 quarts hot water. Cover and soak overnight. Drain well. Discard the liquid and add cold water to cover the beans to about ¹/₂ inch over the top.

Add onions, peppers, celery, ham, salt, cayenne, and black pepper to beans. Bring to a boil. Reduce heat, cover, and simmer 2¹/₂ hours, stirring occasionally. Add onion tops and parsley. Simmer uncovered about 30 minutes, stirring occasionally.

Serve ¹/₂ cup of the hot beans over ¹/₂ cup of the rice per serving. Garnish the beans with a few onion slices, if desired.

Yields 6 cups—12 servings

Nutritive Values Per Serving (including rice)

CAL	CARBS (g)	PRO (g)	TOTAL FAT (g)	SAT. FAT (g)	CHOL (mg)	FIBER (g)	NA (mg)
280	53	14	1	trace	5	4.8	501

Food exchanges per serving: 3 starch, 1 vegetable, 1/3 lean meat.
Low-sodium diets: Omit salt.
Sugar content per serving: None.

Creamy Brown Rice

I never really liked brown rice until Dr. Karen Kuenzel of the Rice Research and Extension Center at the University of Arkansas told me that I wasn't using enough liquid and I wasn't cooking it long enough. She gave me these proportions to use and now I enjoy making and eating it more often.

1 cup brown rice
2½ cups boiling water
½ teaspoon salt

Place rice, water, and salt in a Crock-Pot. Turn on high and cook for about 2 hours or until soft and creamy. Serve hot using 1/3 cup per serving.

Note: If you like brown rice more firm, use less liquid. It can also be cooked in a saucepan over low heat for about 50–60 minutes if you don't like to use the Crock-Pot. Remove the lid and fluff the rice with a fork, cover with a napkin or terry cloth dish towel, and let stand 5–10 minutes to fluff before it is served, using 1/3 cup per serving.

Yields 3 cups—9 servings

Nutritive Values Per Serving

CAL	CARBS (g)	PRO (g)	TOTAL FAT (g)	SAT. FAT (g)	CHOL (mg)	FIBER (g)	NA (mg)
76	16	2	1	trace	0	.7	123

Food exchanges per serving: 1 starch.
Low-sodium diets: Omit salt.
Sugar content per serving: None.

Medium White Sauce

---

2 tablespoons all-purpose flour
¼ cup instant nonfat dry milk
½ teaspoon salt
Dash of white pepper (optional)
1 tablespoon vegetable oil
1 cup cold water

Stir together flour, milk, salt, and pepper until blended. Place oil in a small saucepan. Add the flour mixture and cook and stir over moderate heat until smooth but not browned. Remove from heat.

Add 1 cup water to flour mixture. Return to heat and cook and stir over medium heat until sauce is thickened and smooth. (One cup fat-free chicken broth may be substituted for the cold water, if desired, to make a Velouté sauce with no change in food exchanges. However, the sodium will be increased to 546 mg per serving.) Use for creamed vegetables or meats using ¼ cup per serving.

Yields 1 cup—4 servings

Nutritive Values Per Serving

CAL	CARBS (g)	PRO (g)	TOTAL FAT (g)	SAT. FAT (g)	CHOL (mg)	FIBER (g)	NA (mg)
60	5	2	4	trace	1	trace	297

Food exchanges per serving: ½ skim milk.
Low-sodium diets: Omit salt.
Sugar content per serving: None.

Mock Sour Cream

This recipe from Esther Smith, a home economist from near Wadena, is great on baked potatoes. I also like to add some garlic powder to it and use it as a dip or for salad dressing.

1½ cups well-drained cottage cheese,
  preferably large curd
2 tablespoons dry buttermilk
½ cup skim milk
1 tablespoon lemon juice
½ teaspoon salt

Place all ingredients in bowl of food processor and process until thick and smooth. Refrigerate until needed using ¼ cup as a standard serving.

Yields 2 cups—8 servings

Nutritive Values Per Serving

CAL	CARBS (g)	PRO (g)	TOTAL FAT (g)	SAT. FAT (g)	CHOL (mg)	FIBER (g)	NA (mg)
36	2	6	trace	trace	4	0	158

Food exchanges per serving: 1 very lean meat, ¼ skim milk.
Low-sodium diets: Omit salt.
Sugar content per serving: None.

Blintzes

This recipe is from Anita Kane of Shorewood, Wisconsin. Anita served them with unsweetened applesauce or other fruit. I like them with Cinnamon Shake or Apple Butter (see Index).

FILLING
1 pound well-drained low-fat cottage
  cheese
¼ cup liquid egg substitute
2 teaspoons sugar

PANCAKE
¾ cup liquid egg substitute
1 cup water
¾ cup all-purpose flour
2 tablespoons vegetable oil
Margarine or oil as necessary

Mix cottage cheese, 1/4 cup egg substitute, and sugar together lightly and refrigerate until needed.

Beat together 3/4 cup egg substitute, 1 cup water, flour, and 2 tablespoons oil until smooth.

Heat a little margarine or oil in a 6-inch frying pan (I like oil best). Use a shallow frying pan as you would for frying crepes. Pour about 2 tablespoons batter into the frying pan, tilting the pan so that the batter coats as much of the pan surface as possible. It should make a very thin pancake. Cook over medium heat 1 to 2 minutes or until the bottom of the pancake is lightly browned and the sides are curled up. Carefully turn the pancake out onto a clean dish towel. The pancakes can be stacked like shingles.

When all of the pancakes are cooked, spread about a tablespoon of filling in the center of each pancake. Fold in both sides and then the ends so that you have a neat little package. Place the blintzes seam side down in a baking dish that has been greased with margarine. Brush lightly with melted margarine and bake at 375°F for 30 to 40 minutes or until browned and puffy. Serve hot with fruit, Apple Butter, or Cinnamon Shake (see Index), using three blintzes per serving.

These freeze very well. Put them individually on a cookie sheet until they are frozen and then keep them in a bag in the freezer until you need them. Grease a baking dish well with margarine and let them defrost before you bake them.

Yields 18 blintzes—6 servings

Nutritive Values Per Serving

CAL	CARBS (g)	PRO (g)	TOTAL FAT (g)	SAT. FAT (g)	CHOL (mg)	FIBER (g)	NA (mg)
190	17	16	6	1.5	6	.4	374

Food exchanges per serving: 1 starch, 1 1/2 lean meat, 1/4 skim milk.
Low-sodium diets: Use salt-free margarine.
Sugar content per serving: None.

Stewed Cranberries

1 pound fresh cranberries
1 cup water
Sugar substitute equal to ½ cup sugar

Wash cranberries well under running water. Pick them over and discard any imperfect berries. Place cranberries and water in a small saucepan. Simmer about 5 minutes or until the cranberries have burst.

Remove from heat. Add sugar substitute, mix lightly, and cool to room temperature. Taste for flavor and add more sugar substitute, if desired. Refrigerate until used, using ½ cup per serving.

Yields 3 cups—6 servings

Nutritive Values Per Serving

CAL	CARBS (g)	PRO (g)	TOTAL FAT (g)	SAT. FAT (g)	CHOL (mg)	FIBER (g)	NA (mg)
45	12	trace	trace	0	0	2.8	61

Food exchanges per serving: ³/4 fruit (2 tablespoons may be considered free).
Low-sodium diets: May be used as written.
Sugar content per serving: None.

14

Salads and Salad Dressings

Salads add interest and nutrients to any diet. A chef's salad is easy to order when you are eating out, and a bowl of lettuce added to your lunch or dinner makes you feel as though you have dined well—which you have. Salads offer bulk, fiber, vitamins and minerals, satisfaction, and good taste, all of which are very important. However, you need to be careful even when ordering or making a salad because some salads can hide a lot of cholesterol and carbohydrate, and the most innocent-looking fruit salad can hide a lot of fat in the dressing. So always analyze a salad (quietly to yourself, of course) before you eat it.

Some salad ingredients are so low in calories that you can eat up to a cup without counting them, so I always try to include them in salads whenever possible. They include chinese cabbage, cucumbers, endive, escarole, lettuce, parsley, dill pickles, radishes, and watercress.

A good tossed salad begins with clean, crisp greens. They lose texture and nutrients even when properly refrigerated so it is best to be careful when you are preparing them. They are also fragile and must be stored carefully. It is a good idea not to wash them until shortly before they are used. Everyone has different ideas about how to keep greens fresh. I like to clean them and remove as much of the water as possible, and then store them in a plastic container in the refrigerator until I need them. Some cooks like to wash them and wrap them in a damp towel and refrigerate them until used. If they are wilted you can sometimes bring greens back to a manageable state by soaking them in cold water for a short time and then drying them before they are used. Remember, you shouldn't add the dressing until just before the salad is served because the dressing will wilt the greens.

Hard-cooked egg yolks should not be used in a salad on a low-cholesterol diabetic diet because of the cholesterol in the egg yolks. If you want chopped whole eggs in your salad, you can cook liquid egg substitute in the microwave oven or the top of a double boiler, let it return to room temperature, and then chop it into cubes for use in salads. I generally just hard-cook the eggs, discard the egg yolks, and chop the whites for salad. You can use the egg yolks to garnish the salad, and anyone who doesn't need to watch their cholesterol intake can eat them. Don't feel guilty if you throw away the yolks. Just tell yourself you are discarding cholesterol and it gets easier every time you do it.

There are some good low-calorie salad dressings on the market that are suitable for a low-cholesterol diabetic recipe. However, they hardly ever contain vegetable oil because of the calories, and you do need some polyunsaturated vegetable oils in your diet. Anyone on a low-cholesterol diabetic diet has a hard time balancing the amount of vegetable oil needed for a low-cholesterol diet with the number of fat exchanges on the diabetic diet. Talk to your doctor about it and see which is the most important—getting the polyunsaturated vegetable oil or restricting your fat intake.

Sour cream is also a no-no on a low-cholesterol diet and a lot of very good dressings contain sour cream. You can generally substitute low-fat yogurt for sour cream in most recipes with good results. Again, it is a good idea to read the list of ingredients on the container before you buy salad dressing to be sure they don't contain anything that shouldn't be used on a low-cholesterol diet—as well as honey or sugar, or other things that shouldn't be used on a diabetic diet. If you are in doubt about your favorite dressing, read the label; you may be happily surprised.

Fruits and vegetables—except for coconut and coconut oil and palm oil—do not have any cholesterol. You are free to use any fruits and vegetables in a salad that will fit into your diabetic diet. I haven't used any avocados in the recipes because they are so high in fat exchanges that they are hard to fit into a diabetic diet pattern. However, if you like them well enough that you are willing to use your fat exchanges for them, feel perfectly free to do so; they are a good source of fiber, which is a plus. I also have not used grapefruit or oranges because I feel that most diabetics use them so often and are so used to eating them that I should concentrate on salads that might be a little different. Grapefruit sections or orange sections on a lettuce leaf is a perfect salad for both the low-cholesterol and diabetic diets.

Equal (aspartame) sugar substitute has been used a great deal in this chapter because I like to use it whenever possible, but feel free to use your own favorite sugar substitute. Each packet of Equal is equal to 2 teaspoons sugar—use your own favorite sugar substitute accordingly.

Basic Salad Gelatin

This gelatin base is free and doesn't need to be counted. However, you will need to count any other ingredients that you add to the gelatin unless they, too, are free.

> 1³/₄ cups water
> 1 ¹/₄-ounce packet Knox Unflavored
>   Gelatine
> 2 tablespoons lemon juice or white vinegar
> Sugar substitute equal to 2 tablespoons
>   sugar

Place 1 cup water in pan. Sprinkle gelatin over it and let stand for 5 minutes. Heat and stir over low heat until clear and gelatin is dissolved. Remove from heat.

Add remaining ³/₄ cup water, lemon juice or vinegar, and sweetener to gelatin mixture. Stir to dissolve sugar substitute, if necessary. Pour into mold or dish and refrigerate until firm. Serve about ¹/₂ cup per serving. (Up to 1¹/₂ cups vegetables or fruit may be added to the gelatin. First chill the gelatin until it is the consistency of unbeaten egg whites. Then fold in vegetables and pour into mold or bowl. Chill until firm.)

Yields about 2 cups—4 servings

Nutritive Values Per Serving

CAL	CARBS (g)	PRO (g)	TOTAL FAT (g)	SAT. FAT (g)	CHOL (mg)	FIBER (g)	NA (mg)
11	1	2	trace	0	0	0	28

Food exchanges per serving: May be considered free.
Low-sodium diets: May be used as written.
Sugar content per serving: None.

Fruit-Flavored Gelatin

You can use any flavor unsweetened drink mix with this recipe, but we prefer strawberry or cherry. Of course, you will have to calculate any fruit or other ingredients you add to the gelatin. If you add 1 cup drained, unsweetened fruit to the gelatin, each serving will be a half fruit exchange.

> 1 1/4-ounce packet Knox Unflavored
>   Gelatine
> 2 cups water
> 1 .20-ounce packet Wyler's unsweetened
>   flavored soft drink mix or Kool-Aid
>   unsweetened soft drink mix
> 8 1-gram packets Equal (aspartame) sugar
>   substitute

Sprinkle gelatin over water. Heat over low heat or in the microwave oven until water is hot and gelatin is dissolved. Add drink mix and sweetener to hot gelatin mixture and stir until dissolved. Pour into mold or dish and refrigerate until firm. Serve 1/2 cup per serving.

Yields 2 cups—4 servings

Nutritive Values Per Serving

CAL	CARBS (g)	PRO (g)	TOTAL FAT (g)	SAT. FAT (g)	CHOL (mg)	FIBER (g)	NA (mg)
14	1	3	0	0	0	0	62

Food exchanges per serving: May be considered free.
Low-sodium diets: May be used as written.
Sugar content per serving: None.

Apple Salad

This recipe is from Kay Knochel of Phoenix, Arizona.

> **Sugar-free lemon gelatin to prepare 2 cups**
>   **gelatin**
> **1¾ cups water**
> **½ cup low-fat cottage cheese**
> **2 small (4 to the pound) tart apples**
> **½ cup chopped nuts**

Prepare gelatin according to directions, using 1¾ cups water instead of 2 cups. Refrigerate until it begins to thicken. Drain cottage cheese well and mash with the back of a large spoon. Fold into slightly thickened gelatin. Wash and core apples but do not peel them. Cut into small pieces and stir into the gelatin.

Stir nuts into gelatin and pour into a 9-inch square pan that has been rinsed with cold water. Chill until firm. Cut 3 × 4 into 12 equal portions. Serve one portion on a lettuce leaf per serving. The salad may be garnished with 1 tablespoon Kay's Cooked Dressing (see Index) without adding any exchanges, if desired.

Yields 1 9-inch square pan—12 servings

Nutritive Values Per Serving

CAL	CARBS (g)	PRO (g)	TOTAL FAT (g)	SAT. FAT (g)	CHOL (mg)	FIBER (g)	NA (mg)
54	4	2	3	trace	trace	.6	57

Food exchanges per serving: ¼ fruit, ½ fat.
Low-sodium diets: Use low-sodium variation of the salad dressing.
Sugar content per serving: None.

Molded Spicy Apricot Salad

This salad is excellent for buffets. It is colorful, and the surprising, spicy taste is a good accent to cold roast meats, chicken, and turkey.

> 1 16-ounce can apricot halves in light
>   syrup
> ¼ cup white vinegar
> 2 tablespoons sugar
> 1 stick cinnamon
> 4 whole cloves
> Water
> 1 .3-ounce package apricot or peach sugar-
>   free gelatin
> 3 1-gram packets Equal (aspartame) sugar
>   substitute

Drain apricots well and reserve liquid. Refrigerate apricots. Combine apricot juice, vinegar, sugar, cinnamon, and cloves. Add enough water to yield 2 cups liquid. Pour into a saucepan, cover, and simmer for 10 minutes. Immediately strain spices from liquid and dissolve gelatin in liquid while still hot. Add enough cold water to total 2 cups, if necessary. Stir Equal into gelatin mixture and mix lightly. Cool until syrupy, add apricots, mix lightly, and pour into an 8-inch-square glass dish and refrigerate until set. Cut into six equal portions, using one portion per serving. (The gelatin can also be molded and ½ cup of the salad used per serving.)

Yields 1 8-inch square—6 servings

Nutritive Values Per Serving

CAL	CARBS (g)	PRO (g)	TOTAL FAT (g)	SAT. FAT (g)	CHOL (mg)	FIBER (g)	NA (mg)
73	18	1	trace	0	0	0	44

Food exchanges per serving: 1 fruit.
Low-sodium diets: May be used as written.
Sugar content per serving: .5 teaspoon.

Nectarine Salad

If nectarines aren't available, you can use ¹/₂ cup well-drained, sliced, juice-packed peaches instead.

¹/₄ cup Miracle Whip salad dressing
¹/₄ cup 2% milk
1 1-gram packet Equal (aspartame) sugar substitute
2 cups diced crisp, fresh apples (about 2 medium-size)
1 cup sliced, washed but not peeled, fresh nectarine (about 1 medium)
1 cup diced celery

Place Miracle Whip, milk, and Equal in a bowl and mix until smooth. Let sit at room temperature for 15 minutes to thicken. Add apples, nectarine, and celery. Mix lightly and refrigerate. Serve cold, using ¹/₂ cup per serving.

Yields 3 cups—6 servings

Nutritive Values Per Serving

CAL	CARBS (g)	PRO (g)	TOTAL FAT (g)	SAT. FAT (g)	CHOL (mg)	FIBER (g)	NA (mg)
89	11	1	5	.8	4	1.5	79

Food exchanges per serving: ²/₃ fruit, 1 fat.
Low-sodium diets: May be used as written.
Sugar content per serving: None.

Cranberry Gelatin Salad

Sugar-free strawberry gelatin to yield 4 cups gelatin
1³/₄ cups water
1¹/₄ cups cooked cranberries, unsweetened

> ½ cup finely chopped celery
> ¼ cup Kay's Cooked Dressing (see Index)
> ¼ cup chopped nuts
> Sugar substitute

Prepare gelatin as directed on the package, but use only 1¾ cups water. Cool for 5 minutes. Add cranberries, celery, dressing, and nuts to gelatin mixture. Mix lightly.

Add sweetener to salad to taste. Pour salad into a 9-inch square glass pan. Refrigerate until firm. Cut 3 × 4 into 12 equal portions. Serve one square on a lettuce leaf per serving. The salad may be garnished with 1 teaspoon Kay's Cooked Dressing without changing the exchange values.

Yields 1 9-inch square mold—12 servings

Nutritive Values Per Serving

CAL	CARBS (g)	PRO (g)	TOTAL FAT (g)	SAT. FAT (g)	CHOL (mg)	FIBER (g)	NA (mg)
34	2	1	2	trace	0	.6	53

Food exchanges per serving: One serving may be considered free.
Low-sodium diets: Use low-sodium variation of the salad dressing.
Sugar content per serving: None.

Molded Cabbage Salad

I know it sounds unusual but I like to serve this salad with stir-fry meals. The tartness of the salad complements the sauce on the stir-fry food.

> 1 .3-ounce package sugar-free lemon
>   gelatin
> 1¼ cups boiling water
> 2 tablespoons Kay's Cooked Dressing (see
>   Index)
> 2 tablespoons white vinegar
> 1 tablespoon instant nonfat dry milk
> ¼ teaspoon salt

1 cup finely chopped cabbage
¼ cup finely chopped celery
¼ cup finely chopped onions
2 tablespoons finely chopped fresh green
  peppers

Dissolve gelatin in water and let cool to room temperature. Add salad dressing, vinegar, dry milk, and salt to gelatin and refrigerate until syrupy. Beat with a whip at medium speed until thickened, creamy, and slightly increased in volume. Stir cabbage, celery, onions, and peppers into the gelatin mixture and pour into a shallow 1-quart casserole or mold. Chill until firm and then cut into six equal portions. Use one portion per serving.

Yields 1 mold—6 servings

Nutritive Values Per Serving

CAL	CARBS (g)	PRO (g)	TOTAL FAT (g)	SAT. FAT (g)	CHOL (mg)	FIBER (g)	NA (mg)
21	2	1	trace	trace	trace	.5	149

Food exchanges per serving: ½ vegetable.
Low-sodium diets: Omit salt.
Sugar content per serving: None.

Broccoli Salad

This recipe is based on one from Esther Smith.

2 cups sliced fresh cauliflower
2 cups sliced fresh broccoli
⅓ cup sliced Bermuda onions
1 teaspoon garlic salt
1 cup sliced fresh mushrooms
3 tablespoons Miracle Whip salad dressing
1 tablespoon skim milk

Clean the cauliflower, broccoli, and onion and slice them evenly. I like to trim the skin from the stalks of the broccoli and use the stalks, saving the flowerets for a vegetable. However, I do use the cauliflower flowerets, slicing them lengthwise—they look so pretty together that way.

Sprinkle the garlic salt over the vegetables. Toss them lightly and refrigerate overnight in a covered container.

Drain broccoli mixture well and add sliced mushrooms. Thoroughly mix together salad dressing and milk and pour over the vegetables. Mix lightly and serve ½ cup per serving.

Yields 4½ cups—9 servings

Nutritive Values Per Serving

CAL	CARBS (g)	PRO (g)	TOTAL FAT (g)	SAT. FAT (g)	CHOL (mg)	FIBER (g)	NA (mg)
39	4	1	3	.4	2	1.3	199

Food exchanges per serving: 1 vegetable, ½ fat.
Low-sodium diets: Omit garlic salt. Sprinkle vegetables with ½ teaspoon garlic powder before placing them in the refrigerator overnight.
Sugar content per serving: None.

Marinated Broccoli and Mushrooms

My godchild, Vicki Glastetter, from Redlands, California, shared this recipe with me. She arranges the broccoli flowerets around the edge of the platter and piles the mushrooms in the center for an appetizer that she says she and her friends enjoy. I use it as a salad because it is so pretty and tastes so good. She uses ½ teaspoon pepper, but I use only ⅛ teaspoon pepper. Our taste buds aren't used to the hot Southwestern food that she and her friends enjoy.

> 1½ pounds fresh broccoli
> 8 ounces fresh mushrooms
> ½ cup tarragon vinegar
> 1 tablespoon chopped parsley
> ⅛–½ teaspoon pepper
> ½ teaspoon salt
> 1 tablespoon lemon juice

¼ **cup vegetable oil**
1 **tablespoon sugar**
2 **large cloves garlic**

Wash broccoli and cut into bite-size pieces. Place in a plastic or stainless-steel refrigerator container that has a tight cover. Wash or wipe off mushrooms, thinly slice them, and place on top of broccoli.

In a separate bowl, combine vinegar, parsley, pepper, salt, lemon juice, oil, and sugar. Mash or chop garlic very fine and add to dressing. Mix well and pour over vegetables. Cover container tightly and refrigerate, turning container over several times a day, for 2 or 3 days. Drain well and serve, using ¾ cup as a standard serving.

Yields 6 cups—8 servings

Nutritive Values Per Serving

CAL	CARBS (g)	PRO (g)	TOTAL FAT (g)	SAT. FAT (g)	CHOL (mg)	FIBER (g)	NA (mg)
102	9	3	7	.9	0	2.8	162

Food exchanges per serving: 2 vegetable, 1 fat.
Low-sodium diets: Omit salt.
Sugar content per serving: .4 teaspoon.

Special Broccoli Salad

This is another broccoli salad from Esther Smith.

¼ **cup Miracle Whip salad dressing**
¼ **cup skim milk**
1 **tablespoon white vinegar**
3 **1-gram packets Equal (aspartame) sugar
　substitute**
¼ **teaspoon salt**
1 **quart fresh broccoli flowerets and sliced,
　peeled stems**
2 **tablespoons raisins**

2 tablespoons salted sunflower kernels
1/2 cup chopped onions

Combine Miracle Whip and milk in a mixing bowl and stir until smooth. Add vinegar, sugar substitute, and salt and mix well. Let sit at room temperature for 15–30 minutes.

Prepare broccoli and set aside. Add raisins, sunflower kernels, and onions to Miracle Whip mixture. Mix lightly, pour over broccoli, mix lightly again, and refrigerate 2–8 hours before serving. Serve chilled using 2/3 cup salad per serving.

Yields 4²/₃ cups—7 servings

Nutritive Values Per Serving

CAL	CARBS (g)	PRO (g)	TOTAL FAT (g)	SAT. FAT (g)	CHOL (mg)	FIBER (g)	NA (mg)
85	8	3	5	.7	3	2	162

Food exchanges per serving: 1 vegetable, 1 fat.
Low-sodium diets: Omit salt, use unsalted sunflower kernels.
Sugar content per serving: None.

Chef's Salad

1 cup chopped or shredded fresh crisp lettuce
1/4 medium-size fresh tomato, washed, cored, and sliced or diced
1/4 cup chopped celery
1/4 cup chopped onions
1/2 cup sliced fresh cauliflower
1 ounce (about 3 tablespoons) diced or chopped cooked chicken with all visible fat removed
1 ounce (about 3 tablespoons) diced or chopped lean ham with all visible fat removed
1/4 cup Creamy Garlic Dressing (see Index)

Place lettuce evenly in the bottom of a shallow salad bowl. (I often use a shallow soup bowl for my salad.) Sprinkle tomato, celery, onions, and cauliflower evenly over chopped lettuce.

Sprinkle chicken and ham evenly over chopped vegetables. (You can use sliced chicken and ham, if desired, and cut the slices into strips instead of dicing them.) Pour dressing evenly over salad, or keep on the side and use as needed. Serve salad chilled. Serve all of the salad for one serving.

Yields 1 salad—1 serving

Nutritive Values Per Serving

CAL	CARBS (g)	PRO (g)	TOTAL FAT (g)	SAT. FAT (g)	CHOL (mg)	FIBER (g)	NA (mg)
192	15	20	6	1.7	42	3.3	504

Food exchanges per serving: 2 lean meat, 3 vegetable.
Low-sodium diets: Delete ham and use 2 ounces chicken, and use low-sodium
   variation of the salad dressing.
Sugar content per serving: None.

Carrot and Pineapple Salad

2 cups shredded carrots
¹/₂ cup canned unsweetened crushed
   pineapple with juice
1 tablespoon raisins
¹/₄ cup Kay's Cooked Dressing (see Index)
1 tablespoon lemon juice
¹/₈ teaspoon salt
1 1-gram packet Equal (aspartame) sugar
   substitute

Place carrots, pineapple, and raisins in small mixing bowl.

Stir together dressing, lemon juice, salt, and sweetener to blend and add to carrot mixture. Toss lightly to coat carrot mixture with dressing and refrigerate until served. Serve a quarter of the salad (about ¹/₂ cup) for each serving.

Yields about 2 cups—4 servings

Nutritive Values Per Serving

CAL	CARBS (g)	PRO (g)	TOTAL FAT (g)	SAT. FAT (g)	CHOL (mg)	FIBER (g)	NA (mg)
65	14	2	1	trace	0	2	126

Food exchanges per serving: 1 vegetable, 1/2 fruit.
Low-sodium diets: Omit salt. Use low-sodium variation of the salad dressing.
Sugar content per serving: None.

Coleslaw

Coleslaw has always been a favorite of ours so I generally make a pretty good-sized batch of it. You can make it the day before a party or a picnic because it is even better the second day.

> 1 1/2 pounds cabbage, cleaned, cored, and
>   shredded (about 3 quarts)
> 1 1/2 cups shredded carrots
> 1/4 cup chopped fresh green peppers
> 1/4 cup finely chopped onions
> 2 tablespoons chopped parsley
> 3/4 cup Kay's Cooked Dressing (see Index)
> 1/4 cup vinegar
> 1 tablespoon celery seed
> 2 teaspoons salt
> Sugar substitute equal to 1/3 cup sugar

Place cabbage in the bottom of a big mixing bowl. Add remaining vegetables and toss lightly.

Mix together dressing, vinegar, celery seed, salt, and sweetener until smooth and pour over the vegetables. Mix lightly, cover, and refrigerate at least 2 hours. Toss salad and dressing again just before it is served. Drain excess liquid from the salad and allow 1/2 cup salad per serving.

Yields about 1 1/2 quarts—12 servings

Nutritive Values Per Serving

CAL	CARBS (g)	PRO (g)	TOTAL FAT (g)	SAT. FAT (g)	CHOL (mg)	FIBER (g)	NA (mg)
44	8	2	1	trace	0	2.2	442

Food exchanges per serving: 1 1/2 vegetable.
Low-sodium diets: Omit salt. Use low-sodium variation of the salad dressing.
Sugar content per serving: None.

Traditional Cabbage Salad

This recipe is from M. J. Smith, a registered dietitian from Guttenberg, Iowa, a lovely little town on the Mississippi. She has published several good low-fat cookbooks.

> 1 1/2 teaspoons salad mustard
> Dry sugar substitute equal to 1/4 cup sugar
> 1 tablespoon vegetable oil
> 1/4 teaspoon salt
> 1/4 teaspoon celery seed
> 2 tablespoons white vinegar
> 3 cups shredded cabbage
> 1 1/2 cups shredded carrots
> 1/4 cup shredded onions
> 1/2 cup chopped fresh green peppers

Combine mustard, sugar substitute, oil, salt, celery seed, and vinegar in a jar and set aside.

Place cabbage, carrots, onions, and green peppers in a mixing bowl. Shake dressing well and pour over vegetables. Mix lightly and refrigerate. Serve cold using 2/3 cup per serving.

Yields 4 cups—6 servings

Nutritive Values Per Serving

CAL	CARBS (g)	PRO (g)	TOTAL FAT (g)	SAT. FAT (g)	CHOL (mg)	FIBER (g)	NA (mg)
51	7	1	3	trace	0	2	153

Food exchanges per serving: 1 vegetable, 1/2 fat.
Low-sodium diets: Omit salt.
Sugar content per serving: None.

Snappy Coleslaw

2 quarts shredded cabbage
$1/2$ cup shredded carrots
$1/2$ cup shredded red onions
$1/2$ cup finely chopped jalapeño peppers
$1/2$ cup vegetable oil
$1/4$ cup white vinegar
1 tablespoon sugar
2 teaspoons salt
$1/2$ teaspoon celery seed
$1/4$ teaspoon black pepper

Place cabbage, carrots, onions, and jalapeño peppers in a bowl and toss lightly to mix well. In a separate bowl, stir together oil, vinegar, sugar, salt, celery seed, and black pepper to mix well. Add to vegetables and toss again. Cover and refrigerate for 3 hours before serving. Drain well and serve, using $1/2$ cup per serving.

Yields 1 quart—8 servings

Nutritive Values Per Serving

CAL	CARBS (g)	PRO (g)	TOTAL FAT (g)	SAT. FAT (g)	CHOL (mg)	FIBER (g)	NA (mg)
96	8	1	7	.8	trace	2	567

Food exchanges per serving: $1^{1}/2$ vegetable, 1 fat.
Low-sodium diets: Omit salt.
Sugar content per serving: .4 teaspoon.

Cucumber Salad

Frances Sonitzky, who gave me this recipe, says it is a basic Hungarian recipe. You can add a little more or less onion, make it a little sweeter, or add a whisper of white pepper according to your tastes.

2 small cucumbers (6–7 inches long)
³/₄ teaspoon salt
2 tablespoons finely chopped onions
2 tablespoons white vinegar
2 tablespoons evaporated skim milk
2 1-gram packets Equal (aspartame) sugar
   substitute
Paprika

Slice cucumbers as thin as possible. Sprinkle with salt and let stand at room temperature for 1–2 hours. Drain well, and then with your hands, squeeze out as much juice as possible from the cucumbers.

Mix onions, vinegar, milk, and sweetener together lightly. Add cucumbers and mix lightly. Refrigerate until ready to serve, using about ²/₃ cup (a third of the finished recipe) per serving. Sprinkle each portion with paprika just before it is served.

Yields about 2 cups—3 servings

Nutritive Values Per Serving

CAL	CARBS (g)	PRO (g)	TOTAL FAT (g)	SAT. FAT (g)	CHOL (mg)	FIBER (g)	NA (mg)
30	6	2	trace	trace	trace	1.3	292

Food exchanges per serving: 1 vegetable.
Low-sodium diets: Press as much of the juice out of the cucumbers as you can to eliminate as much of the salt as possible.
Sugar content per serving: None.

Farmer's Salad

I like to use warm, freshly cooked potatoes and green beans for this salad. They seem to absorb the flavor of the dressing better that way.

1 pound new potatoes
1 pound fresh green beans cut into 1-inch
   pieces

½ cup Vinaigrette Dressing (see Index)
1½ cups (6 ounces) lean cubed cooked
   beef with all visible fat removed
Fresh crisp lettuce leaves as necessary
3 medium-size ripe red tomatoes cut into
   wedges
½ cup sliced sweet onions

Cook potatoes and green beans. Peel potatoes and slice them into about ¼-inch-thick slices. Place both potatoes and green beans in a mixing bowl. Pour dressing over potatoes and beans. Mix lightly, cover, and let sit about ½ hour at room temperature. Toss beef with marinated vegetables.

Line a round serving plate with lettuce leaves. Mound the vegetable and meat mixture in the center of the plate and surround it with tomato wedges and onions. Refrigerate if not served immediately (but it is better if served immediately). Serve a sixth of the salad per serving.

Yields about 7½ cups—6 servings

Nutritive Values Per Serving

CAL	CARBS (g)	PRO (g)	TOTAL FAT (g)	SAT. FAT (g)	CHOL (mg)	FIBER (g)	NA (mg)
185	24	12	5	1.1	23	3.6	75

Food exchanges per serving: 1 starch, 1 lean meat, 2 vegetable, ½ fat.
Low-sodium diets: Cook potatoes and beans without salt and use low-sodium variation of the salad dressing.
Sugar content per serving: None.

Garden Cottage Cheese Salad

½ cup thinly sliced radishes
½ cup finely chopped onions
½ cup finely chopped celery
¼ cup finely chopped fresh green peppers
½ cup thinly sliced cucumbers

2 tablespoons Kay's Cooked Dressing (see Index)
1 teaspoon salt
1½ pounds low-fat cottage cheese

Combine vegetables and toss lightly. Combine dressing and salt and stir into vegetables.

Drain cottage cheese well and add to vegetable mixture. Mix lightly and refrigerate until served. Drain off any liquid before it is served, using ½ cup of the mixture per serving. This should be prepared as close to serving time as possible.

Note: You can use the same amounts of any other fresh raw vegetables you might prefer—such as chives, slivers of fresh cauliflower, or broccoli—without changing the exchange values.

Yields 5 cups—10 servings

Nutritive Values Per Serving

CAL	CARBS (g)	PRO (g)	TOTAL FAT (g)	SAT. FAT (g)	CHOL (mg)	FIBER (g)	NA (mg)
70	4	10	2	.9	5	trace	511

Food exchanges per serving: 1 lean meat, 1 vegetable.
Low-sodium diets: Omit salt. Use low-sodium variation of the salad dressing.
Sugar content per serving: None.

Individual Beef Salad

2 ounces (about ⅓ cup) chopped or cubed cooked lean beef with all visible fat removed
¼ cup chopped or sliced fresh sweet onions
¼ cup chopped fresh green peppers
2 tablespoons Spicy Tomato Dressing (see Index)
1 large tomato
Lettuce leaf
½ teaspoon fresh parsley (optional)

Mix beef, onions, peppers, and dressing lightly in a small bowl. Cover and refrigerate 1–8 hours. Wash and core tomato. Cut into cubes or wedges. Add to marinated meat and dressing mixture and toss to coat tomato with dressing.

Line a salad bowl with lettuce. Mound salad in center of the lettuce. Sprinkle parsley on top of salad and serve immediately. Serve all of the salad for one serving.

Yields 1 salad—1 serving

Nutritive Values Per Serving

CAL	CARBS (g)	PRO (g)	TOTAL FAT (g)	SAT. FAT (g)	CHOL (mg)	FIBER (g)	NA (mg)
168	14	19	5	1.4	46	3.3	230

Food exchanges per serving: 2 lean meat, 3 vegetable.
Low-sodium diets: Use low-sodium variation of the salad dressing.
Sugar content per serving: None.

Kidney Bean Salad

The idea of adding apple to a bean or pea salad came from my cousin LaVerle Sniffin of Waterloo, Iowa. We all think it really improves the salad.

> ⅓ cup Kay's Cooked Dressing (see Index)
> 1 tablespoon chopped pimiento
> ¼ cup finely chopped Mrs. Riley's Pickles
>   (see Index) or dill pickles
> ¼ cup finely chopped onions (optional)
> 1 cup thinly sliced celery
> 4 chopped hard-cooked large egg whites
> 1 cup washed and drained canned kidney
>   beans
> 1 small (4 to a pound) tart apple

Place dressing, pimiento, pickles, onions, celery, and egg whites in a mixing bowl and mix lightly. (In order to get the hard-cooked egg whites, I hard-cook 4 eggs and then discard the yolks, or use them to garnish the salad of someone who doesn't need to worry about cholesterol.) Add kidney beans to dressing mix.

Wash, core, and slice apple. Add to salad. Toss lightly and serve ½ cup per serving.

Yields 3 cups—6 servings

Nutritive Values Per Serving

CAL	CARBS (g)	PRO (g)	TOTAL FAT (g)	SAT. FAT (g)	CHOL (mg)	FIBER (g)	NA (mg)
72	10	6	1	trace	0	2.6	242

Food exchanges per serving: 2 vegetable.
Low-sodium diets: Use only 2 tablespoons chopped pickles and low-sodium variation of the salad dressing.
Sugar content per serving: None.

Taco Salad

This recipe makes six salads, but I generally just make two at a time. I freeze the remaining meat in portions and then reheat them as needed in the microwave. This salad is best when the meat is slightly warm when added to the vegetables.

> 1 tablespoon vegetable oil
> 1 pound lean ground beef
> 2 quarts hot water
> 1 cup taco sauce
> 6 cups shredded lettuce
> 2 cups cubed fresh tomatoes
> ½ cup thinly sliced onions
> ½ cup diced fresh green peppers
> ¾ cup Spicy Tomato Dressing (see Index)
> 6 large pitted black olives

Preheat a frying pan over medium heat for 1 minute. Swirl oil around bottom of pan, add meat, and cook and stir over medium heat until meat is well browned and separated.

Place meat in a colander and drain off as much fat as possible. Pour hot water over meat and then discard that liquid also. Rinse the frying pan with hot water, wipe it dry, and return meat to pan. Add taco sauce and cook, stirring frequently, over medium heat until sauce has evaporated. Remove from heat and keep warm until used or refrigerate until needed and then warm again.

Fill six salad bowls with one cup lettuce each. Divide cooked meat into six equal portions and place on top of lettuce. Add ⅓ cup tomato cubes to each salad, and sprinkle each bowl with a sixth of the onions, peppers, and Spicy Tomato Dressing. Slice each olive into thin slices and use as garnish for each salad. Serve as soon as possible using one salad per serving.

Yields 6 salads—6 servings

Nutritive Values Per Serving

CAL	CARBS (g)	PRO (g)	TOTAL FAT (g)	SAT. FAT (g)	CHOL (mg)	FIBER (g)	NA (mg)
226	13	16	13	4.5	48	2.1	562

Food exchanges per serving: 2 medium-fat meat, 2 vegetable, ½ fat.
Low-sodium diets: Use low-sodium taco sauce and low-sodium variation of the salad dressing.
Sugar content per serving: None.

Frijole Salad

¾ cup rinsed and drained kidney beans
⅔ cup Spicy Tomato Dressing (see Index)
4 cups shredded cabbage
½ cup thinly sliced sweet onions or green onions and tops
1 cup diced tomatoes (1 medium-size tomato)
½ cup peeled and thinly sliced cucumbers

Combine beans and dressing, mix lightly, cover, and refrigerate overnight.

Place cabbage in the bottom of a mixing bowl. Place beans with dressing, onions, tomatoes, and cucumbers over the cabbage. Toss lightly just before serving, using ½ cup per serving. Lettuce may be substituted for cabbage, if desired, without changing the exchange values.

Yields about 6 cups—12 servings

Nutritive Values Per Serving

CAL	CARBS (g)	PRO (g)	TOTAL FAT (g)	SAT. FAT (g)	CHOL (mg)	FIBER (g)	NA (mg)
29	6	2	trace	0	0	1.7	107

Food exchanges per serving: 1 vegetable.
Low-sodium diets: Use low-sodium variation of the salad dressing.
Sugar content per serving: None.

Marinated Vegetable Salad

1 cup water
1 tablespoon cornstarch
1 tablespoon prepared mustard
¼ cup lemon juice
6 1-gram packets Equal (aspartame) sugar
   substitute
2 cups broccoli flowerets
2 cups cauliflower flowerets
1 cup sliced celery
¼ cup chopped fresh green peppers
¼ cup chopped onions
½ cup drained and chopped pimientos
½ cup cooked and drained red beans
9 lettuce leaves

Stir water and cornstarch together until smooth in a small saucepan. Add mustard and cook and stir over moderate heat until thickened. Continue to cook and stir for 2 minutes. Remove from heat. Cool to room temperature. Add lemon juice and sweetener to sauce. Mix lightly and set aside for later use.

Put broccoli, cauliflower, and celery in boiling salted water; cook exactly 6 minutes after the water has returned to a boil. Drain immediately and cool to room temperature. Place in the bottom of a refrigerated bowl. Add peppers, onions, pimientos, and beans to broccoli, cauliflower, and celery. Pour reserved dressing over the vegetables and mix lightly. Refrigerate overnight or all day. Toss lightly again just before serving.

Line each salad bowl with a crisp lettuce leaf. Add ¾ cup marinated vegetables per serving and serve chilled.

Yields 7 cups—9 servings

Nutritive Values Per Serving

CAL	CARBS (g)	PRO (g)	TOTAL FAT (g)	SAT. FAT (g)	CHOL (mg)	FIBER (g)	NA (mg)
45	9	3	trace	trace	0	2.4	51

Food exchanges per serving: 2 vegetable.
Low-sodium diets: Cook vegetables without salt.
Sugar content per serving: None.

Cucumber and Lettuce Salad

This salad is light with a delicate flavor, a good accompaniment to a strongly flavored casserole.

> 1 small cucumber (6–7 inches long)
> ½ teaspoon salt
> 1 tablespoon chopped parsley
> 2 tablespoons low-fat yogurt
> ¼ cup Kay's Cooked Dressing (see Index)
> 2 tablespoons skim milk
> 6 cups fresh crisp lettuce

Peel cucumber and grate coarsely. Sprinkle with salt and refrigerate for ½ hour. Drain well, pressing as much juice as possible out of the cucumber. Combine parsley, yogurt, dressing, and milk with drained cucumbers and mix lightly.

Tear lettuce into bite-size pieces. Toss with cucumber mixture just before it is served, using about 1 cup lettuce per serving.

Yields about 6 cups—6 servings

Nutritive Values Per Serving

CAL	CARBS (g)	PRO (g)	TOTAL FAT (g)	SAT. FAT (g)	CHOL (mg)	FIBER (g)	NA (mg)
27	4	2	1	trace	trace	.7	127

Food exchanges per serving: 1 vegetable.
Low-sodium diets: Press as much of the juice out of the cucumbers as you can to eliminate as much of the salt as possible.
Sugar content per serving: None.

Potato Salad

I like to make this several hours before I want to use it so the flavors can develop as the salad marinates.

> **1 cup Kay's Cooked Dressing (see Index)**
> **1 teaspoon salad mustard**
> **1 1-gram packet Equal (aspartame) sugar substitute**
> **½ teaspoon salt**
> **Whisper of white pepper**
> **1 tablespoon chopped parsley**
> **¼ cup chopped Mrs. Riley's Pickles (see Index) or dill pickles**
> **¼ cup finely chopped onions (optional)**
> **¼ cup chopped pimientos**
> **½ cup finely chopped celery**
> **4 chopped hard-cooked egg whites**
> **3 cups cooked, peeled, and diced potatoes**

Place dressing, mustard, sweetener, salt, pepper, and parsley in mixing bowl and mix lightly. Add pickles, onions, pimientos, celery, and egg whites to dressing and mix lightly. (That's right, don't use the egg yolks. Hard-cook the eggs, separate the yolks and whites, and add the whites to the salad. I use the yolks as a garnish, and those who can have the egg yolks add them to their salad.)

Add potatoes and toss lightly to coat the potatoes well. Refrigerate until needed, serving ½ cup per serving.

Yields 4 cups—8 servings

Nutritive Values Per Serving

CAL	CARBS (g)	PRO (g)	TOTAL FAT (g)	SAT. FAT (g)	CHOL (mg)	FIBER (g)	NA (mg)
92	15	4	2	trace	0	1	401

Food exchanges per serving: 1 starch.
Low-sodium diets: Omit salt. Use low-sodium variation of the salad dressing and cook the potatoes without salt.
Sugar content per serving: Negligible.

Sauerkraut Salad

This recipe is based on one from my cousin Ruth Clapper of Clear Lake, Iowa. I rinse the sauerkraut to make it milder but you can use it without rinsing if you like a stronger flavor.

3½ cups (29-ounce can) sauerkraut
⅓ cup white vinegar
3 tablespoons vegetable oil
½ cup water
8 1-gram packets Equal (aspartame) sugar
    substitute
½ cup chopped fresh green peppers
½ cup chopped onions
½ cup chopped and drained canned
    pimientos
1 cup thinly sliced celery

Drain sauerkraut well. Rinse with cold water and set aside to drain for later use.

Combine vinegar, oil, and water in a small saucepan. Bring to a boil and remove from heat. Add sweetener to hot vinegar and mix lightly.

Place drained sauerkraut in mixing bowl. Add remaining vegetables and mix lightly. Pour hot liquid over vegetables and mix again. Place in container, cover tightly, and refrigerate at least overnight before it is served. Serve ½ cup per serving.

Yields 6 cups—12 servings

Nutritive Values Per Serving

CAL	CARBS (g)	PRO (g)	TOTAL FAT (g)	SAT. FAT (g)	CHOL (mg)	FIBER (g)	NA (mg)
47	4	1	4	trace	0	1.2	164

Food exchanges per serving: 1 vegetable, 1 fat.
Low-sodium diets: Rinse sauerkraut well.
Sugar content per serving: None.

Sweet Coleslaw

This recipe came from Gena LeVan of Royalton, Illinois. It keeps well in the refrigerator, so I make it ahead of time to take to potluck dinners.

2¾ cups ice water
1½ tablespoons salt
1 quart shredded cabbage
½ cup shredded fresh green peppers
¾ cup vinegar
1½ teaspoons mustard seed
2 cups thinly sliced celery
7 1-gram packets Equal (aspartame) sugar
    substitute
½ cup chopped, canned, drained pimientos

Place 2 cups ice water and salt in bowl and stir to dissolve salt. Add cabbage and peppers, mix well, and let stand ½ to 1 hour.

Place vinegar, ¾ cup water, and mustard seed in a small saucepan and bring to a boil. Remove from heat. Immediately add celery to hot vinegar mixture. Cover and let cool to room temperature. Drain well, reserving liquid. Add sweetener to cool vinegar liquid.

Drain cabbage mixture well. Combine cabbage mixture, pimientos, and celery and vinegar mixture. Mix well. Refrigerate until needed. Serve ½ cup per serving.

Yields 5 cups—10 servings

Nutritive Values Per Serving

CAL	CARBS (g)	PRO (g)	TOTAL FAT (g)	SAT. FAT (g)	CHOL (mg)	FIBER (g)	NA (mg)
22	5	1	trace	0	0	1.1	248

Food exchanges per serving: 1 vegetable.
Low-sodium diets: Wash cabbage very well to remove as much salt as possible.
Sugar content per serving: None.

Three-Bean Salad

Dried beans are high in fiber and we should try to eat a lot of them. However, they are also high in carbohydrate, so I generally try to mix them with something else that isn't all that high in carbohydrate. This salad recipe comes from my very good friend, Jan Franks, who is a nurse and is very much interested in good nutrition for herself and her family.

> 2 cups (16-ounce can) cooked, drained
>   yellow wax beans cut into 1-inch lengths
> 2 cups (16-ounce can) cooked, drained
>   green beans cut into 1-inch lengths
> ½ cup washed and drained cooked kidney
>   beans
> 1 cup thinly sliced onions

**1 cup coarsely chopped fresh green
  peppers**
1 cup thinly sliced celery
1 cup vinegar
⅛ teaspoon salt
Sugar substitute equal to ½ cup sugar

Place beans, onions, peppers, and celery in mixing bowl. Mix
together vinegar, salt, and sweetener and pour over vegetables.
Mix lightly, cover, and refrigerate at least overnight before serving ½ cup per serving.

Yields 7 cups—14 servings

Nutritive Values Per Serving

CAL	CARBS (g)	PRO (g)	TOTAL FAT (g)	SAT. FAT (g)	CHOL (mg)	FIBER (g)	NA (mg)
29	7	1	trace	0	0	1.1	149

Food exchanges per serving: 1 vegetable.
Low-sodium diets: Omit salt. Use low-sodium canned vegetables or fresh or
  frozen vegetables cooked without salt.
Sugar content per serving: None.

Walnut Wild Rice

*This recipe from Jacalyn Hill of Rancho Palos Verde, California,
may be used as a salad or a potato substitute. We like it as a potato
substitute with chicken, in which case I serve it lukewarm without chilling it.*

**1 6-ounce package Uncle Ben's long-grain
  and wild rice**
1 cup thinly sliced celery
2 tablespoons chopped celery leaves
1 cup shredded carrots
4 tablespoons vegetable oil, divided
¼ cup chopped English walnuts

2 tablespoons red wine vinegar
1 1-gram packet Equal (aspartame) sugar
  substitute
1 teaspoon salt

Prepare rice according to the directions on the package, omitting
the butter. Transfer rice to a large bowl and cool to room temperature. Stir celery, celery leaves, and carrots into cooked rice.

   Place 2 tablespoons oil in a small frying pan. Add walnuts
and cook and stir over medium heat until walnuts are golden and
toasted. Remove from heat. Combine 2 tablespoons oil, vinegar,
sweetener, and salt. Add to walnuts; mix lightly and pour over rice
mixture. Toss lightly to blend well. Cover and chill well. Serve as
a potato substitute or salad using ½ cup per serving.

Yields 5 cups—10 servings

Nutritive Values Per Serving

CAL	CARBS (g)	PRO (g)	TOTAL FAT (g)	SAT. FAT (g)	CHOL (mg)	FIBER (g)	NA (mg)
134	15	3	8	.9	0	1	426

Food exchanges per serving: 1 starch, 1½ fat.
Low-sodium diets: Omit salt.
Sugar content per serving: None.

Zucchini Salad

*This recipe from Thelma VanLaningham of Independence, Iowa,
is a delicious way to use those zucchini that grow so profusely in
all our gardens.*

   ⅔ cup cider vinegar
   2 tablespoons wine vinegar
   2 tablespoons vegetable oil
   ½ teaspoon pepper
   1 teaspoon salt
   Liquid sugar substitute equal to ½ cup
     sugar
   ½ cup diced onions

½ cup diced celery
½ cup diced fresh green peppers
6 medium (about 6–7 inches) zucchini,
    washed and sliced

Combine vinegars, oil, pepper, salt, and sweetener and set aside. Place vegetables in a mixing bowl and toss lightly. Add dressing and toss again. Cover and allow to marinate in the refrigerator at least 4 hours or overnight before it is served, using ½ cup per serving.

Yields about 2 quarts—16 servings

Nutritive Values Per Serving

CAL	CARBS (g)	PRO (g)	TOTAL FAT (g)	SAT. FAT (g)	CHOL (mg)	FIBER (g)	NA (mg)
29	3	1	2	.2	0	.5	143

Food exchanges per serving: 1 vegetable.
Low-sodium diets: Omit salt.
Sugar content per serving: None.

Kay's Cooked Dressing

This creamy cooked dressing is from Kay Knochel of Phoenix, Arizona. Kay gave it to me when we were roommates in Chicago.

2 tablespoons cornstarch
2 teaspoons dry mustard
1 cup water
½ cup liquid egg substitute
¼ teaspoon salt
2 tablespoons margarine
½ cup white wine vinegar
6 1-gram packets Equal (aspartame) sugar
    substitute

Stir cornstarch, mustard, and water together until smooth in a 2-quart heavy saucepan. Add egg substitute, salt, and margarine to liquid in saucepan and mix well. Cook, stirring constantly, over low heat until thickened and smooth. Continue to simmer for 1 more minute, stirring constantly. Remove from heat.

Add vinegar and sweetener to dressing and mix well. Cover and refrigerate until used. Serve 2 tablespoons per serving.

Yields 1¾ cups—14 servings

Nutritive Values Per Serving

CAL	CARBS (g)	PRO (g)	TOTAL FAT (g)	SAT. FAT (g)	CHOL (mg)	FIBER (g)	NA (mg)
27	2	1	2	.3	0	trace	72

Food exchanges per serving: Up to 2 tablespoons may be considered free. ¼ cup is 1 vegetable and 1 fat.
Low-sodium diets: Omit salt. Use salt-free margarine.
Sugar content per serving: None.

Creamy Garlic Dressing

You can vary the amount of garlic powder used according to how much you like the taste of garlic. This is rather mild.

½ cup Kay's Cooked Dressing (see Index)
½ cup plain low-fat yogurt
2 tablespoons skim milk
½ teaspoon garlic powder

Place all ingredients in a bowl and mix with a fork until smooth. Refrigerate in a covered container until served. Use 2 tablespoons per serving.

Yields 1 cup—8 servings

Nutritive Values Per Serving

CAL	CARBS (g)	PRO (g)	TOTAL FAT (g)	SAT. FAT (g)	CHOL (mg)	FIBER (g)	NA (mg)
25	2	2	1	.3	1	trace	48

Food exchanges per serving: Up to 2 tablespoons may be considered free. ¼ cup is 1 vegetable.
Low-sodium diets: Use low-sodium variation of Kay's Cooked Dressing.
Sugar content per serving: None.

French Dressing

---

1 cup vinegar
1 cup water
¼ cup vegetable oil
1 tablespoon paprika
1 teaspoon Worcestershire sauce
1 teaspoon A-1 sauce
½ teaspoon celery seed
1 teaspoon onion powder

Place all ingredients in a bowl and beat with a beater for ½ minute. Pour into a container, cover, and refrigerate until used. Bring back to room temperature and shake well before using. Allow 2 tablespoons per serving.

Yields 2¼ cups—18 servings

Nutritive Values Per Serving

CAL	CARBS (g)	PRO (g)	TOTAL FAT (g)	SAT. FAT (g)	CHOL (mg)	FIBER (g)	NA (mg)
31	1	trace	3	.4	0	0	8

Food exchanges per serving: ½ fat.
Low-sodium diets: May be used as written.
Sugar content per serving: None.

Chef's French Dressing

This recipe came from Walter Marion, who was executive chef for the Swift and Co. general office food service for many years.

⅓ cup ketchup
¼ cup white vinegar
½ cup water
1 tablespoon vegetable oil

**Sugar substitute equal to 2 tablespoons
  sugar**
¹/₂ teaspoon onion salt
¹/₂ teaspoon garlic salt
1 teaspoon paprika
Sprinkle of cayenne pepper

Place ketchup, vinegar, water, oil, sugar substitute, onion salt, garlic salt, paprika, and pepper in a jar and shake vigorously to blend well. Refrigerate until needed. Serve the dressing at room temperature and shake it well just before it is served using 2 tablespoons per serving.

Yields 1¹/₄ cups—10 servings

Nutritive Values Per Serving

CAL	CARBS (g)	PRO (g)	TOTAL FAT (g)	SAT. FAT (g)	CHOL (mg)	FIBER (g)	NA (mg)
19	2	trace	1	trace	0	trace	195

Food exchanges per serving: 2 tablespoons may be considered free. ¹/₄ cup is 1 vegetable.
Low-sodium diets: Omit onion and garlic salts. Add ¹/₄ teaspoon garlic powder and 1 tablespoon dehydrated onions.
Sugar content per serving: None.

Spicy Tomato Dressing

This recipe is based on one from Anita Kane of Shorewood, Wisconsin. It is excellent on vegetables or lettuce and keeps well. If I intend to keep it more than a few days, however, I strain it to take out the dill weed and the onion.

1 cup (8 ounces) canned tomato sauce
¹/₂ teaspoon garlic salt
¹/₂ cup white vinegar
1 teaspoon dill weed
¹/₄ teaspoon Tabasco sauce
2 tablespoons grated onions

3 1-gram packets Equal (aspartame) sugar substitute

Place all ingredients in a small bowl and beat with a wire whip to blend. Refrigerate until needed but bring back to room temperature before it is used. Shake well before using and serve 2 tablespoons per serving.

Yields 1½ cups—12 servings

Nutritive Values Per Serving

CAL	CARBS (g)	PRO (g)	TOTAL FAT (g)	SAT. FAT (g)	CHOL (mg)	FIBER (g)	NA (mg)
9	2	trace	trace	0	0	trace	175

Food exchanges per serving: 2 tablespoons may be considered free. ¼ cup is 1 vegetable.
Low-sodium diets: Omit garlic salt. Use low-sodium tomato sauce and ¼ teaspoon garlic powder instead of the garlic salt.
Sugar content per serving: None.

Thousand-Island Dressing

½ cup Kay's Cooked Dressing (see Index)
¼ cup chopped, drained canned pimientos
½ cup chopped, drained dill pickles
2 tablespoons chopped fresh green peppers
¼ cup chili sauce
¼ cup ketchup
4 1-gram packets Equal (aspartame) sugar substitute

Place all ingredients in a bowl and mix with a fork until smooth. Place in a covered container and refrigerate until served using 2 tablespoons per serving.

Yields 2¼ cups—18 servings

Nutritive Values Per Serving

CAL	CARBS (g)	PRO (g)	TOTAL FAT (g)	SAT. FAT (g)	CHOL (mg)	FIBER (g)	NA (mg)
16	3	1	trace	trace	0	trace	162

Food exchanges per serving: ¹/₂ vegetable.
Low-sodium diets: Use low-sodium ketchup and chili sauce. Use low-sodium
  variation of Kay's Cooked Dressing.
Sugar content per serving: None.

Vinaigrette Dressing

*This recipe, which Frances Nielsen made often, is a great favorite
with our families. It is good on tossed salads, vegetables, cold
meats, and fish. It is best if you make it fresh when you need it,
but it can be refrigerated and then brought back to room temperature for serving, if that is more convenient for you.*

> ¹/₂ **cup vegetable oil**
> **1 cup vinegar**
> **1 tablespoon soy sauce**
> **1 tablespoon chopped parsley**
> **1 tablespoon chopped celery**
> ¹/₃ **cup finely chopped onions**
> **1 cup water**
> **Sugar substitute equal to** ¹/₂ **cup sugar**
> ¹/₂ **teaspoon vanilla**
> ¹/₄ **teaspoon garlic powder**

Place all ingredients in a 1-quart container and shake well to mix.
Shake well before using. Serve 2 tablespoons per serving.

Yields 3 cups—24 servings

Nutritive Values Per Serving

CAL	CARBS (g)	PRO (g)	TOTAL FAT (g)	SAT. FAT (g)	CHOL (mg)	FIBER (g)	NA (mg)
45	1	trace	5	.6	0	trace	59

Food exchanges per serving: 1 fat.
Low-sodium diets: Use low-sodium soy sauce.
Sugar content per serving: None.

Vinegar and Oil Dressing

You can change the seasonings in this dressing with no change in the exchange values but I like the ones I have included. It tastes like there is a lot of oil in it instead of less than ½ teaspoon per serving.

½ cup cider or white vinegar
½ cup water
1 tablespoon vegetable oil
3 1-gram envelopes sugar substitute
1 teaspoon paprika
¼ teaspoon onion salt
¼ teaspoon garlic salt
Whisper of black pepper

Place vinegar, water, oil, sugar substitute, paprika, onion salt, garlic salt, and pepper in a jar and shake vigorously to blend well. Refrigerate when not in use but return to room temperature and shake vigorously when used, using 2 tablespoons per serving.

Yields 1 cup—8 servings

Nutritive Values Per Serving

CAL	CARBS (g)	PRO (g)	TOTAL FAT (g)	SAT. FAT (g)	CHOL (mg)	FIBER (g)	NA (mg)
20	1	trace	2	trace	0	0	81

Food exchanges per serving: Up to 2 tablespoons may be considered free. ¼ cup is 1 fat.
Low-sodium diets: Omit onion and garlic salts. Add ¼ teaspoon garlic powder and 1 tablespoon dehydrated onions.
Sugar content per serving: None.

Yogurt Topping

My friend Jan Franks gave me this recipe and it is a good dip, a good salad dressing, and makes a tasty topping for baked potatoes. It is easy to make and keeps well in the refrigerator for a week or more.

2 teaspoons dehydrated minced onions
½ teaspoon salt
1 tablespoon dried parsley flakes
⅛ teaspoon garlic powder
1 cup (8 ounces) plain low-fat yogurt
¼ cup Kay's Cooked Dressing (see Index)

Stir together onions, salt, parsley, and garlic powder to blend well in a small bowl. Add yogurt and dressing to dry ingredients and mix lightly but thoroughly. Refrigerate until needed. Serve with fresh vegetables as a dip or a dressing, or as a topping for baked potatoes. Serve 2 tablespoons per serving.

Yields 1¼ cups—10 servings

Nutritive Values Per Serving

CAL	CARBS (g)	PRO (g)	TOTAL FAT (g)	SAT. FAT (g)	CHOL (mg)	FIBER (g)	NA (mg)
21	2	2	1	trace	1	0	140

Food exchanges per serving: 2 tablespoons may be considered free. ¼ cup is 1 vegetable.
Low-sodium diets: Omit salt. Use low-sodium variation of the salad dressing.
Sugar content per serving: None.

15

Breads

It isn't terribly difficult to find a good bread when you are diabetic, but if it must also be suitable for a low-cholesterol diet, you need to be more careful in your selection. You want to be sure that the bread you buy doesn't include any whole milk, egg yolks, butter, or most shortenings. French, Italian, and Vienna bread are traditionally suitable because they are generally made of flour, oil, water, and a little salt.

It isn't advisable to buy many of the specialty breads in bakeries if you are on a low-cholesterol diet, because most bakeries won't give you a list of the ingredients in their specialty breads. They may not have sugar in them but they might have egg yolks or other hidden fats. Many of the light commercial breads are a good choice because they contain dry milk and oil for reasons of cost, but if you do buy them be sure to read the list of ingredients on the wrapper. Remember, the ingredients are listed in the order of their importance, so the first ingredients on the list are always the ones that form the greatest percentage of the final product.

If you need salt-free bread, it is easy to make one of your favorite recipes using oil or salt-free margarine for the fat, and without salt and other ingredients such as milk and cheese that are high in sodium. Most of the breads in this chapter are low in sodium, and those that aren't can easily be adapted for a low-sodium diet. Salt gives flavor to bread but you can always use salt substitute or add some flavoring such as herbs, spices, or seeds like caraway or sesame if you feel the need for more flavor. Or add a little cinnamon to low-sodium whole grain bread—not enough to make it taste like cinnamon, but just enough to give it a little flavor, about ¼ teaspoon per loaf. You can also add some sugar substitute to give it a slightly sweet taste that helps compensate for not using salt.

Making bread isn't all that difficult, but it is important to pay close attention to correct temperatures and ingredients. Use a thermometer every time you make bread to check the temperature of the liquid in which you dissolve the yeast. Using liquid that is too hot or too cold can spoil a batch of bread very quickly. I have a friend (who shall be nameless) who could never make good bread. She used water that was just barely lukewarm, as her mother always had—and that explained her failures. Her mother had used the old-fashioned yeast cake and my friend was using active dry yeast. Once we got that straightened out, my friend started using a thermometer to check the temperature of the water before she added the yeast and began making excellent bread.

Flour is a very important part of making bread, and it is a good idea to use a good quality flour. I keep all-purpose and bread flour at room temperature because I use them up fast. However, I keep an assortment of whole grain flours in the refrigerator or freezer, taking care to bring them back to room temperature before I use them, because I don't always use them all that quickly. Use bread flour because of its high gluten content, which helps compensate for the lower gluten content of the whole grain flours. However, it does take more liquid than all-purpose flour, and therefore you need to use a recipe specifically written for the bread flour or do some experimenting with it when you are adapting your own recipes. Use whole grain flours whenever possible because a high-fiber regime is good for anyone on a low-cholesterol or diabetic diet.

Instant nonfat dry milk is used in many recipes because it is convenient, economical, easy to use, and easy to store. Also, using dry milk means you don't need to scald it before you add it to the bread, and that is a timesaver. It is free of butterfat and therefore good for a low-cholesterol diet. I also use dehydrated buttermilk in many of the recipes in this book for the same reasons. I very seldom reconstitute the milk when using it for breads because it can be added very easily along with other dry ingredients, and you get the same results as if you had added water to it and then added it to the dough or batter.

It is also very convenient to use liquid egg substitute instead of egg yolks for the low-cholesterol diet. It can get a little expensive if you use a lot of it so I try to use egg whites whenever possible, but there are some recipes that really need those whole eggs. It is wonderful to have the liquid egg substitute to use when egg whites just can't replace those cholesterol-rich whole eggs.

Many people think yeast needs sugar to grow, but it will thrive without any sugar in the recipe. If you have a recipe that you feel absolutely has to have a couple of tablespoons of sugar, go ahead and use it, but be sure to include the sugar in your nutritive calculations.

If you want to use your own recipes for baking bread, you can use them if you calculate them according to the information in Chapter 3. You will probably find you will have to adjust the number of slices in each loaf, but you shouldn't have any other difficulties unless you are using ingredients that are not suitable on a low-sodium or low-cholesterol diet.

I find that I can make a much better loaf of bread using the dough hook on my electric mixer. If you don't have a dough hook, you can do the first step in the regular mixer and then put it all in a big bowl to add the final flour to the batter by hand—or you can do the whole process by hand. If you are doing it by hand, you should knead the dough for several minutes to develop the gluten, since you aren't developing it with the dough hook in the mixer.

If you have a bread maker, follow the directions that came with your bread machine. Most of them provide good recipes that you can use if they don't contain egg yolks, other high-cholesterol foods, or sugar in large amounts. Liquid egg substitutes may be used instead of whole eggs, using 1/4 cup of most substitutes to replace each egg. If there is a recipe that looks good to you, analyze it according to the directions in Chapter 3 to see if it can fit into your diet.

The number of loaves and the slices per loaf are shown with each recipe. This is very important because it is an essential part of the information used to calculate the food exchanges per serving. The diabetic calculations are accurate only if you follow the recipes exactly and then cut the finished product into the number of servings shown on the recipe.

Any loaf of bread can be used to make rolls, if you roll the dough out into a long roll and then cut it into the same number of pieces that you would cut for a finished loaf. Then each portion can be used to make a roll with the same nutritive values as each slice of bread would have contained. If you want larger rolls, cut the bread dough into half the number of pieces you would cut for a finished loaf, and then shape and bake, with each roll having twice the nutritive values of a slice of bread.

Homemade bread has always been a special treat. I believe in providing myself and my guests with fresh homemade bread whenever possible. I hope you feel the same way and that you will enjoy preparing these breads.

Cinnamon Applesauce Muffins

I like to have a variety of oat and wheat bran muffins in the freezer so that I can have a different kind to pop in the microwave for breakfast each morning or with a salad or soup for lunch.

1 cup 100% Bran
2 large egg whites
¼ cup vegetable oil
1 cup unsweetened applesauce
2 tablespoons brown sugar
2 tablespoons water
1 cup all-purpose flour
2 tablespoons Splenda No Calorie
   Sweetener (optional)
1 teaspoon baking soda

2 tablespoons dry buttermilk
½ teaspoon salt
1 teaspoon ground cinnamon

Place bran, egg whites, oil, applesauce, brown sugar, and water in mixer bowl. Mix lightly to blend and let sit at room temperature for 30 to 45 minutes.

Stir flour, sugar substitute, soda, dry buttermilk, salt, and cinnamon together to blend well. Add to bran mixture and mix at medium speed only until all flour is moistened. Grease muffin tins with margarine or line with paper cups. Fill tins half full (level No. 20 dipper) and bake at 400°F for 20 minutes, or until muffins spring back when touched in the center. Serve hot if possible, using one muffin per serving.

Yields 12 muffins—12 servings

Nutritive Values Per Serving

CAL	CARBS (g)	PRO (g)	TOTAL FAT (g)	SAT. FAT (g)	CHOL (mg)	FIBER (g)	NA (mg)
127	17	3	6	.8	1	2.2	263

Food exchanges per serving: 1 starch, 1 fat.
Low-sodium diets: Omit salt.
Sugar content per serving: .5 teaspoon.

Bran Nut Muffins

1 cup water
1 cup All Bran, Bran Buds, or 100% Bran
Dry sugar substitute equal to 3
  tablespoons sugar (optional)
2 large egg whites at room temperature
⅓ cup (⅔ stick) margarine at room
  temperature
1¼ cups all-purpose flour
¼ cup instant nonfat dry milk
4 teaspoons baking powder
¼ cup chopped nuts

Combine water, bran, sweetener, and egg whites and let sit for 5 to 10 minutes.

Cream margarine at medium speed until light and fluffy.

Stir flour, dry milk, baking powder, and nuts to blend well and add to creamed margarine along with bran mixture. Mix at medium speed only until flour is moistened. Do not overmix. Grease muffin tins with margarine or line with paper liners. Fill muffin tins half full (level No. 20 dipper) and bake at 400°F for 20 to 25 minutes, or until muffins spring back when touched in the center. Serve hot, if possible. Serve one muffin per serving.

Yields 12 muffins—12 servings

Nutritive Values Per Serving

CAL	CARBS (g)	PRO (g)	TOTAL FAT (g)	SAT. FAT (g)	CHOL (mg)	FIBER (g)	NA (mg)
139	15	3	8	1.1	trace	2	297

Food exchanges per serving: 1 starch, 1½ fat.
Low-sodium diets: Use salt-free margarine and low-sodium baking powder.
Sugar content per serving: None.

Dark Bran Muffins

---

1 cup all-purpose flour
1 teaspoon baking soda
1 cup All Bran, Bran Buds, 100% Bran, or
   oat bran
¼ cup dry buttermilk
1 cup water
2 large egg whites at room temperature
2 tablespoons vegetable oil
Liquid sugar substitute equal to 3
   tablespoons sugar (optional)
¼ cup dark molasses

Place flour, soda, bran, and dry buttermilk in mixer bowl and mix at low speed to blend.

Combine water, egg whites, oil, sweetener, and molasses and stir with a fork to blend. Add to flour mixture and mix at medium speed only until flour is moistened. Grease muffin tins with margarine or line with paper liners. Fill muffin tins half full (level No. 20 dipper) and bake at 400°F for 20–25 minutes, or until muffins spring back when touched in the center. Serve hot, if possible. Serve one muffin per serving.

Yields 12 muffins—12 servings

Nutritive Values Per Serving

CAL	CARBS (g)	PRO (g)	TOTAL FAT (g)	SAT. FAT (g)	CHOL (mg)	FIBER (g)	NA (mg)
108	17	3	4	.5	2	2	189

Food exchanges per serving: 1 starch, 1 fat.
Low-sodium diets: May be used as written.
Sugar content per serving: 1 teaspoon.

Refrigerator Bran Muffins

This recipe is based on one from Doris Walker of Grinnell, Iowa. I like to keep this batter on hand and generally bake six muffins at a time. They are dark, rich muffins that I often serve to friends without telling them that it's a low-sugar recipe.

> **3 cups Bran Buds, All Bran, or 100% Bran cereal**
> **3 cups water**
> **1/3 cup vegetable oil**
> **4 large egg whites**
> **Liquid sugar substitute equal to 1/3 cup sugar**
> **2 1/2 cups all-purpose flour**
> **1/2 cup dry buttermilk**
> **1/4 cup sugar**
> **1 tablespoon baking soda**
> **1/2 teaspoon salt**

Place bran, water, oil, egg whites, and sweetener in mixer bowl and mix at low speed to blend.

Stir remaining dry ingredients together to blend well. Add to bran mixture and mix at medium speed only to blend. Line 30 muffin tins with paper cups or spray with cooking spray. Fill muffin tins half full (level No. 20 dipper) and bake at 375°F for about 20 minutes, or until they spring back when touched in the center. Serve hot if possible, one muffin per serving.

Muffins can be baked immediately or batter can be covered and kept in the refrigerator for up to 3 weeks. The batter does not need to be brought to room temperature when it is used. If the batter gets too thick, it can be thinned with a little hot water.

Yields 30 muffins—30 servings

Nutritive Values Per Serving

CAL	CARBS (g)	PRO (g)	TOTAL FAT (g)	SAT. FAT (g)	CHOL (mg)	FIBER (g)	NA (mg)
97	17	3	3	.4	1	2.6	232

Food exchanges per serving: 1 starch, 1/2 fat.
Low-sodium diets: Omit salt.
Sugar content per serving: .4 teaspoon.

Raisin Bran Muffins

1 cup water
2 large egg whites at room temperature
1/4 cup vegetable oil
1/4 cup instant nonfat dry milk
1 cup all-purpose flour
1 tablespoon baking powder
1 cup All Bran, Bran Buds, 100% Bran, or
   oat bran
1/4 cup raisins

Place water, egg whites, oil, and dry milk in mixer bowl and mix at low speed to blend.

Stir together flour and baking powder to blend.

Add bran and raisins to liquid along with flour mixture. Mix at medium speed only until flour is moistened. Do not overmix. Grease muffin tins with margarine or line with paper liners. Fill muffin tins half full (level No. 20 dipper) and bake at 400°F for 20–25 minutes, or until muffins spring back when touched in the center. Serve hot, if possible. Serve one muffin per serving.

Yields 12 muffins—12 servings

Nutritive Values Per Serving

CAL	CARBS (g)	PRO (g)	TOTAL FAT (g)	SAT. FAT (g)	CHOL (mg)	FIBER (g)	NA (mg)
117	15	3	6	.7	trace	2.1	197

Food exchanges per serving: 1 starch, 1 fat.
Low-sodium diets: Use low-sodium baking powder.
Sugar content per serving: None.

Applesauce Oat Bran Muffins

1 cup bread flour
1 cup oat bran
¼ cup packed brown sugar
4 teaspoons baking powder
1 teaspoon ground cinnamon or pumpkin
   pie spice
½ cup unsweetened applesauce
½ cup water
¼ cup vegetable oil
2 large egg whites

Place flour, oat bran, brown sugar, baking powder, and cinnamon or pumpkin pie spice in bowl and mix well at low speed. In a separate bowl combine applesauce, water, oil, and egg whites and beat with a fork to blend.

Add applesauce mixture to flour mixture and mix at medium speed only until all flour is moistened. Grease muffin tins with margarine or line with paper cups. Fill muffin tins half full (level No. 20 dipper) and bake at 400°F for about 20 minutes, or until muffins are browned and spring back when touched in the center. Serve hot, if possible, using one muffin per serving.

Yields 12 muffins—12 servings

Nutritive Values Per Serving

CAL	CARBS (g)	PRO (g)	TOTAL FAT (g)	SAT. FAT (g)	CHOL (mg)	FIBER (g)	NA (mg)
132	19	3	6	.8	0	1.7	186

Food exchanges per serving: 1 starch, 1 fat, 1/4 other carbohydrate.
Low-sodium diets: Use low-sodium baking powder.
Sugar content per serving: 1 teaspoon.

Oat Bran Muffins

This muffin isn't very big, and it is plain but very good. The bread flour provides the gluten, which the oat bran needs to give the muffins a good texture.

> 1 cup bread flour
> 1 cup oat bran cereal
> 2 tablespoons sugar
> 2 tablespoons instant nonfat dry milk
> 1 tablespoon baking powder
> Dry sugar substitute equal to 1/3 cup sugar
> 1 cup water
> 1/2 cup egg whites or liquid egg substitute
> 1/4 cup vegetable oil
> 1 teaspoon vanilla

Place bread flour, oat bran, sugar, dry milk, baking powder, and sugar substitute in mixer bowl and mix at low speed to blend well. Stir water, egg whites or liquid egg substitute, oil, and vanilla together to blend and add to the flour mixture. Mix at medium speed only until the flour is moistened. Fill muffin cups that have been greased or lined with paper liners half full (level No. 20 dipper) and bake at 400°F for 20–25 minutes or until lightly browned. Serve hot, if possible, using one muffin per serving.

Yields 12 muffins—12 servings

Nutritive Values Per Serving

CAL	CARBS (g)	PRO (g)	TOTAL FAT (g)	SAT. FAT (g)	CHOL (mg)	FIBER (g)	NA (mg)
130	17	4	6	.8	trace	1.4	174

Food exchanges per serving: 1 starch, 1 fat.
Low-sodium diets: Use low-sodium baking powder.
Sugar content per serving: .5 teaspoon.

Chocolate Oat Bran Muffins

These muffins can add more variety to the oat bran muffins you take along to work for coffee breaks. If you want them sweeter, you can add 2 teaspoons dry Weight Watchers Low Calorie Sweetener along with the flour without changing the food exchange value.

> 1 cup bread flour
> 1 cup oat bran
> 1/3 cup cocoa
> 1/4 cup sugar
> 1 tablespoon baking powder
> 1/2 teaspoon salt
> 1 cup plus 2 tablespoons water at room
>   temperature
> 1/4 cup vegetable oil
> 2 large egg whites
> 1 teaspoon vanilla

Place flour, oat bran, cocoa, sugar, baking powder, and salt in a mixer bowl and mix well at low speed. Combine water, oil, egg whites, and vanilla and stir with a fork to blend.

Add liquid mixture to flour mixture and mix at low speed only until all flour is moistened. Grease muffin tins with margarine or line with paper cups. Fill muffin tins half full (level No. 20 dipper) and bake at 400°F for about 20 minutes, or until muffins spring back when touched in the center. Serve hot, if possible, using one muffin per serving.

Yields 12 muffins—12 servings

Nutritive Values Per Serving

CAL	CARBS (g)	PRO (g)	TOTAL FAT (g)	SAT. FAT (g)	CHOL (mg)	FIBER (g)	NA (mg)
132	19	4	7	1	0	2.2	234

Food exchanges per serving: 1 starch, 1 fat.
Low-sodium diets: Omit salt. Use low-sodium baking powder.
Sugar content per serving: 1 teaspoon.

Pineapple Bran Muffins

These are a favorite of my sister Shirley, and I try to keep them on hand when she comes to visit me.

> 1 cup all-purpose flour
> 1 tablespoon baking powder
> 1/2 teaspoon baking soda
> 2 tablespoons instant nonfat dry milk
> 2 tablespoons sugar
> Sugar substitute equal to 1/4 cup sugar
> 2 large egg whites or 1/4 cup liquid egg substitute
> 1/2 cup water at room temperature
> 1/4 cup vegetable oil
> 1 cup All Bran, Bran Buds, 100% Bran, or oat bran
> 1 cup well drained, unsweetened crushed pineapple

Place flour, baking powder, soda, dry milk, sugar, and sugar substitute in a bowl and mix at low speed to blend well. Stir egg whites or liquid egg substitute, water, and oil together to mix well and add to the flour mixture along with the bran and pineapple. Mix at medium speed only until the flour is moistened. Grease muffin tins with margarine, spray with cooking spray, or line with paper liners. Fill muffin tins half full (level No. 20 dipper) and bake at 400°F 20–25 minutes or until lightly browned and firm. Serve hot, if possible, using one muffin per serving.

Yields 12 muffins—12 servings

Nutritive Values Per Serving

CAL	CARBS (g)	PRO (g)	TOTAL FAT (g)	SAT. FAT (g)	CHOL (mg)	FIBER (g)	NA (mg)
128	18	3	6	.7	trace	2	260

Food exchanges per serving: 1 starch, 1 fat.
Low-sodium diets: Use low-sodium baking powder.
Sugar content per serving: .5 teaspoon.

Rye Muffins

You can vary the amount of caraway seed without changing the exchange values of the muffins. I like 1½ tablespoonfuls of them but you might like 1 or 2 tablespoonfuls depending upon your own taste.

> 1 cup bread flour
> 1 cup rye flour
> 2 tablespoons brown sugar
> 1 tablespoon baking powder
> ¼ teaspoon salt
> 1–2 tablespoons caraway seed
> 1 cup water at room temperature
> 4 large egg whites or ½ cup liquid egg
>   substitute at room temperature
> ¼ cup vegetable oil

Stir flours, brown sugar, baking powder, salt, and caraway seed together at low speed to blend. Beat water, egg whites or egg substitute, and oil together with a fork to blend and add to the flour mixture. Mix at medium speed only until the flour is moistened. Grease muffin tins with margarine, spray with cooking spray, or line with paper liners. Fill muffin tins half full (level No. 20 dipper) and bake at 400°F for 20–25 minutes or until lightly browned and firm. Serve hot, if possible, using one muffin per serving.

Yields 12 muffins—12 servings

Nutritive Values Per Serving

CAL	CARBS (g)	PRO (g)	TOTAL FAT (g)	SAT. FAT (g)	CHOL (mg)	FIBER (g)	NA (mg)
131	17	3	6	.7	0	1.5	197

Food exchanges per serving: 1 starch, 1 fat.
Low-sodium diets: Omit salt and use low-sodium baking powder.
Sugar content per serving: .5 teaspoon.

Yankee Cornbread

If you like your cornbread thicker, bake it in an 8-inch square pan. I like it thinner and crustier so I bake it in a 9-inch square pan.

> 1 cup cornmeal
> 1 cup all-purpose flour
> 4 teaspoons baking powder
> 1/4 cup sugar
> 1/4 cup instant nonfat dry milk
> 1/4 teaspoon salt
> 1 cup water at room temperature
> 1/4 cup liquid egg substitute at room
>   temperature
> 1/4 cup vegetable oil

Place dry ingredients in mixer bowl and mix at low speed to blend well. (I find that I get much better results mixing it in a mixer than I do when I mix it by hand.)

Beat together water, egg substitute, and oil with a fork and add all at once to the flour mixture. Beat at low speed only until the flour is moistened. Pour into an 8- or 9-inch square pan that has been greased with margarine. Bake at 400°F for about 25 minutes for a 9-inch pan or 30–35 minutes for an 8-inch pan. Serve hot, if possible. Cut 4 × 4 to yield 16 squares. Serve one square as a standard serving.

Yields 1 8- or 9-inch square—16 servings

Nutritive Values Per Serving

CAL	CARBS (g)	PRO (g)	TOTAL FAT (g)	SAT. FAT (g)	CHOL (mg)	FIBER (g)	NA (mg)
109	17	2	4	.5	trace	.7	127

Food exchanges per serving: 1 starch, 1 fat.
Low-sodium diets: Omit salt. Use low-sodium baking powder.
Sugar content per serving: .8 teaspoon.

Applesauce Nut Bread

⅓ cup (⅔ stick) margarine at room
    temperature
3 tablespoons sugar
3 large egg whites at room temperature
1 cup all-purpose flour
⅔ cup graham flour
1 teaspoon pumpkin pie spice
1 tablespoon baking powder
½ teaspoon baking soda
½ teaspoon salt
1 cup unsweetened applesauce
Liquid sugar substitute equal to 3
    tablespoons sugar
½ cup chopped nuts

Cream margarine and sugar together until light and fluffy. Add egg whites to creamed mixture and beat at medium speed for ½ minute.

Stir together flours, spice, baking powder, soda, and salt until well blended.

Add applesauce, sweetener, and nuts, along with flour mixture to creamed mixture. Mix at medium speed only until the flour is moistened. Do not overbeat. Spread evenly in a 9″ × 5″ × 3″ loaf pan that has been greased with margarine. Bake at 375°F for 45 minutes, or until a cake tester comes out clean from the center and the bread pulls away from the sides of the pan. Cool 10 minutes in the pan and turn out onto a wire rack to cool to room temperature. Cut into 16 equal slices. Serve one slice per serving.

Yields 1 loaf—16 servings

Nutritive Values Per Serving

CAL	CARBS (g)	PRO (g)	TOTAL FAT (g)	SAT. FAT (g)	CHOL (mg)	FIBER (g)	NA (mg)
126	15	3	7	.9	0	1.2	266

Food exchanges per serving: 1 starch, 1 fat.
Low-sodium diets: Omit salt. Use salt-free margarine and low-sodium baking powder.
Sugar content per serving: .6 teaspoon.

Banana Nut Bread

This recipe is based on one from Florence Jennings.

> ½ cup (1 stick) margarine at room temperature
> 2 tablespoons sugar
> ½ cup liquid egg substitute at room temperature
> Dry sugar substitute equal to ⅓ cup sugar
> 1 cup all-purpose flour
> ¾ cup oat bran
> 2 teaspoons baking powder
> ½ teaspoon baking soda

**1 cup mashed bananas (3 medium
 bananas)**
¼ cup chopped nuts

Cream together margarine and sugar at medium speed until light and fluffy. Add egg substitute and sweetener to creamed mixture and beat at medium speed for 1 minute.

Stir together flour, oat bran, baking powder, and soda to blend well. Add bananas to creamed mixture along with the flour mixture and beat 1 minute at medium speed.

Add nuts to batter and mix lightly. Spread evenly in a 9″ × 5″ × 3″ loaf pan that has been greased with margarine.

Bake at 375°F for 45 minutes, or until a cake tester comes out clean from the center of the loaf and the loaf starts to pull away from the sides of the pan. Cool in the pan for 10 minutes. Turn out onto a wire rack and cool to room temperature. Cut into 14 equal slices and serve at room temperature. Serve one slice per serving.

Yields 1 loaf—14 servings

Nutritive Values Per Serving

CAL	CARBS (g)	PRO (g)	TOTAL FAT (g)	SAT. FAT (g)	CHOL (mg)	FIBER (g)	NA (mg)
146	17	3	9	1.3	0	1.4	209

Food exchanges per serving: 1 starch, 1³/4 fat.
Low-sodium diets: Use salt-free margarine and low-sodium baking powder.
Sugar content per serving: .4 teaspoon.

Zucchini Bread

This recipe is based on one from Delores LeMaster of Strawberry Point, Iowa. Delores, who also has diabetes, works at the nursing home where I worked as a dietary consultant. She is quite clever about adapting recipes for her own use and she often shares them with me.

2 cups all-purpose flour
1½ teaspoons cinnamon
¼ teaspoon salt
1 teaspoon baking soda
½ teaspoon baking powder
3 large egg whites
⅓ cup vegetable oil
1½ teaspoons vanilla
Dry sugar substitute equal to ¾ cup sugar
1½ cups well-packed shredded fresh
   zucchini

Place flour, cinnamon, salt, soda, and baking powder in a mixer bowl and mix at low speed to blend well.

Place egg whites, oil, vanilla, and sweetener in a cup and mix well with a fork to blend.

Add zucchini to flour mixture along with oil mixture and mix at medium speed until well blended and creamy. Pour into a 9″ × 5″ × 3″ loaf pan that has been greased with margarine. Bake at 375°F for 45 minutes, or until a cake tester comes out clean from the center and the bread pulls away from the sides of the pan. Cool in the pan for 10 minutes. Turn out onto a wire rack and cool to room temperature. Cut into 18 equal slices and serve one slice per serving.

Yields 1 loaf—18 servings

Nutritive Values Per Serving

CAL	CARBS (g)	PRO (g)	TOTAL FAT (g)	SAT. FAT (g)	CHOL (mg)	FIBER (g)	NA (mg)
99	13	2	4	.6	0	.5	156

Food exchanges per serving: 1 starch, 1 fat.
Low-sodium diets: Omit salt. Use low-sodium baking powder.
Sugar content per serving: None.

Chocolate Nut Bread

If you are a chocoholic (and it seems to me that most diabetics are), this bread is for you. Even nondiabetics love it. I like to serve it with peanut butter.

> 1³/4 cups all-purpose flour
> 1/3 cup cocoa
> 1/4 cup dry buttermilk
> 1/4 cup sugar
> 1 teaspoon cinnamon
> 1 teaspoon baking soda
> 1 teaspoon baking powder
> 1 cup water
> 1/4 cup vegetable oil
> 1/4 cup liquid egg substitute at room
>   temperature
> Dry sugar substitute equal to 1/3 cup sugar
> 1 teaspoon vanilla
> 1/2 cup chopped nuts

Place first seven ingredients in mixer bowl and mix at low speed to blend well.

Mix water, oil, egg substitute, sweetener, and vanilla with a fork to blend. Add to flour mixture and mix at medium speed only until flour is moistened. Do not overbeat.

Add nuts to dough and spread evenly in a 9″ × 5″ × 3″ loaf pan that has been greased with margarine. Bake at 375°F for 45 minutes, or until a cake tester comes out clean from the center and the bread pulls away from the sides of the pan. Let cool in the pan for 10 minutes and then turn out onto a wire rack to cool to room temperature. Cut into 16 equal slices. Serve one slice per serving.

Yields 1 loaf—16 servings

Nutritive Values Per Serving

CAL	CARBS (g)	PRO (g)	TOTAL FAT (g)	SAT. FAT (g)	CHOL (mg)	FIBER (g)	NA (mg)
135	17	3	6	.9	1	1	144

Food exchanges per serving: 1 starch, 1 fat.
Low-sodium diets: Use low-sodium baking powder.
Sugar content per serving: .8 teaspoon.

Graham Scones

Scones can be, and often are, made from all-white flour, but I like to think that this is more like the way they were made in Scotland before white flour was so readily available.

1 cup graham flour
1 cup all-purpose flour
4 teaspoons baking powder
2 tablespoons brown sugar
1 teaspoon cinnamon
¼ teaspoon salt
½ cup (1 stick) margarine
¼ cup raisins or currants
¼ cup liquid egg substitute at room
    temperature
⅓ cup skim milk

Place flours, baking powder, sugar, cinnamon, and salt in a mixing bowl and stir with a spoon to blend well. Cut margarine into the flour mixture with a pastry blender until it resembles coarse meal. Stir raisins or currants into the flour and margarine mixture to coat them with flour.

Mix together egg substitute and milk and add as much as necessary of the mixture to the flour mixture to make a soft dough like a baking powder biscuit dough. Knead several times in the bowl and then turn out onto a lightly floured working surface. Shape into a 9-inch round and place on a baking sheet that has been lightly greased with margarine. Crease the top of the round about ¼ inch deep to form 16 equal pie-shaped wedges. The scones may be baked as they are or the wedges may be cut through and separated to form a crustier scone. If left whole, the scones should be baked at 400°F for 25–30 minutes then broken apart and served hot. If separated, the wedges should be baked at 400°F about 15 minutes or until browned and crisp. Serve one wedge per serving.

Yields 1 9-inch round—16 servings

Nutritive Values Per Serving

CAL	CARBS (g)	PRO (g)	TOTAL FAT (g)	SAT. FAT (g)	CHOL (mg)	FIBER (g)	NA (mg)
128	16	3	6	1	trace	1	239

Food exchanges per serving: 1 starch, 1 fat.
Low-sodium diets: Omit salt. Use low-sodium baking powder and salt-free margarine.
Sugar content per serving: .4 teaspoon.

Challah

This Jewish bread makes marvelous French toast or bread pudding if you have any of it left over.

> 1⅓ cups water at 110–115°F
> 2 packages (1½ tablespoons) active dry yeast
> 7 cups all-purpose flour, divided
> 1 cup liquid egg substitute at room temperature
> 2 teaspoons salt
> ¼ cup (½ stick) margarine at room temperature
> 1 egg white at room temperature
> ¼ cup water at room temperature
> 2 teaspoons sesame seeds

Place 1¹/₃ cups water and yeast in mixer bowl. Mix lightly and let stand for 5 minutes. Add 3 cups flour to liquid and beat at low speed, using dough hook, for 4 minutes.

Add egg substitute, salt, margarine, and 3 cups flour to dough and mix, using dough hook, at low speed for another 2 minutes or until a smooth dough is formed.

Turn dough out onto a working surface and knead, using as much of the remaining flour as necessary to form a smooth resilient dough. Form into a ball and place in a bowl that has been well greased with margarine. Turn the ball over to cover the top with margarine. Cover and let stand in a warm place until doubled in volume.

Turn the dough out onto a lightly floured working surface. Divide the dough into two equal portions. Round each portion into a ball. Cover with a cloth and let rest for 10 minutes. Divide each ball into three equal portions. Roll each portion gently to form a roll about 14 inches long. Braid three rolls to form a loaf. Place the loaves on one or two cookie sheets that have been greased lightly with margarine. Cover with a cloth and let stand in a warm place until doubled in volume.

Beat egg white and ¹/₄ cup water together with a fork until smooth. Brush each loaf with the egg white mixture and sprinkle with sesame seeds. Bake at 400°F for 30 minutes or until the loaves sound hollow and are lightly browned. Transfer loaves to wire rack to cool to room temperature. Cut each loaf into 20 equal slices and serve one slice per serving.

Yields 2 loaves—40 servings

Nutritive Values Per Serving

CAL	CARBS (g)	PRO (g)	TOTAL FAT (g)	SAT. FAT (g)	CHOL (mg)	FIBER (g)	NA (mg)
98	17	3	2	.3	0	.7	138

Food exchanges per serving: 1 starch.
Low-sodium diets: Omit salt. Use salt-free margarine.
Sugar content per serving: None.

Note: This bread can be baked in regular loaf pans, if desired. If the dough is baked in three equal loaves and each loaf is cut into 14 slices, each slice will provide the following:

Nutritive Values Per Serving

CAL	CARBS (g)	PRO (g)	TOTAL FAT (g)	SAT. FAT (g)	CHOL (mg)	FIBER (g)	NA (mg)
93	16	3	2	.2	0	.7	131

Food exchanges per serving: 1 starch.
Low-sodium diets: Omit salt. Use salt-free margarine.
Sugar content per serving: None.

Whole Wheat Italian Bread

This bread dough makes excellent hard rolls. We like to divide the dough into 18 equal portions, shape it into long hard rolls, and bake them to eat with hot beef sandwiches. Each roll is equal to two bread exchanges with double the nutritive values for each slice of bread.

> **2 cups water at 110–115°F**
> **2 packages (1½ tablespoons) active dry**
>   **yeast**
> **4 cups all-purpose flour**
> **¼ cup vegetable oil**
> **2 teaspoons salt**
> **2 cups whole wheat flour, divided**
> **1 egg white**
> **1 tablespoon cold water**

Combine 2 cups water and yeast and let stand 5 minutes in mixer bowl. Add 4 cups all-purpose flour to liquid and beat 4 minutes at medium speed, using dough hook. Add oil, salt, and 1½ cups whole wheat flour to batter and beat, using dough hook, at low speed for 4 minutes.

Use as much of the remaining flour as necessary to make a smooth, resilient dough. Turn dough out onto a lightly floured working surface and knead a few times. Form into a ball and place in a bowl that has been greased with margarine. Turn the ball over so the top will be greased with the margarine. Cover with a cloth and set in a warm place until doubled in volume.

Turn dough out onto a lightly floured working surface, knead lightly, and divide into two equal portions. Form each portion into a ball and let rest, covered with a cloth, for 10 minutes. Shape each ball into a long, thin loaf tapered at the ends. Place loaves diagonally, seamed side down, on greased baking sheets. Cut slits about 1/8 inch deep, about 2 inches apart on tops of loaves.

Beat egg white and 1 tablespoon water together and brush tops and sides of loaves with this mixture. Cover with a cloth and let rise again until doubled in volume.

Bake at 400°F for 10 minutes; reduce heat to 350°F and bake another 10 minutes. Brush tops and sides of loaves again with egg white mixture. Continue baking for another 30 minutes for a total of 50 minutes, or until loaves are golden brown. Turn out on a wire rack and cool to room temperature. Cut each loaf into 18 equal slices and serve one slice per serving.

Yields 2 loaves—36 servings

Nutritive Values Per Serving

CAL	CARBS (g)	PRO (g)	TOTAL FAT (g)	SAT. FAT (g)	CHOL (mg)	FIBER (g)	NA (mg)
91	16	3	2	.3	0	1.3	127

Food exchanges per serving: 1 starch.
Low-sodium diets: Omit salt.
Sugar content per serving: None.

Raisin Bread

I have always loved raisin bread. I just wish that raisins weren't so high in carbohydrate so we could double the amount of them in the bread.

> 1 1/2 cups hot water
> 1/3 cup instant nonfat dry milk
> 2 packages (1 1/2 tablespoons) active dry
>   yeast
> 5 cups all-purpose flour, divided
> Dry sugar substitute equal to 1/2 cup sugar
>   (optional)

2 teaspoons salt
¼ cup liquid egg substitute at room
    temperature
¼ cup vegetable oil
½ cup raisins

Place water and dry milk in mixer bowl and mix at slow speed only to dissolve milk. Let cool to 110–115°F. Add yeast to liquid and let stand for 5 minutes. Add 2 cups flour to liquid and mix at low speed, using dough hook, for 3 minutes.

Add sweetener, salt, egg substitute, oil, and 2 cups flour to batter and mix at low speed, using dough hook, for another 2 minutes. Add raisins to dough and mix at low speed for another minute.

Turn dough out onto a working surface spread with 1 cup flour and knead, using as much of the remaining flour as necessary to form a smooth, elastic dough. Form dough into a ball and place in a bowl that has been well greased with margarine. Turn the ball over so the top will be greased with the margarine, cover, and let stand in a warm place until doubled in volume.

Turn the dough out onto a lightly floured working surface. Knead lightly. Divide into two equal parts. Form each half into a ball, cover, and let rest for 10 minutes. Form each ball into a loaf and place each loaf in a 9″ × 5″ × 3″ loaf pan that has been greased with margarine. Cover and let rise in a warm place until doubled in volume.

Bake at 375°F for about 45 minutes or until browned. As soon as the bread is removed from the oven, turn it out onto a wire rack and brush it with margarine. Slice each loaf into 18 equal slices and serve one slice per serving.

Yields 2 loaves—36 servings

Nutritive Values Per Serving

CAL	CARBS (g)	PRO (g)	TOTAL FAT (g)	SAT. FAT (g)	CHOL (mg)	FIBER (g)	NA (mg)
91	16	2	2	trace	trace	.7	133

Food exchanges per serving: 1 starch.
Low-sodium diets: Omit salt.
Sugar content per serving: None.

Country Loaf

This bread is also good for a low-sodium diet. Without the salt, it contains only 3 mg sodium per serving.

> 2½ cups hot water
> 2 tablespoons brown sugar
> 1 cup cornmeal
> 2 packages (1½ tablespoons) active dry
>   yeast
> 3½ cups bread flour, divided
> ¼ cup liquid egg substitute
> ¼ cup vegetable oil
> 2 teaspoons salt
> 2 cups graham or whole wheat flour

Place water, sugar, and cornmeal in a mixer bowl. Mix to dissolve the sugar and let cool to 110–115°F. Add yeast to liquid mixture and let stand for 5 minutes. Add 3 cups bread flour to liquid and beat at medium speed, using dough hook, for 4 minutes. Add egg substitute, oil, salt, and 2 cups graham flour to batter and beat at low speed, using dough hook, for another 4 minutes.

Use as much of the remaining bread flour as necessary to make a smooth, resilient loaf. Turn dough out onto a lightly floured working surface and knead a couple of times. Form into a ball and place in a bowl that has been greased with margarine. Turn the ball over to coat the top of it with margarine. Cover with a cloth and set in a warm place until doubled in volume.

Turn dough out onto a lightly floured working surface, knead lightly, and divide into three equal portions. Form each portion into a ball and let rest, covered with a cloth, for 10 minutes. Form each ball into a loaf and place in a 9″ × 5″ × 3″ loaf pan that has been greased with margarine.

Cover and let rise until doubled in volume. Bake at 475°F for 45 minutes or until browned and firm. Turn out onto a wire rack and cool to room temperature. Cut each loaf into 14 equal slices and serve one slice per serving.

Yields 3 loaves—42 servings

Nutritive Values Per Serving

CAL	CARBS (g)	PRO (g)	TOTAL FAT (g)	SAT. FAT (g)	CHOL (mg)	FIBER (g)	NA (mg)
93	16	3	2	trace	0	1.2	112

Food exchanges per serving: 1 starch.
Low-sodium diets: Omit salt.
Sugar content per serving: Trace.

Rich Whole Wheat Bread

This is a good bread for a low-sodium diet. Without the salt, it contains only 3 mg sodium per slice. However, I included the salt because if you aren't on a low-sodium diet, it adds to the flavor of the bread.

> **2 cups hot water**
> **¼ cup brown sugar**
> **2 packages (1½ tablespoons) active dry yeast**
> **3½ cups bread flour, divided**
> **⅓ cup vegetable oil**
> **¼ cup liquid egg substitute**
> **2 teaspoons salt**
> **3 cups whole wheat flour**

Place water and sugar in mixer bowl and stir to dissolve sugar. Cool to 110–115°F. Add yeast to liquid and let stand for 5 minutes. Add 3 cups bread flour to liquid and mix, using dough hook, for 4 minutes at medium speed.

Add oil, egg substitute, salt, and 3 cups whole wheat flour to dough and mix, using dough hook, for 4 minutes at low speed.

Add as much of the remaining bread flour as necessary to the dough to make a smooth, resilient dough. Turn out onto a lightly floured working surface and knead a few times. Form into a ball and place in a bowl that has been greased with margarine. Turn the ball over to coat the top of the ball with margarine. Cover with a cloth and set in a warm place until doubled in volume.

Turn dough out onto a lightly floured working surface, knead lightly, and divide into three equal portions. Form each portion into a ball and let rest, covered with a cloth, for 10 minutes. Form each ball into a loaf and place each loaf in a 9" × 5" × 3" loaf pan that has been greased with margarine. Cover and let rise in a warm place until doubled in volume. Bake at 375°F for 45 minutes, or until browned and firm. Turn bread out onto wire rack and let cool to room temperature. Cut each loaf into 14 equal slices and serve one slice per serving.

Yields 3 loaves—42 servings

Nutritive Values Per Serving

CAL	CARBS (g)	PRO (g)	TOTAL FAT (g)	SAT. FAT (g)	CHOL (mg)	FIBER (g)	NA (mg)
96	16	3	2	trace	0	1.4	113

Food exchanges per serving: 1 starch.
Low-sodium diets: Omit salt.
Sugar content per serving: .3 teaspoon.

Panettone

This bread has been a favorite of mine since Chuck's cousin sent us a loaf from Milan, Italy, as a Christmas gift one year. I tried to duplicate it but couldn't until I added anise flavoring and used bread flour. It is frequently baked in a round shape on a cookie sheet or in a special panettone pan that I have, but it is easier to cut into the right portions when it is baked in a loaf pan.

> **¾ cup water at 110–115°F**
> **2 tablespoons instant nonfat dry milk**
> **1 package (2¼ teaspoons) active dry yeast**
> **2¼ cups bread flour, divided**
> **Dry sugar substitute equal to 3**
>   **tablespoons sugar**

2 drops yellow food coloring
¹/₄ teaspoon anise extract
¹/₈ teaspoon ground ginger
¹/₄ cup liquid egg substitute at room
temperature
¹/₂ teaspoon salt
2 tablespoons margarine at room
temperature
¹/₄ cup chopped candied cherries

Combine water, dry milk, and yeast and let stand for 5 minutes in a mixer bowl. Add 1 cup flour to liquid and beat at low speed, using a dough hook, for 4 minutes.

Add sweetener, food coloring, anise, ginger, egg substitute, salt, margarine, and 1 cup flour to batter and mix at low speed, using a dough hook, for another 4 minutes. Add candied cherries to dough and mix, using a dough hook, only until fruit is mixed into the dough.

Use as much additional flour as necessary to form a smooth, resilient loaf. Turn dough out onto a lightly floured working surface and knead a couple of times. Form into a ball and place in a bowl that has been well greased with margarine. Turn the ball over to coat the top of it with margarine. Cover with a cloth and set in a warm place until doubled in volume.

Turn dough out onto a lightly floured working surface, knead lightly, and form into a ball. Cover with a cloth and let rest for 10 minutes. Form into a loaf and place in a 9″ × 5″ × 3″ loaf pan that has been greased with margarine. Cover and let rise again until doubled in volume. Bake at 375°F for 45 minutes until well browned and firm. Turn out onto a wire rack and cool to room temperature. Cut into 18 equal slices and serve one slice as a standard serving.

Note: It is important to use bread flour in this recipe. However, if you do use all-purpose flour (3¹/₄ cups) and cut the loaf into 18 equal slices, each slice will have a nutritive value of 1¹/₃ bread exchanges (114 calories); or you can cut it into 24 thin slices with a nutritive value of one bread exchange (85 calories) per serving.

Yields 1 loaf—18 servings

Nutritive Values Per Serving

CAL	CARBS (g)	PRO (g)	TOTAL FAT (g)	SAT. FAT (g)	CHOL (mg)	FIBER (g)	NA (mg)
88	15	3	2	trace	trace	.4	87

Food exchanges per serving: 1 starch.
Low-sodium diets: Omit salt. Use salt-free margarine.
Sugar content per serving: Negligible.

Three-Grain Bread

½ cup cornmeal
2 teaspoons salt
¼ cup (½ stick) margarine
2 cups boiling water
2 packages (1½ tablespoons) active dry
    yeast
½ cup water at 110–115°F
3 cups bread flour, divided
1 cup light rye flour
1 cup graham or whole wheat flour

Place cornmeal, salt, margarine, and 2 cups boiling water in mixer bowl and mix at low speed to melt margarine. Cool to room temperature. Stir together yeast and ½ cup warm water and let rest for 5 minutes. Add to cornmeal mixture and mix lightly. Add 2¾ cups bread flour and mix at medium speed, using dough hook, for 4 minutes. Add rye and graham or whole wheat flours to dough and mix, using dough hook, for another 4 minutes at low speed.

Turn dough out onto a lightly floured working surface and knead, using as much of the remaining bread flour as necessary to form a smooth, resilient dough. Form into a ball and place in a bowl that has been greased with margarine, turning the dough so it is greased on top. Cover with a cloth and let rise in a warm place until it is doubled in volume.

Turn the dough out onto a lightly floured working surface. Divide the dough into two equal portions. Round each portion into a ball. Cover with a cloth and let rest for 10 minutes. Shape each ball into a loaf and place each loaf in a 9″ × 5″ × 3″ loaf pan that has been greased with margarine. Cover and let rise until doubled in volume. Bake at 375°F for 45 minutes, or until browned and firm. Turn bread out onto wire rack and let cool to room temperature. Cut each loaf into 18 equal slices and serve one slice per serving.

Note: It is important to use bread flour in this recipe.

Yields 2 loaves—36 servings

Nutritive Values Per Serving

CAL	CARBS (g)	PRO (g)	TOTAL FAT (g)	SAT. FAT (g)	CHOL (mg)	FIBER (g)	NA (mg)
86	15	2	2	trace	0	1.2	142

Food exchanges per serving: 1 starch.
Low-sodium diets: Omit salt. Use salt-free margarine.
Sugar content per serving: None.

Whole Wheat Bread

2½ cups water at 110–115°F
½ cup instant nonfat dry milk
2 packages (1½ tablespoons) active dry
    yeast
3 cups bread flour
¼ cup (½ stick) margarine at room
    temperature
2 teaspoons salt
2¾ cups whole wheat flour, divided

Combine water, dry milk, and yeast and let stand 5 minutes in a mixer bowl. Add 3 cups bread flour to liquid and beat at medium speed, using dough hook, for 4 minutes.

Add margarine, salt, and 2½ cups whole wheat flour to batter and mix at low speed, using the dough hook, for another 4 minutes.

Use as much of the remaining whole wheat flour as necessary to make a smooth, resilient dough. Turn dough out onto a lightly floured working surface and knead a couple of times. Form into a ball and place in a bowl that has been well greased with margarine. Turn the ball over to coat the top of it with margarine. Cover with a cloth and set in a warm place until doubled in volume.

Turn dough out onto a lightly floured working surface, knead lightly, and divide into two equal portions. Form each portion into a ball and let rest, covered with a cloth, for 10 minutes. Form each ball into a loaf and place in a 9″ × 5″ × 3″ loaf pan that has been greased with margarine. Cover and let rise again until doubled in volume. Bake at 375°F for 45 minutes, or until browned and firm. Turn out onto a wire rack and cool to room temperature. Cut each loaf into 18 equal slices and serve one slice per serving.

Note: It is important to use bread flour in this recipe. The gluten in the bread flour helps give texture to the finished loaf of bread.

Yields 2 loaves—36 servings

Nutritive Values Per Serving

CAL	CARBS (g)	PRO (g)	TOTAL FAT (g)	SAT. FAT (g)	CHOL (mg)	FIBER (g)	NA (mg)
92	16	3	2	trace	trace	1.4	147

Food exchanges per serving: 1 starch.
Low-sodium diets: Omit salt. Use salt-free margarine.
Sugar content per serving: None.

Cinnamon Rolls

These rolls are a great favorite of my friend John Franks. I've known him to eat four of them at one time, washed down with a couple of glasses of milk. He knows what he likes for between-meal snacks, and I agree with him that there is nothing like a hot, fresh cinnamon roll, right from the oven.

1 cup water at 110–115°F
1/4 cup instant nonfat dry milk
1 package (2 1/4 teaspoons) active dry yeast
3 1/2 cups all-purpose flour, divided
1/8 teaspoon ground ginger
1/4 cup vegetable oil
1 teaspoon salt
1 teaspoon cinnamon
Dry sugar substitute equal to 2
   tablespoons sugar
1 tablespoon margarine at room
   temperature
1/4 cup brown sugar
Dry brown sugar substitute equal to 1/4 cup
   brown sugar
1/2 teaspoon cinnamon
1 1/2 tablespoons margarine at room
   temperature

Place water, dry milk, and yeast in mixer bowl; mix lightly and let stand for 5 minutes. Add 1 1/2 cups flour to liquid. Mix at medium speed, using dough hook, for 4 minutes. Add ginger, oil, salt, 1 teaspoon cinnamon, dry sugar substitute, and 1 1/2 cups flour and mix at low speed, using the dough hook, for another 4 minutes.

Spread the remaining 1/2 cup flour on a mixing board. Turn the dough out onto the flour and use as much of it as necessary to make a smooth, resilient dough. Shape the dough into a ball and place it in a bowl that has been greased with margarine. Turn the ball over to coat the top of it with margarine. Cover with a cloth and let stand in a warm place until doubled in volume.

Use 1 tablespoon margarine to grease the sides and bottom of a 9″ × 13″ cake pan. Set aside for later use.

Stir brown sugar, brown sugar substitute, and ½ teaspoon cinnamon to blend well and set aside for later use.

Turn dough out onto a lightly floured working surface. Knead lightly and form into a ball. Cover with a cloth and let rest for 10 minutes. Roll dough out to form a 9″ × 13″ rectangle. Spread 1½ tablespoons of margarine evenly over the dough. Sprinkle evenly with the brown sugar mixture. Roll into a long roll like a jelly roll and cut into 24 equal slices. Place the slices, cut side down, in the cake pan, spacing them evenly. Cover with a cloth and let rise until doubled in volume. Bake at 375°F for 25–30 minutes, or until golden brown. Turn rolls out of the pan onto a wire rack and serve warm, if possible. Serve one roll per serving.

Yields 24 rolls—24 servings

Nutritive Values Per Serving

CAL	CARBS (g)	PRO (g)	TOTAL FAT (g)	SAT. FAT (g)	CHOL (mg)	FIBER (g)	NA (mg)
111	17	2	4	.5	trace	.6	111

Food exchanges per serving: 1 starch, 1 fat.
Low-sodium diets: Omit salt. Use salt-free margarine.
Sugar content per serving: ½ teaspoon.

Oat Bran Pancakes

> ½ cup bread flour
> ½ cup oat bran
> 2 tablespoons sugar
> ½ teaspoon baking soda
> ¼ teaspoon salt
> ¼ cup dry buttermilk
> 1 cup water at room temperature

**2 large egg whites or ¼ cup liquid egg
  substitute**
2 tablespoons vegetable oil

Place flour, oat bran, sugar, soda, salt, and dry buttermilk in
mixer bowl and mix well at low speed. Beat water, egg whites or
liquid egg substitute, and oil together with a fork to blend well.
Add to flour mixture and beat until almost smooth.

Lightly grease a griddle and preheat to 375°F (the fat on the
griddle has been included in your fat exchange). Pour ⅓ cup
(level No. 12 dipper) batter onto griddle and cook about 3 minutes on one side, or until bubbles begin to form on surface and
edges of pancake are dry. Turn and cook 2–3 minutes on other
side, or until nicely browned. Repeat with remaining batter and
serve hot using one pancake per serving.

Yields 7 pancakes—7 servings

Nutritive Values Per Serving

CAL	CARBS (g)	PRO (g)	TOTAL FAT (g)	SAT. FAT (g)	CHOL (mg)	FIBER (g)	NA (mg)
130	17	5	6	.9	3	1.3	205

Food exchanges per serving: 1 starch, 1 fat.
Low-sodium diets: Omit salt.
Sugar content per serving: .9 teaspoon.

Buttermilk Pancakes

*Frances Nielsen used to make these as a special treat for Chuck
when we visited her. He ate them with lots of margarine and syrup
but I liked them with unsweetened applesauce sprinkled with cinnamon and sugar substitute.*

2 cups bread flour
1 teaspoon baking powder
1 teaspoon baking soda
1 tablespoon sugar

¼ cup dry buttermilk
2 cups water at room temperature
½ cup liquid egg substitute
½ teaspoon vanilla
2 tablespoons vegetable oil

Stir flour, baking powder, soda, sugar, and dry buttermilk together to blend well. Beat water, egg substitute, vanilla, and oil together and add to the flour and beat with a large spoon until smooth.

Pour ¼ cup (level No. 16 dipper) batter onto a lightly greased griddle that has been preheated to 375°F. Cook about 3 minutes on one side or until bubbles form on the surface and the edges of the pancake are dry. Turn and cook 2–3 minutes on the other side, or until nicely browned. Repeat with remaining batter. Serve hot using one pancake per serving.

Yields 16 pancakes—16 servings

Nutritive Values Per Serving

CAL	CARBS (g)	PRO (g)	TOTAL FAT (g)	SAT. FAT (g)	CHOL (mg)	FIBER (g)	NA (mg)
97	14	3	3	.4	1	.4	132

Food exchanges per serving: 1 starch, ½ fat.
Low-sodium diets: May be used as written.
Sugar content per serving: Trace.

Cinnamon Spread

This counts as a regular fat exchange but it adds something special to toast or hot breads. I keep some in the refrigerator most of the time and I have given it, in a pretty little ceramic pot, to friends for Christmas or birthday presents. You can vary it using other spices but I prefer cinnamon.

8 ounces soft margarine at room
temperature
2 teaspoons ground cinnamon

Granulated sugar substitute equal to ¹/₂ cup sugar

Combine ingredients and mix well. Return to container and refrigerate except when it is being used. Yields 24 servings of 2 teaspoons each.

Yields 1 cup—24 servings

Nutritive Values Per Serving

CAL	CARBS (g)	PRO (g)	TOTAL FAT (g)	SAT. FAT (g)	CHOL (mg)	FIBER (g)	NA (mg)
70	1	trace	8	1.3	0	0	117

Food exchanges per serving: 1¹/₂ fat.
Low-sodium diets: Use salt-free margarine.
Sugar content per serving: None.

Cinnamon Shake

This is good to shake on hot buttered toast, cereal, baked apples, or other fruit, or as directed in recipes in this book.

Granulated sugar substitute equal to ¹/₂ cup sugar
1 teaspoon ground cinnamon

Mix sugar substitute and cinnamon well. Put in a shaker and use as desired.

Yields ¹/₂ cup

Nutritive Values Per Serving

CAL	CARBS (g)	PRO (g)	TOTAL FAT (g)	SAT. FAT (g)	CHOL (mg)	FIBER (g)	NA (mg)
3	1	0	0	0	0	0	23

Food exchanges per serving: May be used as desired without adding any nutritive value.
Low-sodium diets: May be used as written.
Sugar content per serving: None.

Noodles

I call this noodle *dough, the Italians call it* pasta, *and the Polish call it* kluski. *It can be cut wide for lasagna, square for manicotti, thin and narrow for fettucini, or in small squares for some types of southern noodles. I also use it for ravioli or cut it thin and narrow to use with spaghetti sauce.*

Remember, when you're deciding which noodles to use, keep in mind that oat bran noodles are very chewy, and wheat noodles have a nutty taste. These characteristics may keep you from using them in various recipes.

Ingredients	Basic	Oat Bran	Wheat
Bread flour	2¼ cups	2 cups	1 cup
Oat bran cereal	none	1 cup	none
Whole wheat flour	none	none	1 cup
Salt	1 teaspoon for all recipes		
Liquid egg substitute	¾ cup	½ cup	½ cup
Lukewarm water	¼ cup	½ cup	½ cup
Vegetable oil	1 tablespoon for all recipes		
Yellow food coloring	2 drops	2 drops	none
Raw yield	20 ounces	24 ounces	20 ounces
Cooked yield	10 cups	12 cups	10 cups

Place dry ingredients in mixer bowl and mix at low speed for ½ minute to blend well. Beat liquid ingredients together with a fork to blend well. Add to dry ingredients and beat, using dough hook, at medium speed for 4 minutes. Turn out onto lightly floured working surface and knead a few times. Form into a ball, place on lightly floured working surface, cover with a cloth, and let stand for 30 minutes to 1 hour.

Divide dough into three equal portions. Work with one portion at a time, keeping the other two portions covered with the cloth. Roll each portion into a very thin rectangle (I like to use my marble rolling pin) on a floured surface. As you roll out the dough, lightly sprinkle the surface with flour to keep it from sticking to the rolling pin. The dough can be cut immediately with a noodle cutter or allowed to dry flat for about 1 hour and then rolled up like a jelly roll and cut with a sharp knife into noodles as wide as you like. You can also use a noodle machine, as I do, for more uniform noodles. Shake out the strips and lay them on a lightly floured towel if you are not going to use them immediately. If the room is sufficiently warm and dry, they should dry in a few hours or overnight; then they can be used right away or stored in the freezer or an airtight container until you need them.

Noodles can also be frozen without drying first. Spread a layer of noodles on a piece of waxed paper, sprinkle with a little flour, and repeat, stacking layers of waxed paper and noodles on top of one another. Wrap the layers in an airtight package and freeze until needed. *Do not defrost noodles before you use them.* Just drop into boiling liquid, as you would fresh noodles, stir until separated, and cook about 20 minutes, or until tender.

When you are ready to cook the noodles, drop them into boiling water or broth, add 1 tablespoon vegetable oil to the pot, and simmer for 10 to 20 minutes depending on the thickness of the noodles. Drain well. Toss with a little margarine and serve hot, or prepare as directed by recipe in which you are using them.

Nutritive Values Per Cup of Cooked Noodles

VALUES	BASIC	OAT BRAN	WHEAT
CAL	132	115	107
CARBS (g)	24	23	19
PRO (g)	5	5	4
TOTAL FAT (g)	3	3	3
SAT. FAT (g)	trace	trace	trace
CHOL (mg)	0	0	0
FIBER (g)	.5	2.3	2
NA (mg)	238	193	222

Food exchanges per cup of cooked noodles: Basic: 1²/₃ starch; Oat bran: 1²/₃ starch; Wheat: 1¹/₃ starch.
Low-sodium diets: Omit salt.
Sugar content per serving: None.

16

Pies

Man lives not by bread alone. Most people want an occasional piece of pie along with their bread, and if we have to give up some bread to have our pie, well, isn't it worth it once in a while? I, for one, think it is better to enjoy a small piece of pie occasionally and know I can have it once in a while than to feel deprived and think I'll never be able to eat pie again.

It isn't advisable to buy already prepared pie, even if it is advertised as low calorie, because you don't know what kind of fat is used in the crust and filling—and this is very important on a low-cholesterol diet. It is best to make the crust and filling at home and then you will know it is prepared correctly.

It is difficult to make a good crust without a certain amount of fat. We can cut the fat back a little bit, but it still requires a fair amount of fat to have a tender crust. Since the crust is necessarily high in fat and calories, it is better to serve one-crust pies rather than double-crust pies and to use a filling that is lower in calories.

The pie crust recipes in this chapter yield just enough dough for a single crust. If you want to make a double-crust pie, double the recipe and it will be the correct amount of dough for a double crust. It won't be enough for the elaborate edges and fancy decorations that some good cooks like to add to their pies, but it will be enough for a generous crust.

If you want to make a pie filling using your own recipe, you can calculate the exchanges for the filling according to Chapter 3 and then use it in one of the crusts in this chapter. Sometimes you may have to work with your filling a little bit to get it down to where you can afford it, but if it is a family favorite it can be worthwhile to work on it.

Of course, we use unsweetened fruits and sugar substitutes routinely, and don't forget that sugar-free puddings make good pie fillings. You can use a sugar-free pudding and a couple of fresh bananas to make a very good banana pie, and you can always garnish it with a couple of tablespoons of Whipped Topping (see Index).

I have included the exchange values of the pie crust in the pie recipes. If you need to know the values of the filling, you can subtract the values of the crust from the total values of the pie.

Mom's Pie Crust

This is the crust that my mother always made. She used lard until we started following a low-cholesterol meal pattern; then she changed to margarine. She always said that she couldn't make good pie crust until she started using this recipe—and then she never had a failure.

¹/₃ cup (²/₃ stick) margarine
2 tablespoons water
1 cup all-purpose flour
¹/₄ teaspoon baking powder
¹/₄ teaspoon salt
Warm water

Heat margarine and 2 tablespoons water together until margarine is melted. Set aside to cool to room temperature. Place flour, baking powder, and salt in mixing bowl and stir to blend well. Mix margarine mixture with a fork to blend and then add to flour mixture.

Add warm water by the tablespoonful to crust mixture, if necessary. (It will depend upon the type of flour, but I've never needed to add more than 2 tablespoons to any flour that I have used.) Round dough into a ball and let stand, covered, at room temperature for 15–30 minutes. Roll crust out on a lightly floured working surface to form a circle. Fit into 9-inch pie pan and prick the bottom 6 or 7 times with the tines of a fork. Bake at 425°F for 12–15 minutes or until lightly browned. Cool and fill with desired filling; or fill the unbaked crust with desired filling and bake according to directions with the filling.

I use two pie pans when I'm making a single crust. I place the crust in the bottom pan, prick it with a fork, and then put another pan exactly the same size on top of the crust, and bake it about 15 minutes or until lightly browned. I then remove it from the oven and remove the top pan, cool to room temperature, and use as desired.

Serve one-eighth of the crust per serving.

Yields 1 9-inch crust—8 servings

Nutritive Values Per Serving

CAL	CARBS (g)	PRO (g)	TOTAL FAT (g)	SAT. FAT (g)	CHOL (mg)	FIBER (g)	NA (mg)
124	12	2	8	1.3	0	.4	171

Food exchanges per serving: 3/4 starch, 1 1/2 fat.
Low-sodium diets: Omit salt. Use low-sodium baking powder and salt-free margarine.
Sugar content per serving: None.

Graham Cracker Crust

I like to bake this crust because that makes it crisp. If you want a softer crust, refrigerate it after it is prepared instead of baking it.

> **8 crushed graham crackers (2 1/2-inch squares)**
> **3 tablespoons melted margarine**
> **2 tablespoons sugar**

Combine ingredients in 9-inch pie tin and mix well with your fingers. Press crumbs evenly around the edges and on the bottom of the pie tin. Bake at 350°F for 6 minutes. Cool and fill as desired. Cut into eight even portions, using one portion per serving.

Yields 1 9-inch crust—8 servings

Nutritive Values Per Serving

CAL	CARBS (g)	PRO (g)	TOTAL FAT (g)	SAT. FAT (g)	CHOL (mg)	FIBER (g)	NA (mg)
80	9	1	5	.9	0	trace	93

Food exchanges per serving: 1/2 starch, 1 fat.
Low-sodium diets: Use salt-free margarine.
Sugar content per serving: .8 teaspoon.

Southern Pie Crust

This crust isn't as yellow as it is when it is made with egg yolks. If you like the yellow color, you can add a drop or two of yellow food coloring to the ice water when you are mixing the crust.

> 1/2 **cup cake flour**
> 1/2 **cup all-purpose flour**
> 1/3 **cup (2/3 stick) margarine from the**
>   **refrigerator**
> 1/4 **cup ice water**
> 1/4 **teaspoon salt**
> 1 **egg white**
> 1 1/2 **teaspoons white vinegar**

Place flours in bowl and stir to blend. Cut margarine into the flour until the mixture resembles coarse meal.

Combine water, salt, egg white, and vinegar in a cup. Mix well with a fork and then add to the flour mixture. Mix lightly with a fork until you can round the pastry into a ball. Refrigerate, or cover and let stand at room temperature for 15–30 minutes. Roll crust out on a lightly floured working surface to form a circle.

Fit into 9-inch pie tin and prick the bottom 6 or 7 times with the tines of a fork. Bake at 425°F for 12–15 minutes, or until lightly browned. Cool and fill with the desired filling; or fill the unbaked crust with the desired filling and bake according to directions with the filling. Serve one-eighth of the pie per portion.

Yields 1 9-inch crust—8 servings

Nutritive Values Per Serving

CAL	CARBS (g)	PRO (g)	TOTAL FAT (g)	SAT. FAT (g)	CHOL (mg)	FIBER (g)	NA (mg)
123	12	2	8	1.2	0	trace	163

Food exchanges per serving: ³/₄ starch, ¹/₂ fat.
Low-sodium diets: Omit salt. Use salt-free margarine.
Sugar content per serving: None.

Apple Pie

FILLING
7 tart medium (4 to the pound) apples
**³/₄ cup Sugar Twin Brown Sugar
    Replacement**
2 tablespoons flour
¹/₈ teaspoon nutmeg or mace
1 teaspoon cinnamon
¹/₄ teaspoon salt

**2 unbaked 9-inch Mom's Pie Crusts (see
    Index)**
2 tablespoons margarine

Peel and core apples and slice thin. Stir together Sugar Twin, flour, nutmeg or mace, cinnamon, and salt to blend and then mix lightly with apples.

Fill bottom crust evenly with apple mixture. Dot with margarine. Cut slits in upper crust and place over filling. Seal pie crust at the edges and bake at 400°F for 50 minutes, or until pie is browned and well done. Cool to room temperature on wire rack. Cut into eight equal pieces and serve one piece per serving.

Yields 1 9-inch pie—8 servings

Nutritive Values Per Serving

CAL	CARBS (g)	PRO (g)	TOTAL FAT (g)	SAT. FAT (g)	CHOL (mg)	FIBER (g)	NA (mg)
336	40	4	19	3	0	2.5	443

Food exchanges per serving: 1¹/₂ starch, 1 fruit, 3¹/₂ fat.
Low-sodium diets: Omit salt. Use salt-free margarine and low-sodium variation of the pie crust.
Sugar content per serving: None.

Cherry Pie

FILLING
2 16-ounce cans unsweetened red cherries
1 cup liquid from the cherries
1 tablespoon cornstarch
Sugar substitute equal to 1 cup sugar
¹/₄ teaspoon almond flavoring

1 prebaked 9-inch Mom's Pie Crust (see Index)
Whipped Topping (see Index)

Drain cherries well, reserving 1 cup liquid. Set cherries aside and combine 1 cup liquid and cornstarch. Cook and stir over moderate heat until thickened and transparent and the starchy taste is gone. Remove from heat and add sugar substitute, almond flavoring, and cherries. Taste and add more sweetener, if desired. Cool to room temperature.

Spread filling evenly in crust. Let stand at least 15 minutes. Cut into eight equal portions and serve one portion per serving.

Garnish each serving of pie with 1 or 2 tablespoons Whipped Topping, if desired.

Yields 1 9-inch pie—8 servings

Nutritive Values Per Serving

CAL	CARBS (g)	PRO (g)	TOTAL FAT (g)	SAT. FAT (g)	CHOL (mg)	FIBER (g)	NA (mg)
181	26	3	8	1.3	0	.4	269

Food exchanges per serving: 1/4 starch, 1 fruit, 1 1/2 fat.
Low-sodium diets: Use low-sodium variation of the pie crust.
Sugar content per serving: None.

Custard Pie

This recipe is from Vera Wilson, a friend of mine in Wadena. Vera has been a great help to me in writing this—she gave me several recipes.

FILLING
1 cup liquid egg substitute
2 tablespoons sugar
Sugar substitute equal to 1/3 cup sugar
1 teaspoon vanilla
1/4 teaspoon salt
1 teaspoon cornstarch
3/4 cup instant nonfat dry milk
2 cups water

1 unbaked 9-inch Mom's Pie Crust (see Index)
Ground nutmeg as desired

Combine all filling ingredients and mix thoroughly. Pour filling into unbaked pie crust.

Sprinkle nutmeg over filling and bake at 475°F for 10 minutes. Reduce heat to 425°F without opening the oven door and bake another 15 minutes. Test to see if it is done by sticking a knife in the center of the pie—if the knife doesn't come out clean, bake another 5 minutes. (It has always been done for me at the end of 15 minutes but Vera said to be sure and include that caution.) Cool to room temperature out of drafts. Cut into eight pieces and serve one piece per serving.

Yields 1 9-inch pie—8 servings

Nutritive Values Per Serving

CAL	CARBS (g)	PRO (g)	TOTAL FAT (g)	SAT. FAT (g)	CHOL (mg)	FIBER (g)	NA (mg)
181	21	7	8	1.3	1	.4	354

Food exchanges per serving: 1 starch, 1/2 skim milk, 1 fat.
Low-sodium diets: Omit salt. Use low-sodium variation of the pie crust.
Sugar content per serving: .8 teaspoon.

Key Lime Pie

FILLING
1 packet Knox Unflavored Gelatine
3 tablespoons lime juice
1/2 cup boiling water
9 1-gram packets Equal (aspartame) sugar
    substitute
1 cup evaporated skim milk
1 teaspoon vanilla
Juice of 1 1/2 limes
2 drops green food coloring

1 9-inch Graham Cracker Crust (see Index)
Lime zest
Thin lime slices

Sprinkle gelatin over lime juice and let it stand for 1 minute. Add boiling water and sweetener to gelatin mixture and stir until gelatin is dissolved. Refrigerate about 45 minutes or until slightly thickened.

Combine milk and vanilla and freeze 30 minutes. Remove from freezer and whip at high speed until stiff. Stir lime juice and food coloring into whipped milk. (Save remaining ½ lime for garnish.) Slowly blend gelatin mixture into whipped milk.

Spoon pie filling into crust. Chill until firm. Garnish with lime zest and lime slices. Cut into eight even portions and serve one portion per serving.

Yields 1 9-inch pie—8 servings

Nutritive Values Per Serving

CAL	CARBS (g)	PRO (g)	TOTAL FAT (g)	SAT. FAT (g)	CHOL (mg)	FIBER (g)	NA (mg)
117	14	4	5	1	1	trace	132

Food exchanges per serving: 1 starch, 1 fat.
Low-sodium diets: Use low-sodium variation of the pie crust.
Sugar content per serving: .8 teaspoon in the crust.

Lemon Pie

FILLING
2 large egg whites at room temperature
¼ teaspoon cream of tartar
¼ cup sugar
1 cup water
3 tablespoons lemon juice
2 tablespoons cornstarch
Grated rind of 1 lemon
1 tablespoon margarine
3 drops yellow food coloring
8 1-gram packets Equal (aspartame)

1 9-inch Graham Cracker Crust (see Index)

Beat egg whites until frothy. Add cream of tartar and continue to beat at high speed, gradually adding sugar until meringue is stiff.

Combine water, lemon juice, and cornstarch in a small saucepan and stir until smooth. Add lemon rind, margarine, and food coloring to cornstarch mixture and cook and stir over moderate heat until thickened and the starchy taste is gone. Remove from heat. Mix sweetener into hot cooked mixture. Fold hot cooked mixture into meringue and mix lightly but thoroughly.

Pour filling into crust and refrigerate until firm. Cut into eight equal pieces and serve one piece per serving.

Yields 1 9-inch pie—8 servings

Nutritive Values Per Serving

CAL	CARBS (g)	PRO (g)	TOTAL FAT (g)	SAT. FAT (g)	CHOL (mg)	FIBER (g)	NA (mg)
134	18	2	6	1.1	0	trace	124

Food exchanges per serving: 1 starch, 1 fat.
Low-sodium diets: Use salt-free margarine and low-sodium variation of the pie crust.
Sugar content per serving: 2.3 teaspoons including crust.

Pumpkin Pie

Every year when we have our annual church dinner in the fall, I cut and serve the pies, and it keeps me busy. I have noticed that pumpkin and sour cream raisin pies are the most popular, with cherry and apple right behind them. I've really tried, but I can't manage a sour cream raisin pie that fits into our diets—but we can have pumpkin, apple, and cherry, so let's enjoy them!

FILLING
1 16-ounce can solid-pack pumpkin
½ cup liquid egg substitute
2 tablespoons sugar
Sugar substitute equal to ⅓ cup sugar
½ teaspoon salt

2 teaspoons pumpkin pie spice
1²/₃ cups water
¹/₂ cup instant nonfat dry milk

1 unbaked 9-inch Mom's Pie Crust (see Index)

Combine filling ingredients and mix until smooth.

Pour filling into the unbaked pie crust. Be careful to build up the crust around the edges of the pan because the pie will puff while it is baking. Bake at 425°F for 15 minutes. Reduce the temperature of the oven to 350°F without opening the oven door and continue to bake for another 45 minutes, or until a knife inserted in the center of the pie comes out clean. Cool to room temperature. Cut into eight even portions and serve one piece as a standard serving.

Yields 1 9-inch pie—8 servings

Nutritive Values Per Serving

CAL	CARBS (g)	PRO (g)	TOTAL FAT (g)	SAT. FAT (g)	CHOL (mg)	FIBER (g)	NA (mg)
184	24	5	8	1.3	1	1.4	389

Food exchanges per serving: 1 starch, ²/₃ skim milk, 1 fat.
Low-sodium diets: Omit salt. Use low-sodium variation of the pie crust.
Sugar content per serving: .8 teaspoon.

Pumpkin Scotch Pie

This recipe is from Dorothea Odekirk of Fayette, Iowa. Dorothea and I both belong to the Fayette County Branch of the American Association of University Women and she gave me this recipe after I had talked about my new book one night at a meeting.

FILLING
1 2¹/₈-ounce package sugar-free butterscotch pudding
1³/₄ cups skim milk

1 cup precooked canned pumpkin
¼ cup Sugar Twin Brown Sugar
   Replacement
1 teaspoon pumpkin pie spice

1 9-inch Graham Cracker Crust (see Index)
Whipped Topping (see Index)

Empty package of pudding mix into small saucepan. Add milk gradually. Cook and stir over moderate heat until pudding comes to a boil. Remove from heat. Add pumpkin, sweetener, and spice to cooked pudding. Mix well.

Pour filling into prepared crust. Refrigerate until served. Cut into eight equal portions and serve one portion per serving. Garnish with Whipped Topping just before pie is served, if desired (2 tablespoons topping is free).

Yields 1 9-inch pie—8 servings

Nutritive Values Per Serving

CAL	CARBS (g)	PRO (g)	TOTAL FAT (g)	SAT. FAT (g)	CHOL (mg)	FIBER (g)	NA (mg)
124	17	3	5	1	1	.7	292

Food exchanges per serving: 1 starch, 1 fat.
Low-sodium diets: Use low-sodium variation of the pie crust.
Sugar content per serving: .8 teaspoon in crust.

Strawberry Chiffon Pie

This pie is as good as it looks. You can use different flavors of soft drink mix if you like, with different garnishes.

FILLING
1 cup water
1 envelope Knox Unflavored Gelatine

1 .20-ounce packet Wyler's unsweetened
strawberry flavored soft drink mix or
Kool-Aid unsweetened soft drink mix
8 1-gram packets Equal (aspartame) sugar
substitute
1 recipe Whipped Topping (see Index)
2 tablespoons instant nonfat dry milk

1 9-inch Graham Cracker Crust (see Index)
9 fresh strawberries (optional)

Combine water and gelatin. Let stand for 5 minutes and then heat until gelatin is melted. Add soft drink mix and sweetener to gelatin. Mix well and refrigerate until slightly thickened.

Prepare Whipped Topping while gelatin is thickening. Refrigerate until needed. Add dry milk to thickened gelatin and whip at high speed until creamy and stiff. Remove beater and gently fold Whipped Topping into whipped gelatin.

Spread filling evenly in graham cracker crust. Garnish each serving with a fresh strawberry, placing a fresh strawberry in the center of the pie. Refrigerate until firm. Cut into eight equal pieces and serve one piece per serving.

Yields 1 9-inch pie—8 servings

Nutritive Values Per Serving

CAL	CARBS (g)	PRO (g)	TOTAL FAT (g)	SAT. FAT (g)	CHOL (mg)	FIBER (g)	NA (mg)
120	15	4	5	.9	1	trace	154

Food exchanges per serving: 1 starch, 1 fat.
Low-sodium diets: Use low-sodium variation of the pie crust.
Sugar content per serving: .8 teaspoon in crust.

Whipped Topping

This topping may be spread on top of a pie or used as a garnish for pies, puddings, or gelatins. It should be prepared as close to serving time as possible since it loses volume after a period of time.

> ½ cup instant nonfat dry milk
> ⅓ cup cold water
> 2 tablespoons lemon juice
> 2 tablespoons sugar
> Dry sugar substitute equal to ¼ cup sugar
> (optional)
> ½ teaspoon vanilla

Combine dry milk and water and refrigerate for 30 minutes. Beat at high speed for 4 minutes.

Add lemon juice to whipped milk and beat at high speed for 4 minutes. Stir the sugar and sugar substitute together and add gradually to the whipped milk while it is being beaten. Add vanilla to Whipped Topping and refrigerate until used. Yields 24 servings of 2 tablespoons each.

Yields 3 cups topping—24 servings

Nutritive Values Per Serving

CAL	CARBS (g)	PRO (g)	TOTAL FAT (g)	SAT. FAT (g)	CHOL (mg)	FIBER (g)	NA (mg)
10	2	1	trace	0	trace	0	8

Food exchanges per serving: 2 tablespoons may be considered free. ⅓ cup is 1 vegetable exchange.
Low-sodium diets: May be used as written.
Sugar content per serving: .3 teaspoon.

17

Cakes

Many persons with diabetes long for the cakes and cookies that we used to enjoy so much. In fact, when I asked my friends and others with diabetes what recipes they would like to see in this book, most of them started out with, "Some really good cakes and cookies." That is a tough request for a diabetic cookbook and gets even tougher when the recipes also need to be tasty and suitable for a low-cholesterol diet.

We all know that we can't have cake and cookies for every meal, because we need to save the exchanges for more important foods—but there are times such as birthdays when you really would like to be able to eat a piece of cake along with everyone else. Another time I like to have diabetic cake or cookies on hand is when we have unexpected guests and I want to offer them cake or cookies along with their coffee or tea. I also have learned to slip a couple of my diabetic cookies in my purse (well-wrapped, of course) and take them along with me when we are invited out for afternoon coffee. Hostesses don't seem to mind so much if I eat my own cookies as long as I have something.

Let's face it. We will probably never get a really fine-textured cake suitable for a diabetic diet because the percentage of sugar in a cake is very important to the texture of the cake. However, we can get an acceptable cake if we use ingredients at room temperature and follow the directions for making the cake very carefully, using the recipes that follow.

A cake suitable for a low-cholesterol diet needs to avoid whole eggs, butter, cream, lard, and whole milk. Therefore, a cake suitable for a low-cholesterol diabetic diet needs to be made with margarine or oil, egg whites or liquid egg substitute, fat-free milk, and last but not least, very little sugar or other sweetener.

I have managed to develop some cakes suitable for the low-cholesterol diabetic diet using approved ingredients which I think you will like. I found that cocoa used with buttermilk and baking soda gives a good texture. I also managed to develop several other good cakes, including some with syrup or molasses. I used the regular corn syrup, but you can use fructose syrup if you like sweeter cakes. I did use a little sugar or syrup, which I counted when I analyzed the recipes. You might discuss the use of either with your doctor before preparing these recipes, but since both are part of the carbohydrate allowance, most doctors feel that it is permissible to use them.

Instant nonfat dry milk and dry buttermilk are used in these recipes because I find them so convenient. They are generally lower in cost than the fresh skim milk or buttermilk made with skim milk and they can be kept unopened on the shelf or in the refrigerator after they are opened, if you like, for a fairly long period of time. It isn't all that easy in our area to get fresh buttermilk made with skim milk and for that reason also I like to keep the powdered buttermilk on hand. It is nationally available so if your store doesn't carry it, I'm sure they can get it for you.

Technique, or the way you mix the cake, is very important when you are making a cake, and even more so when you are working with very little sugar. Because of the high proportion of flour to sugar, it is easy to mix the flour too much, which develops the gluten in the flour. That is all to the good when you are making bread, but can be a disaster when you are making a cake. When the gluten in the cake has been developed too much, you get a very tough cake with large air holes. Therefore, it is important to cream the fat and the little bit of sugar very well—but to add the flour mixture very carefully and mix it only as much as is absolutely necessary.

I hope that you will use these recipes as a basis for your own needs. Add fruit to them for a shortcake, garnish them with a couple of tablespoons of Whipped Topping (see Index), layer them with diabetic jelly between the layers, and sprinkle them with

Sugar Twin instead of powdered sugar—or add various flavorings to the cakes to vary their flavor. They can be the basis for lots of interesting desserts.

I have used a minimum of sugar substitute in these recipes because that is how we prefer them. If you want an increased amount, feel free to vary the amount according to your own tastes; it won't affect the final recipe if used within normal bounds. I have also shown the amount according to the sugar equivalents because that is how people tell me they prefer to have recipes written.

Of course, when you are making a low-cholesterol diabetic cake, you need to follow all of the suggestions for a good cake made with the ordinary amount of sugar:

1. Have all ingredients at room temperature unless the directions state otherwise. This is particularly important for the liquid egg substitute. Don't use it right from the refrigerator in a cake or cookies.

2. Use stick margarine unless the recipe specifies soft margarine.

3. Always read the recipe thoroughly before you start to prepare it to be sure that you understand it and that you have all of the ingredients on hand. I like to get out all of the ingredients and prepare the pans before I start mixing the cake. These recipes also presume that the oven will be preheated, so I generally start the oven when I start to mix the cake.

4. Always use regulation-size measuring cups and spoons and bake cakes in the size pan specified in the recipe. An otherwise good cake can be ruined if baked in the wrong size pan. If you want to bake a cake in a smaller pan, fill the pan two-thirds full of batter and bake any remaining batter as cupcakes.

5. Don't sift the flour unless the recipe directs you to do so. Sifting changes the amount of flour in a cup. I never sift flour. I always combine the ingredients and stir them together. This is much simpler and yields the same results.

6. Follow the recipe exactly the first time. Then you can change it if you like after you are sure that you want to make a change in it. Don't forget that if you add nuts or raisins or other goodies to a recipe, you need to count those added ingredients in your diet.

7. Use margarine, not oil, to grease your pans. I like to use the margarine wrapper with a little bit of the margarine left on it to grease the pan for a cake that includes margarine as an ingredient.

8. These cakes were all tested in metal pans. If you use a glass baking dish, decrease the baking temperature 25°F.

9. When you want to defrost a cake that has been frozen, it should be unwrapped and placed in a refrigerator until it is defrosted. If you try to defrost it at room temperature in the wrappings it will get sticky, and if you defrost it unwrapped at room temperature it will collect moisture and be soggy. I always had a rough time trying to get a cake defrosted without ruining it until Thelma Richburg of Columbia, South Carolina, told me how to do it successfully, and it really works this way. She is the mother of Olivia Sniffin, one of my favorite cousins-in-law. Mrs. Richburg bakes a lot of cakes and decorates them for special occasions and really knows how to bake good cakes—and how to take care of them after they are baked.

Chocolate Cake

---

³/₄ cup (1¹/₂ sticks) margarine at room
   temperature
¹/₄ cup sugar
¹/₂ cup liquid egg substitute at room
   temperature
Dry sugar substitute equal to ¹/₃ cup sugar
2 teaspoons vanilla
2 cups cake flour
2 teaspoons baking powder
¹/₄ cup instant nonfat dry milk
¹/₃ cup cocoa
1 cup water at room temperature

Cream together margarine and sugar at medium speed until light and fluffy. Add egg substitute, sweetener, and vanilla to creamed mixture and beat at medium speed for ¹/₂ minute.

Stir together flour, baking powder, dry milk, and cocoa to blend.

Add 1 cup water to creamed mixture along with flour mixture and mix at medium speed only until smooth. Spread evenly in a 9-inch square pan that has been greased with margarine. Bake at 350°F for 30–35 minutes, or until a cake tester comes out clean and the cake pulls away from the sides of the pan. Cool to room temperature and cut 4 × 4 to yield 16 equal servings.

Yields 1 cake—16 servings

Nutritive Values Per Serving

CAL	CARBS (g)	PRO (g)	TOTAL FAT (g)	SAT. FAT (g)	CHOL (mg)	FIBER (g)	NA (mg)
154	16	3	9	1.6	trace	.5	183

Food exchanges per serving: 1 starch, 2 fat.
Low-sodium diets: Use salt-free margarine and low-sodium baking powder.
Sugar content per serving: .8 teaspoon.

Cocoa Cake

This recipe is based on one from Lois Erickson.

> ½ cup cocoa
> ½ cup boiling water
> ¾ cup (1½ sticks) margarine at room
>   temperature
> Dry sugar substitute equal to ½ cup sugar
> 2 teaspoons vanilla
> 3 large egg whites at room temperature
> ½ teaspoon cream of tartar
> ⅓ cup sugar
> 2½ cups cake flour
> 1 teaspoon baking soda
> 2 teaspoons baking powder
> ¼ teaspoon salt
> ½ teaspoon cinnamon
> 1 cup cool water

Mix together cocoa and boiling water to blend and set aside to cool to room temperature. Cream margarine at medium speed until light and fluffy. Add sweetener and vanilla to creamed margarine, along with cooled cocoa mixture. Mix at medium speed until well blended.

Beat egg whites at medium speed until foamy. Add cream of tartar and beat at high speed, gradually adding sugar, to form a meringue. Set aside for later use. Stir together flour, soda, baking powder, salt, and cinnamon to blend well.

Add 1 cup water to creamed mixture along with flour mixture. Beat at medium speed for 1–2 minutes or until well blended. Stir batter carefully into the meringue. Spread half of the batter evenly in each of two 9-inch cake layer pans that have been greased with margarine and lined on the bottom with wax paper. Bake at 350°F for 30–35 minutes, or until a cake tester comes out clean from the center of the cake and the cake pulls away from the sides of the pan. Turn cakes out onto a rack, remove the paper, and cool to room temperature.

Put diabetic jelly between the cake layers and frost at the last minute with Fluffy Frosting (see Index). Cut cake into 16 equal servings.

Yields 1 2-layer cake—16 servings

Nutritive Values Per Serving

CAL	CARBS (g)	PRO (g)	TOTAL FAT (g)	SAT. FAT (g)	CHOL (mg)	FIBER (g)	NA (mg)
170	19	3	10	1.7	0	.8	291

Food exchanges per serving: 1 starch, 1 vegetable, 2 fat.
Low-sodium diets: Omit salt. Use salt-free margarine and low-sodium baking powder.
Sugar content per serving: 1 teaspoon.

Banana Bran Cake

Please don't avoid this cake because there is bran in it. It is delicious, as well as good for you, and I think you'll like it.

> **1 cup All Bran, Bran Buds, or 100% Bran**
> **1/3 cup vegetable oil**
> **1/2 cup egg whites or liquid egg substitute**
> **3/4 cup water**
> **1 teaspoon vanilla**
> **1 teaspoon banana flavoring**
> **1 1/4 cups all-purpose flour**
> **1/4 cup sugar**
> **2 tablespoons dry buttermilk**
> **1 teaspoon baking soda**
> **Dry sugar substitute equal to 1/2 cup sugar**
> **2 medium-size ripe bananas**

Place bran, oil, egg whites or liquid egg substitute, water, and flavorings in mixer bowl and mix at low speed for 30 seconds. Let the bran mixture stand for 30–45 minutes. (This timing is very important.)

Stir flour, sugar, dry buttermilk, soda, and sugar substitute together to blend well and set aside.

At the end of 30–45 minutes, slice the bananas into the bran mixture and mix at medium speed until the bananas are dissolved and the mixture is creamy. Add the flour mixture and mix to blend. Spread the batter evenly in a 9-inch-square cake pan that has been greased with margarine or sprayed with cooking spray and bake at 350°F for 25–30 minutes, or until the cake pulls away from the sides of the pan and a cake tester comes out clean from the center of the cake. Cool to room temperature and cut 3 × 4 to yield 12 servings.

Yields 1 cake—12 servings

Nutritive Values Per Serving

CAL	CARBS (g)	PRO (g)	TOTAL FAT (g)	SAT. FAT (g)	CHOL (mg)	FIBER (g)	NA (mg)
166	24	4	7	.9	.9	2.3	208

Food exchanges per serving: 1½ starch, 1 fat.
Low-sodium diets: May be used as written.
Sugar content per serving: 1 teaspoon.

Raisin Cake

This cake from Ruth Schoephoerster of Oelwein, Iowa, tastes like the fruitcake my mother used to make when I was a child.

1 cup raisins
Boiling water as necessary
Dry sugar substitute equal to ¾ cup sugar
3 large egg whites
½ cup oil
1½ teaspoons vanilla
1 cup unsweetened applesauce
2 cups all-purpose flour
1 teaspoon baking soda
1 teaspoon baking powder
1¼ teaspoons cinnamon

¹/₂ **teaspoon nutmeg**
¹/₂ **teaspoon salt**

Cover raisins with water. Let stand 5 minutes. Drain well and place the raisins in a mixer bowl. Discard the liquid. Add sweetener, egg whites, oil, vanilla, and applesauce to raisins and mix at medium speed for a few seconds to blend.

Blend remaining dry ingredients well and add to raisin mixture. Mix at medium speed to blend. Spread evenly in a 9" × 13" cake pan that has been greased with margarine. Bake at 350°F for 35–40 minutes, or until well browned and the cake has drawn away from the sides of the pan. Cut 4 × 5 to yield 20 pieces. Serve one piece per serving.

Yields 1 cake—20 servings

Nutritive Values Per Serving

CAL	CARBS (g)	PRO (g)	TOTAL FAT (g)	SAT. FAT (g)	CHOL (mg)	FIBER (g)	NA (mg)
127	17	2	6	.8	0	.9	154

Food exchanges per serving: 1 starch, 1 fat.
Low-sodium diets: Omit salt. Use low-sodium baking powder.
Sugar content per serving: None.

Devil's Food Cake

¹/₂ **cup cocoa**
¹/₂ **cup boiling water**
2 **cups cake flour**
¹/₂ **teaspoon baking soda**
1¹/₂ **teaspoons baking powder**
¹/₈ **teaspoon salt**
¹/₃ **cup sugar**
³/₄ **cup liquid egg substitute at room**
    temperature
Dry sugar substitute equal to ³/₄ cup sugar
1 **teaspoon vanilla**

**½ cup (1 stick) margarine at room
    temperature**

Stir together cocoa and boiling water until smooth. Set aside to
cool to room temperature.

Place flour, soda, baking powder, salt, and sugar in mixer
bowl and mix at low speed about 1 minute to blend.

Add egg substitute, sweetener, and vanilla to cocoa mixture
and mix well.

Add margarine to dry ingredients along with cocoa mixture
and mix at medium speed about 1 minute or until well blended.
Pour into a 9-inch square (for thicker cake) or 9" × 13" pan
greased with margarine. Bake at 350°F for about 30 minutes, or
until a cake tester comes out clean and the cake pulls away from
the sides of the pan. Cool in the pan and cut 6 × 3 to yield 18
pieces. Serve cold with a tablespoon of Whipped Topping (see
Index) or warm with some Chocolate Sauce (see Index). Allow one
piece per serving.

Yields 1 cake—18 servings

Nutritive Values Per Serving

CAL	CARBS (g)	PRO (g)	TOTAL FAT (g)	SAT. FAT (g)	CHOL (mg)	FIBER (g)	NA (mg)
117	15	3	6	1	0	.7	170

Food exchanges per serving: 1 starch, 1 fat.
Low-sodium diets: Omit salt. Use low-sodium baking powder and salt-free
    margarine.
Sugar content per serving: .9 teaspoon.

Spice Cupcakes

2 cups cake flour
⅓ cup brown sugar
1 teaspoon cinnamon
1½ teaspoons baking powder
½ cup water at room temperature
Dry sugar substitute equal to ⅓ cup sugar

¹/₂ cup liquid egg substitute at room
 temperature
¹/₃ cup vegetable oil
2 teaspoons vanilla

Place flour, sugar, cinnamon, and baking powder in mixer bowl and mix at low speed to blend well.

Mix together ¹/₂ cup water, sweetener, egg substitute, oil, and vanilla with a fork. Add to flour mixture and mix with a spoon only until well blended. Grease nine muffin tins with margarine or line with paper. Fill muffin tins about half full and bake at 375°F for 20–25 minutes, or until well browned. Serve one cupcake per serving.

Yields 9 cupcakes—9 servings

Nutritive Values Per Serving

CAL	CARBS (g)	PRO (g)	TOTAL FAT (g)	SAT. FAT (g)	CHOL (mg)	FIBER (g)	NA (mg)
207	28	3	9	1.2	0	0	117

Food exchanges per serving: 1 starch, 1 other carbohydrate, 1 fat.
Low-sodium diets: Use low-sodium baking powder.
Sugar content per serving: 1.8 teaspoon.

Wacky Cupcakes

My sister has been making this cake ever since she was a little girl. The original recipe said to put the dry ingredients in the pan and then add the rest and mix it in the pan you bake it in, but I like this way better.

1¹/₂ cups cake flour
¹/₄ cup sugar
¹/₄ cup cocoa
1 teaspoon baking soda
¹/₂ teaspoon salt
1 cup water at room temperature

Dry sugar substitute equal to ½ cup sugar
1 tablespoon vinegar
2 teaspoons vanilla
½ cup vegetable oil

Place flour, sugar, cocoa, soda, and salt in mixer bowl and mix at low speed to blend.

Beat together remaining ingredients with a fork to blend. Add all at once to dry ingredients and beat at medium speed until smooth. Paper-line 12 muffin tins or grease with margarine and flour. Fill muffin tins about half full and bake at 350°F for about 30 minutes, or until a cake tester comes out clean from the center of the cupcake. Serve one cupcake per serving.

Yields 12 cupcakes—12 servings

Nutritive Values Per Serving

CAL	CARBS (g)	PRO (g)	TOTAL FAT (g)	SAT. FAT (g)	CHOL (mg)	FIBER (g)	NA (mg)
153	16	2	10	1.3	0	.5	197

Food exchanges per serving: 1 starch, 2 fat.
Low-sodium diets: Omit salt.
Sugar content per serving: 1 teaspoon.

White Cake

This recipe is based on one from Margaret Foxwell of Elgin, Iowa. It has the texture of a firm European cake.

½ cup (1 stick) margarine at room
    temperature
¼ cup white corn syrup
Dry sugar substitute equal to ⅓ cup sugar
2 teaspoons vanilla
3 large egg whites at room temperature
2 cups cake flour
1 tablespoon baking powder
2 tablespoons instant nonfat dry milk
½ cup water at room temperature

Beat margarine, corn syrup, sweetener, vanilla, and egg whites at medium speed about 1 minute or until blended.

Stir together flour, baking powder, and dry milk until well blended.

Add flour mixture and ½ cup water to creamed mixture and stir with a large spoon until well mixed. Do not overbeat. Spread evenly in a 9-inch square pan that has been greased with margarine, and bake at 350°F for 30–35 minutes or until lightly browned and it pulls away from the sides of the pan. Cool and cut 4 × 4 into 16 equal servings.

Yields 1 cake—16 servings

Nutritive Values Per Serving

CAL	CARBS (g)	PRO (g)	TOTAL FAT (g)	SAT. FAT (g)	CHOL (mg)	FIBER (g)	NA (mg)
124	15	2	6	1	trace	0	181

Food exchanges per serving: 1 starch, 1 fat.
Low-sodium diets: Use salt-free margarine and low-sodium baking powder.
Sugar content per serving: .8 teaspoon.

Yellow Cake

2 cups cake flour
½ teaspoon baking soda
1½ teaspoons baking powder
½ cup sugar
3 tablespoons dry buttermilk
¾ cup water at room temperature
⅓ cup vegetable oil
Dry sugar substitute equal to ¼ cup sugar
2 teaspoons vanilla
½ cup liquid egg substitute at room
    temperature
¼ cup (½ stick) margarine at room
    temperature

Place dry ingredients in mixer bowl and mix at low speed until they are blended.

Combine ³⁄₄ cup water, oil, sweetener, vanilla, and egg substitute and mix with a fork to blend. Add margarine to flour mixture along with liquid mixture and mix with a spoon only until well blended. Spread evenly in a 9-inch square pan that has been greased with margarine. Bake 30–35 minutes at 375°F, or until a cake tester comes out clean and the cake pulls away from the sides of the pan. Cool to room temperature and cut 4 × 4 to yield 16 equal servings.

Yields 1 cake—16 servings

Nutritive Values Per Serving

CAL	CARBS (g)	PRO (g)	TOTAL FAT (g)	SAT. FAT (g)	CHOL (mg)	FIBER (g)	NA (mg)
144	16	2	8	1	1	0	141

Food exchanges per serving: 1 starch, 1¹⁄₂ fat.
Low-sodium diets: Use low-sodium baking powder and salt-free margarine.
Sugar content per serving: 1 teaspoon.

Butter Cream Frosting

You'll be surprised how good this frosting tastes. The recipe was developed by my friend Patsy Spies, who wanted it as a special treat for her grandmother who was diabetic.

> ¹⁄₂ cup water
> 2 tablespoons instant nonfat dry milk
> 2¹⁄₂ tablespoons all-purpose flour
> ¹⁄₂ cup (1 stick) margarine at room
>   temperature
> 10 1-gram packets Equal sugar substitute
> ¹⁄₂ teaspoon vanilla, lemon, almond, or
>   other flavoring

Combine water, dry milk, and flour and stir until smooth. Cook, stirring constantly, over medium heat until thick and smooth, or cook in a microwave oven on high for 2 minutes, stirring every 30 seconds. Place container in cool water and stir until cool. Set aside. Cream margarine and sugar substitute together until light and fluffy. Add cooled sauce 1 tablespoon at a time while beating at medium speed. Add vanilla or other flavoring and beat at high speed until light and fluffy. Refrigerate until used. Use 1 tablespoon per portion (¾ cup for a 12-portion cake or 1 cup for a 16-portion cake). Return to room temperature before spreading the frosting on a cool cake.

Yields 1¼ cups—20 servings

Nutritive Values Per Serving

CAL	CARBS (g)	PRO (g)	TOTAL FAT (g)	SAT. FAT (g)	CHOL (mg)	FIBER (g)	NA (mg)
48	1	1	5	.7	trace	trace	56

Food exchanges per serving: 1 fat.
Low-sodium diets: Use salt-free margarine.
Sugar content per serving: None.

Fluffy Frosting

This recipe from the makers of Sweet'n Low reminds me of the seven-minute frosting my mother used to make. You can change the frosting easily by adding a couple of drops of food coloring and some flavoring, such as 2 drops of red coloring and some peppermint flavoring.

> ½ cup sugar
> 2 tablespoons water
> 2 packets Sweet'n Low
> 2 large egg whites
> ¼ teaspoon cream of tartar
> ½ teaspoon vanilla

Combine sugar, water, Sweet'n Low, egg whites, and cream of tartar in top of a double boiler and beat at high speed for 1 minute. Set over simmering water in the bottom of the double boiler. Continue to beat at high speed for 4–5 minutes or until soft peaks form. Remove from heat.

Add vanilla to frosting and continue beating at high speed 1–2 minutes or until thick enough to spread on a cooled cake. Use about 3 tablespoons per portion if frosting individually; or use entire recipe to frost a two-layer cake or a 9-inch square cake, both of which would then be cut into 16 equal servings.

Yields about 3 cups—16 servings

Nutritive Values Per Serving

CAL	CARBS (g)	PRO (g)	TOTAL FAT (g)	SAT. FAT (g)	CHOL (mg)	FIBER (g)	NA (mg)
27	7	trace	0	0	0	0	7

Food exchanges per serving: 1 vegetable.
Low-sodium diets: May be used as written.
Sugar content per serving: 1.5 teaspoon.

Lemon Sauce

This sauce adds a lot to a plain or spice cake—either warm or at room temperature.

> 2 cups water
> 2 tablespoons cornstarch
> ⅛ teaspoon salt
> 2 tablespoons margarine
> 2 tablespoons lemon juice
> Grated rind of 1 lemon
> 1 drop yellow food coloring
> 8 1-gram packets Equal (aspartame) sugar
>   substitute

Combine water, cornstarch, and salt and stir until smooth in a small saucepan. Cook and stir over moderate heat until thickened and clear and then continue to simmer, stirring constantly, for another 2 minutes. Remove from heat.

Add remaining ingredients to sauce and stir lightly to mix well. Serve warm, if possible, over cake or pudding. Serve ¼ cup per serving.

Yields 2 cups—8 servings

Nutritive Values Per Serving

CAL	CARBS (g)	PRO (g)	TOTAL FAT (g)	SAT. FAT (g)	CHOL (mg)	FIBER (g)	NA (mg)
38	3	1	3	.5	0	trace	69

Food exchanges per serving: ½ fat, ½ vegetable.
Low-sodium diets: Omit salt.
Sugar content per serving: None.

Chocolate Sauce

This is good on ice milk or as a topping for cake or pudding.

> 3 tablespoons cocoa
> 4 teaspoons cornstarch
> ⅓ cup instant nonfat dry milk
> ⅛ teaspoon salt
> 1½ cups water
> 1 tablespoon margarine
> 2 teaspoons vanilla
> 10 1-gram packets Equal (aspartame)
>   sugar substitute

Stir together cocoa, cornstarch, dry milk, and salt to blend in a small saucepan. Stir water into dry mixture until smooth. Add margarine and cook and stir over low heat. Bring to a boil and simmer for 2 minutes, stirring constantly. Remove from heat.

Add vanilla and sweetener to sauce. Stir lightly to mix. Pour into a glass jar and refrigerate until used. Return to room temperature before serving over ice cream, or it may be heated again to serve on cake or pudding. Serve 2 tablespoons per serving.

Yields 1½ cups—12 servings

Nutritive Values Per Serving

CAL	CARBS (g)	PRO (g)	TOTAL FAT (g)	SAT. FAT (g)	CHOL (mg)	FIBER (g)	NA (mg)
28	3	1	1	trace	trace	trace	45

Food exchanges per serving: ½ vegetable.
Low-sodium diets: Omit salt.
Sugar content per serving: None.

18

Cookies

A friend of mine commented when I started this book that she would like me to include some crisp cookies. She said that she was so tired of the soft cookies, which were all she knew how to make. I've never been too fond of those, either, so I tried to work on some rather crisp cookies. Sugar helps, but since we can't have much of that we need something else to give us that crisp texture. Egg whites also help, so I used those in several recipes; and believe it or not, just letting the cookies sit on a tray at room temperature for a couple of days does the trick. The buttermilk cookies in this chapter become much more crisp after you let them stay out for a couple of days.

I like to have cookies on hand for special occasions and therefore I generally try to keep some cookies in the freezer. All of the cookies in this chapter freeze well. If I'm having company and they don't need diabetic cookies, I always include some of my own cookies on the tray so I can have a cookie or two without comment—although it is amazing how many people tell me they would like to cut down on sugar and choose to eat my cookies instead of the ones with lots of sugar and fat in them.

Since our cookies need to be low cholesterol as well as low carbohydrate, we need to make them without butter, cream, whole milk, egg yolks, lard, chocolate, and coconut. I'm glad we can have cocoa, nuts, raisins, applesauce, and other fruits, even if we do have to count them, because we can use all of those to make our cookies more interesting. Cookies can't be frosted with powdered sugar frosting or rolled in powdered sugar, but they can be rolled in granular sugar substitute, which works rather well.

Of course, while we are making our diabetic low-cholesterol cookies, we still need to observe the fundamentals of good cookie-making. I have found that following these guidelines helps me to have better cookies:

1. Read the recipe to be sure you understand it before you start. Get out all of the ingredients and any equipment you will need to make the cookies before you start mixing any ingredients. I generally start preheating the oven after I am sure I have everything ready to go, since I need to preheat my oven for 10 minutes and that is about the length of time it takes me to mix up a batch of cookies.

2. Use good quality ingredients and don't substitute ingredients without regard to the proper substitution rates.

3. Don't sift flour unless the recipe tells you to do so because sifted and unsifted flours measure differently. Flour is sifted to mix it with other ingredients and to make it lighter, and both of these are accomplished when it is stirred.

4. Always use regulation measuring cups and spoons. Cakes and cookies are delicately balanced formulas and won't respond well to irregular measurements.

5. It is important that ingredients be at room temperature if the recipe so indicates. This is especially important for liquid egg substitute and margarine.

6. All cookies on the same baking sheet should be the same size and thickness so they will bake evenly. If there is not enough dough for a full pan of cookies, bake them on a smaller pan or in the center of the larger pan you have been using.

7. Cookies should be placed on a cool pan before they are put in the oven. A hot pan will start them baking before they go in the oven and will generally result in imperfectly baked cookies. Cookies should also be loosened from hot pans and

put on a wire rack to cool so they won't continue baking after they are removed from the oven.

8. Cookies should be defrosted in the container in which they were frozen or in another airtight container so they don't pick up moisture from the air, which softens them. If they are to be defrosted on a plate, the plate should be refrigerated so they can defrost at the temperature in the refrigerator and not at room temperature.

Chocolate Date Cookies

You can substitute raisins for the dates, if you like, without changing the exchange values, but we like dates for a change.

**¹/₂ cup (1 stick) margarine at room
temperature**
¹/₃ cup sugar
¹/₃ cup brown sugar
¹/₂ cup egg whites or liquid egg substitute
2 teaspoons vanilla
2¹/₄ cups all-purpose flour
¹/₃ cup cocoa
1 teaspoon baking powder
Sugar substitute equal to ¹/₂ cup sugar
³/₄ cup chopped pitted dates
¹/₃ cup water at room temperature

Cream together margarine and sugars at medium speed until light and fluffy. Add egg whites or liquid egg substitute and vanilla and mix until smooth. Stir flour, cocoa, baking powder, sugar substitute, and dates together to blend and add with the water to the creamed mixture. Mix only until blended and then drop by 1¹/₂ tablespoonfuls (level No. 40 dipper) onto cookie sheets that have been lined with aluminum foil or sprayed with cooking spray.

Press down lightly with your fingers or the back of a spoon dipped in water. Bake at 350°F for 12–15 minutes or until the cookie springs back when touched in the center. Remove from the hot cookie sheets onto a wire rack and cool to room temperature. Serve one cookie per serving.

Yields 2¹/₂ dozen cookies—30 servings

Nutritive Values Per Serving

CAL	CARBS (g)	PRO (g)	TOTAL FAT (g)	SAT. FAT (g)	CHOL (mg)	FIBER (g)	NA (mg)
98	16	2	3	.6	0	.8	72

Food exchanges per serving: 1 starch, ¹/₂ fat.
Low-sodium diets: Use salt-free margarine and low-sodium baking powder.
Sugar content per serving: 1.1 teaspoons.

Chocolate Bars

I'm a chocoholic so you know I tried very hard to develop a recipe for chocolate bars that I could eat. We like these best made with the black walnuts that grow so abundantly in this area, but they are also good with pecans or other types of nuts.

> ¹/₂ **cup cocoa**
> ¹/₃ **cup boiling water**
> **2 cups all-purpose flour**
> **1 teaspoon baking soda**
> ¹/₂ **teaspoon salt**
> **4 large egg whites at room temperature**
> **2 teaspoons vanilla**
> **Liquid sugar substitute equal to ¹/₂ cup sugar**
> ¹/₂ **cup white corn syrup**
> **1 cup (2 sticks) margarine at room temperature**
> **1 cup chopped nuts**

Mix together cocoa and boiling water with a teaspoon until smooth and set aside to cool to room temperature. Place flour, soda, and salt in mixer bowl and mix at low speed about 1 minute to blend well. Add egg whites, vanilla, sugar substitute, and corn syrup to cocoa mixture and mix with a spoon to blend. Add margarine to flour mixture along with cocoa mixture and mix at medium speed about 1 minute or until well blended. Do not overmix the dough.

Add nuts to dough. Spread dough evenly (this is very important) in an 11" × 15" jelly roll pan that has been greased with margarine or sprayed with cooking spray. Bake at 350°F for about 20 minutes, or until the bars start to pull away from the sides of the pan. Cool to room temperature and cut 4 × 6 to yield 24 squares. Serve one square per serving.

Yields 2 dozen squares—24 servings

Nutritive Values Per Serving

CAL	CARBS (g)	PRO (g)	TOTAL FAT (g)	SAT. FAT (g)	CHOL (mg)	FIBER (g)	NA (mg)
167	15	3	11	1.7	0	1	208

Food exchanges per serving: 1 starch, 2 fat.
Low-sodium diets: Omit salt. Use salt-free margarine and unsalted nuts.
Sugar content per serving: 1 teaspoon.

Chocolate Balls

This cookie, based on a recipe from Frances Nielsen, is one of my sister Shirley's favorites.

> ½ cup (1 stick) margarine at room
>   temperature
> 2 tablespoons sugar
> 2 teaspoons vanilla
> Liquid sugar substitute equal to ⅓ cup
>   sugar
> 1¼ cups all-purpose flour

3 tablespoons cocoa
½ teaspoon salt
¼ cup chopped nuts
2 tablespoons raisins
Sprinkle Sweet granulated sugar substitute
   as necessary

Cream together margarine and sugar until light and fluffy. Add vanilla and sugar substitute to creamed mixture. Beat at medium speed for ½ minute. Stir together flour, cocoa, and salt to blend. Add to creamed mixture and mix at low speed about 1 minute or until blended.

Add nuts and raisins to dough. Mix lightly. Shape into balls using 1 tablespoonful (level No. 60 dipper) of dough per ball. Place balls on a cookie sheet that has been lined with aluminum foil or sprayed with cooking spray. Bake at 325°F for 20–25 minutes or until slightly firm. Remove from oven and cool slightly.

Roll lukewarm balls in Sprinkle Sweet. Cool to room temperature, and serve two balls per serving.

Variation:
CHOCOLATE MINT BALLS

Add ½ teaspoon peppermint flavoring along with 1 teaspoon vanilla instead of the 2 teaspoons vanilla.

Yields 20 cookies—10 servings

Nutritive Values Per Serving

CAL	CARBS (g)	PRO (g)	TOTAL FAT (g)	SAT. FAT (g)	CHOL (mg)	FIBER (g)	NA (mg)
179	18	3	11	1.8	0	1.1	218

Food exchanges per serving: 1 starch, 2 fat.
Low-sodium diets: Omit salt. Use salt-free margarine and unsalted nuts.
Sugar content per serving: .6 teaspoon.

Chocolate Raisin Nut Cookies

This cookie has a soft cakelike texture that many people enjoy.

2 cups all-purpose flour
1/2 cup sugar
1/2 cup brown sugar
1/3 cup cocoa
1 teaspoon baking soda
1/2 teaspoon salt
1/2 cup vegetable oil
1/2 cup egg whites or liquid egg substitute
2 tablespoons water
2 teaspoons vanilla
1/2 cup chopped walnuts
1/4 cup raisins

Place flour, sugars, cocoa, soda, and salt in mixer bowl and mix at low speed to blend well. Add oil, egg whites or egg substitute, water, and vanilla and mix at medium speed until blended. Add nuts and raisins and drop by 1 1/2 tablespoonfuls (level No. 40 dipper) onto cookie sheets that have been sprayed with cooking spray or lined with aluminum foil. Bake at 350°F for 10–12 minutes or until firm. Remove to wire racks to cool to room temperature. These cookies should not be baked too long since they will get too hard if overbaked. Serve one cookie per serving.

Yields 2 1/3 dozen cookies—28 servings

Nutritive Values Per Serving

CAL	CARBS (g)	PRO (g)	TOTAL FAT (g)	SAT. FAT (g)	CHOL (mg)	FIBER (g)	NA (mg)
119	16	2	6	.7	0	.7	94

Food exchanges per serving: 1 starch, 1 fat.
Low-sodium diets: Omit salt.
Sugar content per serving: 1.7 teaspoons.

Chocolate Chip Cookies

1 cup (2 sticks) margarine at room
   temperature
1/4 cup sugar
3/4 cup Sugar Twin Brown Sugar
   Replacement
3 large egg whites at room temperature
1 tablespoon vanilla
2 cups all-purpose flour
1 teaspoon baking soda
1/4 teaspoon salt
1/4 cup water at room temperature
1/2 cup mini semisweet chocolate chips

Cream margarine, sugar, and sugar substitute at medium speed
until light and fluffy. Add egg whites and vanilla to creamed mixture and beat at medium speed for 1 minute.

Stir together flour, soda, and salt to blend well. Add 1/4 cup
water to creamed mixture along with the flour mixture and mix
at medium speed for 1 minute or until smooth.

Add chocolate chips to dough and mix lightly. Drop by 1
tablespoonful (level no. 60 dipper) onto cookie sheets that have
been lined with aluminum foil or sprayed with cooking spray.
Press down lightly with fingers dipped in cold water to form a
circle about 2 inches across. Bake at 375°F for about 12 minutes
or until browned. (The cookies won't be crisp unless they are
browned.) Remove cookies from hot cookie sheets to wire racks
to cool to room temperature. Allow two cookies per serving.

Variation:
CHOCOLATE CHIP BARS

Instead of dropping dough onto cookie sheets, spread dough
evenly in a jelly roll pan (11″ × 15″) that has been greased with
margarine or sprayed with cooking spray. Bake at 375°F for 20–25
minutes, or until lightly browned and the bars pull away from the

sides of the pan. Cool to room temperature and cut 9 × 4 to yield 36 bars. Serve two bars per serving.

Yields 3 dozen cookies—18 servings

Nutritive Values Per Serving

CAL	CARBS (g)	PRO (g)	TOTAL FAT (g)	SAT. FAT (g)	CHOL (mg)	FIBER (g)	NA (mg)
182	18	2	12	2.4	trace	trace	229

Food exchanges per serving: 1 starch, 2 fat (exchanges remain the same for the variation of the basic recipe).
Low-sodium diets: Omit salt. Use salt-free margarine.
Sugar content per serving: .7 teaspoon.

Mocha Cookies

These cookies are a favorite of my friend Jan Franks.

1 tablespoon instant or freeze-dried coffee
¼ cup hot water
1 cup (2 sticks) margarine at room
 temperature
⅔ cup sugar
½ cup egg whites or liquid egg substitute
2 teaspoons vanilla
2½ cups all-purpose flour
⅓ cup cocoa
Sugar substitute equal to ½ cup sugar
1½ teaspoons baking powder
¾ cup raisins

Combine coffee and water. Stir to mix well and set aside.

Cream together margarine and sugar until light and fluffy. Add egg whites or egg substitute and vanilla and mix until smooth. Stir flour, cocoa, sugar substitute, baking powder, and raisins together to blend. Add to creamed mixture along with the coffee mixture and mix at medium speed only until blended. Drop by 1½ tablespoonfuls (level No. 40 dipper) onto a cookie sheet lined with aluminum foil or sprayed with cooking spray.

Press down lightly with your fingers or the back of a spoon dipped in cold water. Bake at 375°F about 12 minutes or until the cookies spring back when touched. Transfer from the hot cookie sheets onto a wire rack and cool to room temperature. Serve one cookie per serving.

Yields 2½ dozen cookies—30 servings

Nutritive Values Per Serving

CAL	CARBS (g)	PRO (g)	TOTAL FAT (g)	SAT. FAT (g)	CHOL (mg)	FIBER (g)	NA (mg)
128	17	2	6	1	0	.8	115

Food exchanges per serving: 1 starch, 1 fat.
Low-sodium diets: Use salt-free margarine and low-sodium baking powder.
Sugar content per serving: 1.1 teaspoons.

Date Graham Cookies

---

1 cup graham flour
½ cup all-purpose flour
3 tablespoons dry buttermilk
½ teaspoon baking soda
½ teaspoon salt
½ cup brown sugar
½ cup Sugar Twin Brown Sugar
**   Replacement**
2 large egg whites at room temperature
¼ cup dark molasses
½ cup (1 stick) margarine at room
**   temperature**
½ cup chopped pitted dates

Place flours, dry buttermilk, soda, salt, brown sugar, and sugar substitute in mixer bowl and mix at low speed for about 1 minute to mix well. Add egg whites, molasses, and margarine to flour mixture and mix at medium speed for about 1 minute or until well blended.

Add dates to dough and mix lightly. Drop by tablespoonfuls (level No. 60 dipper) onto cookie sheets that have been lined with aluminum foil or sprayed with cooking spray. Bake at 375°F for 10–12 minutes, or until lightly browned. Remove from hot cookie sheets onto wire rack to cool to room temperature. Serve one cookie per serving.

Yields 2 dozen cookies—24 servings

Nutritive Values Per Serving

CAL	CARBS (g)	PRO (g)	TOTAL FAT (g)	SAT. FAT (g)	CHOL (mg)	FIBER (g)	NA (mg)
102	16	2	4	1	.7	.9	130

Food exchanges per serving: 1 starch, 1 fat.
Low-sodium diets: Omit salt. Use salt-free margarine.
Sugar content per serving: 1 teaspoon.

Buttermilk Cookies

These cookies are based on a recipe for buttermilk cookies that Vera Wilson made for years. I have always loved them, and she used to save some of them for me whenever she or her daughter Mary made them. I hated to give them up when I developed diabetes, but I feel better about it now that I have developed a cookie suitable for my diet that is almost like the original.

¹/₂ cup (1 stick) margarine at room temperature
¹/₄ cup sugar
2 teaspoons vanilla
Dry sugar substitute equal to ¹/₃ cup sugar
¹/₂ cup liquid egg substitute at room temperature
2 cups all-purpose flour
¹/₂ teaspoon baking soda
¹/₂ teaspoon baking powder
2 tablespoons dry buttermilk
1 to 2 tablespoons water

Cream together margarine and sugar until light and fluffy. Add vanilla, sugar substitute, and egg substitute to creamed mixture and beat at medium speed for 1 minute. Stir together flour, soda, baking powder, and dry buttermilk to blend and add to creamed mixture.

Add to creamed and flour mixture as much of the water as necessary to make a soft dough. While adding, beat at low speed. Roll out on a lightly floured working surface to about ¼ inch thick. Cut with a 3-inch cookie cutter and place on cookie sheets that have been lined with aluminum foil or sprayed with cooking spray. Sprinkle with Cinnamon Shake (see Index) if desired and bake at 350°F for 12–15 minutes or until lightly browned. (The cookies need to be browned on the bottom to develop their best flavor.) Remove from hot cookie sheets to wire rack and cool to room temperature. Serve two cookies to a serving.

Variations:
SPICE COOKIES

Add 1 teaspoon pumpkin pie spice, apple pie spice, or cinnamon along with the flour.

CHOCOLATE COOKIES

Use ¼ cup cocoa and 1¾ cups all-purpose flour instead of the 2 cups all-purpose flour in the basic recipe.

PASTEL COOKIES

Substitute ¼ cup fruit-flavored regular, nondiabetic gelatin for the ¼ cup sugar in the basic recipe.

Yields 30 cookies—15 servings

Nutritive Values Per Serving

CAL	CARBS (g)	PRO (g)	TOTAL FAT (g)	SAT. FAT (g)	CHOL (mg)	FIBER (g)	NA (mg)
138	17	3	6	1	.7	.5	148

Food exchanges per serving: 1 starch, 1 fat (exchanges remain the same for the variations of the basic recipe).
Low-sodium diets: Use salt-free margarine and low-sodium baking powder.
Sugar content per serving: .8 teaspoon.

Oatmeal Cookies

Vera Wilson said that this cookie (with lots more sugar in it, of course) was one that she made ever since her oldest daughter Donna was just a baby. I like it especially well because it reminds me of the oatmeal cookies that my mother used to make when we were children. She also used to send them to me at college, and later to my sister and me when we were living in Chicago.

> ½ cup raisins
> ¾ cup boiling water
> ⅔ cup sugar
> Dry sugar substitute equal to ½ cup sugar
> 1 cup (2 sticks) margarine at room temperature
> ½ cup liquid egg substitute at room temperature
> 1 teaspoon vanilla
> 2 cups all-purpose flour
> 1 teaspoon cinnamon
> 1 teaspoon baking powder
> ½ teaspoon baking soda
> 2 cups rolled oats or rolled wheat
> ½ cup chopped nuts

Combine raisins and boiling water and set aside to cool to room temperature.

Cream together sugar, sugar substitute, and margarine at medium speed until light and fluffy. Add egg substitute and vanilla to creamed mixture and mix at low speed for 1 minute.

Stir together flour, cinnamon, baking powder, and soda to blend well.

Add oats and nuts to creamed mixture along with flour mixture, raisins, and liquid in which raisins were soaked. Mix at medium speed until flour is moistened. Drop by 1½ tablespoonfuls (level No. 40 dipper) onto cookie sheets that have been lined with aluminum foil or sprayed with cooking spray. Press down lightly with fingers dipped in cold water to form circles about 2 inches across; bake at 375°F for 10–12 minutes. Remove from hot cookie sheet to wire rack to cool to room temperature. Serve one cookie per serving.

Yields 3 dozen cookies—36 servings

Nutritive Values Per Serving

CAL	CARBS (g)	PRO (g)	TOTAL FAT (g)	SAT. FAT (g)	CHOL (mg)	FIBER (g)	NA (mg)
123	15	2	6	1	0	8	107

Food exchanges per serving: 1 starch, 1 fat.
Low-sodium diets: Use salt-free margarine, low-sodium baking powder, and
    unsalted nuts.
Sugar content per serving: .9 teaspoon.

Peanut Butter Cookies

This recipe from Frances Nielsen can be made with smooth peanut butter, but we prefer chunky.

> ½ cup chunky peanut butter at room
>   temperature
> ⅓ cup (⅔ stick) margarine at room
>   temperature
> ¼ cup dark molasses
> 2 teaspoons liquid sugar substitute
> 3 large egg whites at room temperature
> 1¼ cups all-purpose flour
> ½ teaspoon baking soda
> ⅛ teaspoon salt

Cream together peanut butter, margarine, molasses, and sugar substitute at medium speed until smooth. Add egg whites to creamed mixture and beat at medium speed until smooth.

Stir together flour, soda, and salt to blend and add to creamed mixture. Mix at medium speed until smooth. Drop by table-spoonfuls (level No. 60 dipper) onto a cookie sheet that has been lined with aluminum foil or sprayed with cooking spray. Press down lightly with fingers dipped in cold water to form circles about 2 inches wide. Bake at 375°F for 10–12 minutes, or until lightly browned. Remove from hot cookie sheet to wire rack and cool to room temperature. Serve two cookies per serving.

Yields 30 cookies—15 servings

Nutritive Values Per Serving

CAL	CARBS (g)	PRO (g)	TOTAL FAT (g)	SAT. FAT (g)	CHOL (mg)	FIBER (g)	NA (mg)
141	13	4	8	1.5	0	.8	163

Food exchanges per serving: 1 starch, 1¹/₂ fat.
Low-sodium diets: Omit salt. Use salt-free peanut butter.
Sugar content per serving: .8 teaspoon.

Whole Wheat Spice Cookies

---

¹/₂ cup (1 stick) margarine at room
    temperature
¹/₂ cup brown sugar
2 teaspoons vanilla
Liquid sugar substitute equal to ¹/₃ cup
    sugar
3 large egg whites at room temperature
2 tablespoons water at room temperature
²/₃ cup whole wheat flour
1¹/₃ cups all-purpose flour
¹/₂ teaspoon baking soda
¹/₂ teaspoon baking powder
¹/₄ teaspoon salt
1 teaspoon cinnamon
¹/₂ teaspoon nutmeg
2 tablespoons dry buttermilk

Cream together margarine and sugar until light and fluffy. Add vanilla, sugar substitute, egg whites, and water to creamed mixture and mix 2 minutes at medium speed.

Stir together remaining dry ingredients to blend well. Add to creamed mixture and mix at low speed to blend. Roll on a lightly floured working surface to ¼-inch thickness. Cut with a 3-inch cookie cutter and place on cookie sheets that have been lined with aluminum foil or sprayed with cooking spray. Bake at 350°F for 12–15 minutes, or until lightly browned. Remove from hot cookie sheet to wire rack and cool to room temperature. Serve one cookie per serving.

Yields 2 dozen cookies—24 servings

Nutritive Values Per Serving

CAL	CARBS (g)	PRO (g)	TOTAL FAT (g)	SAT. FAT (g)	CHOL (mg)	FIBER (g)	NA (mg)
94	13	2	4	.7	trace	.6	116

Food exchanges per serving: 1 starch, 1 fat.
Low-sodium diets: Omit salt. Use salt-free margarine and low-sodium baking powder.
Sugar content per serving: 1 teaspoon.

Hermits

These soft spice cookies are good with fruit for a snack or as dessert at a picnic.

> **1 teaspoon instant or freeze-dried coffee**
> **½ cup very hot water**
> **½ cup (1 stick) margarine at room temperature**
> **½ cup brown sugar**
> **Sugar substitute equal to ½ cup sugar**
> **2 large egg whites at room temperature**
> **2¼ cups all-purpose flour**
> **2 tablespoons dry buttermilk**
> **½ teaspoon baking powder**
> **½ teaspoon baking soda**
> **1 teaspoon cinnamon**
> **½ teaspoon nutmeg**
> **¼ teaspoon cloves**

¼ **cup raisins**
¼ **cup chopped walnuts**

Combine coffee and water. Stir to mix well and set aside.

Combine margarine, brown sugar, and sugar substitute and cream at medium speed until light and fluffy. Add egg whites and mix well.

Stir flour, dry buttermilk, baking powder, soda, cinnamon, nutmeg, cloves, and raisins together to blend. Add to creamed mixture along with the nuts and the coffee mixture. Mix at medium speed to blend and then drop by 1½ tablespoonfuls (level No. 40 dipper) onto cookie sheets that have been sprayed with cooking spray or lined with aluminum foil.

Bake at 375°F for 10–12 minutes or until firm. Remove from hot cookie sheets to wire rack to cool to room temperature. Serve one cookie per serving.

Yields 2 dozen cookies—24 servings

Nutritive Values Per Serving

CAL	CARBS (g)	PRO (g)	TOTAL FAT (g)	SAT. FAT (g)	CHOL (mg)	FIBER (g)	NA (mg)
114	16	2	5	.7	trace	.5	106

Food exchanges per serving: 1 starch, 1 fat.
Low-sodium diets: Use salt-free margarine and low-sodium baking powder.
Sugar content per serving: 1 teaspoon.

High-Fiber Cookies

These cookies, which provide 1.4 grams of dietary fiber each, aren't terribly sweet. We like them this way, but if you prefer them sweeter, you can add 1 tablespoon of Weight Watchers Low Calorie Sweetener or Splenda when you add the sugar without changing the nutritive values.

1 cup oat bran
1 cup rolled oats
1 cup Fiber One cereal
1 cup Kellogg's Bran Flakes

1 cup raisins
1 cup chopped English walnuts
¾ cup sugar
¾ cup brown sugar
1 cup (2 sticks) margarine at room
   temperature
2 large egg whites
2 teaspoons vanilla
2 cups all-purpose flour
1 teaspoon baking powder
1 teaspoon baking soda
½ teaspoon salt
½ cup water at room temperature

Place oat bran, rolled oats, Fiber One, Bran Flakes, raisins, and walnuts in a bowl. Mix lightly and set aside.

Place sugars and margarine in mixer bowl and mix at medium speed until light and fluffy. Add egg whites and vanilla and mix lightly, scraping down the bowl before and after adding egg whites and vanilla.

In a separate bowl combine flour, baking powder, soda, and salt and mix at low speed about ½ minute to blend well. Add flour mixture and water to sugar mixture and mix at medium speed only until flour is moistened. Add bran mixture and mix at medium speed until well blended.

Drop by 1½ tablespoonfuls (level No. 40 dipper) onto a cookie sheet that has been sprayed with cooking spray or lined with aluminum foil. Bake at 375°F for 12–14 minutes or until lightly browned. Remove from oven and let sit for 1 minute. Remove cookies to a wire rack and cool to room temperature. Serve one cookie per serving.

Yields 4 dozen cookies—48 servings

Nutritive Values Per Serving

CAL	CARBS (g)	PRO (g)	TOTAL FAT (g)	SAT. FAT (g)	CHOL (mg)	FIBER (g)	NA (mg)
121	17	2	6	.8	0	1.4	122

Food exchanges per serving: 1 starch, 1 fat.
Low-sodium diets: Use salt-free margarine and low-sodium baking powder.
Sugar content per serving: 1.3 teaspoons.

Nut Slices

This recipe is based on one from Anita Kane of Shorewood, Wisconsin. We traded recipes frequently and hers were always good. I always felt safe giving away a copy of one of her recipes without testing it, because I knew she tested it thoroughly before giving it to me.

> ½ cup (1 stick) margarine at room
>   temperature
> 2 tablespoons sugar
> 4 large egg whites at room temperature
> Dry sugar substitute equal to ⅓ cup sugar
> 1 teaspoon vanilla
> ½ teaspoon almond flavoring
> 2 cups all-purpose flour
> 1 teaspoon baking powder
> ½ teaspoon salt
> ½ cup chopped almonds

Cream together margarine and sugar until light and fluffy. Add egg whites, sugar substitute, vanilla, and almond flavoring to creamed mixture and mix at medium speed about 1 minute to blend. Add flour, baking powder, and salt to creamed mixture and mix at medium speed for 1 minute or until well blended.

Add almonds to dough. Turn out onto a lightly floured working surface and form into a roll about 2 inches wide and 12 inches long. Flatten the top of the roll, keeping it the same size, and place on a cookie sheet that has been lined with aluminum foil or sprayed with cooking spray. Bake at 350°F for 25 minutes. Remove roll from hot cookie sheet onto a working surface. As soon as you can handle the roll, slice with a serrated knife into 24 slices about ½ inch thick. Place the slices flat on the cookie sheet and return to the 350°F oven. Bake 5 minutes on one side and then about the same on the other side. Remove from hot cookie sheet to a cooling rack and cool to room temperature. Serve one slice per serving.

Note: If another kind of nut is used other than almonds, use another flavoring instead of the almond flavoring. We use black walnuts in this area and I'm sure that everyone has their own favorites.

Yields 2 dozen cookies—24 servings

Nutritive Values Per Serving

CAL	CARBS (g)	PRO (g)	TOTAL FAT (g)	SAT. FAT (g)	CHOL (mg)	FIBER (g)	NA (mg)
96	10	2	5	8	0	6	120

Food exchanges per serving: 2/3 starch, 1 fat.
Low-sodium diets: Omit salt. Use salt-free margarine, low-sodium baking powder, and unsalted nuts.
Sugar content per serving: .3 teaspoon.

Mexican Wedding Cookies

These cookies are based on a recipe from Frances Nielsen. They freeze beautifully and look so nice when they are rolled in the Sprinkle Sweet.

> 1½ cups (3 sticks) margarine at room
>   temperature
> ½ cup powdered sugar
> 2 teaspoons vanilla
> Dry sugar substitute equal to ⅓ cup sugar
> 3 cups all-purpose flour
> ¾ cup chopped nuts
> Sprinkle Sweet granulated sugar substitute
>   as necessary

Cream together margarine and powdered sugar at medium speed until light and fluffy. Add vanilla, sugar substitute, and flour to creamed mixture and mix at medium speed about 2 minutes or until well blended.

Add nuts to dough and mix at low speed only until nuts are blended into the dough. Form dough into balls using 1½ tablespoons (level No. 40 dipper) of dough for each ball. Bake on cookie sheets lined with aluminum foil or sprayed with cooking spray at 350°F for about 20 minutes, or until lightly browned. Remove from heat.

Roll cookies in Sprinkle Sweet while they are warm but not hot. Serve one cookie per serving.

Yields 3 dozen cookies—36 servings

Nutritive Values Per Serving

CAL	CARBS (g)	PRO (g)	TOTAL FAT (g)	SAT. FAT (g)	CHOL (mg)	FIBER (g)	NA (mg)
129	10	2	9	1.4	0	trace	90

Food exchanges per serving: ⅔ starch, 2 fat.
Low-sodium diets: Use salt-free margarine and unsalted nuts.
Sugar content per serving: .3 teaspoon.

Raisin Bars

This recipe is based on one from Vera Wilson. Her recipe is richer and is frosted, but I'm sure you will like this version, too.

⅓ cup raisins
1 cup water
¾ cup (1½ sticks) margarine at room
   temperature
¼ cup sugar
3 large egg whites at room temperature
Dry sugar substitute equal to ½ cup sugar
2¼ cups all-purpose flour
1 teaspoon baking soda
½ teaspoon salt
1 teaspoon cinnamon

Combine raisins and water in a small saucepan. Bring to a boil, cover, and remove from heat. Cool to room temperature.

Cream together margarine and sugar until light and fluffy. Add egg whites and sugar substitute to creamed mixture and mix at medium speed for 1 minute.

Stir together flour, soda, salt, and cinnamon to blend well. Add to creamed mixture along with the raisins and the liquid in which they were cooked. Mix at medium speed about 1 minute or until well blended. Spread evenly in a 9″ × 13″ cake pan that has been well greased with margarine. Bake at 350°F for 25–30 minutes or until browned and the bars pull away from the sides of the pan. Cut 4 × 5 to yield 20 squares. Serve one square per serving.

Yields 20 squares—20 servings

Nutritive Values Per Serving

CAL	CARBS (g)	PRO (g)	TOTAL FAT (g)	SAT. FAT (g)	CHOL (mg)	FIBER (g)	NA (mg)
134	15	2	7	1.2	0	.5	209

Food exchanges per serving: 1 starch, 1 fat.
Low-sodium diets: Omit salt and use salt-free margarine.
Sugar content per serving: .6 teaspoon.

Applesauce Bran Squares

This recipe is based on one from Betty Jane Walter of Jackson, Michigan. Betty Jane is a dietary consultant who has diabetes herself, and we often discuss our work as well as our favorite recipes. She has been very active in the American Heart Association program in her area and is concerned about low-cholesterol diets as well as diabetic diets.

> 1 cup all-purpose flour
> ²/₃ cup Bran Buds, All Bran, or 100% Bran
> ¹/₂ cup rolled oats
> ¹/₃ cup brown sugar

¹/₂ teaspoon salt
¹/₂ teaspoon baking soda
1 teaspoon baking powder
1 teaspoon cinnamon
¹/₄ teaspoon ground cloves or nutmeg
**¹/₂ cup (1 stick) margarine at room
temperature**
2 large egg whites at room temperature
1 teaspoon vanilla
Dry sugar substitute equal to ¹/₂ cup sugar
¹/₃ cup chopped nuts
**1 cup unsweetened applesauce at room
temperature**

Place dry ingredients in mixer bowl and mix at low speed for 1 minute.

Add margarine, egg whites, vanilla, sugar substitute, nuts, and applesauce to flour mixture and mix at medium speed for ¹/₂ minute or until blended. Spread evenly in a 9″ × 13″ cake pan that has been greased with margarine or sprayed with cooking spray. Bake at 375°F for 25–30 minutes or until browned and it starts to pull away from the sides of the pan. Cut 3 × 5 into 15 squares and serve warm or at room temperature. Serve one square per serving.

Yields 15 squares—15 servings

Nutritive Values Per Serving

CAL	CARBS (g)	PRO (g)	TOTAL FAT (g)	SAT. FAT (g)	CHOL (mg)	FIBER (g)	NA (mg)
153	18	3	8	1.2	0	1.9	255

Food exchanges per serving: 1 starch, 1¹/₂ fat.
Low-sodium diets: Omit salt. Use salt-free margarine, low-sodium baking powder, and unsalted nuts.
Sugar content per serving: 1.1 teaspoons.

19

Mixes

One thing I missed after I developed diabetes was those convenient cake mixes that I had been using. I could still use angel food mix, and frequently did, but I missed some of the other mixes such as the basic mixes for white, yellow, and chocolate cakes. I hadn't used bread mixes and only occasionally used muffin or cookie mixes so I didn't miss them all that much, but I really missed my cake mixes.

I still remember how I jumped at the suggestion the day my neighbor, Jan Franks, suggested I do as she did and create my own mixes. It was such a simple solution. I had never thought about doing it but it didn't take me long to start making my own mixes.

Jan's method was to make an extra mix every time she made a cake, muffins, or cookies. She measured equal amounts of the dry ingredients in each of two bowls. She finished the recipe using the ingredients in one of the bowls and put the dry ingredients from the other bowl in a plastic bag. She labeled the bag, added a note to herself telling her how to finish the recipe, and put it in the cupboard. Most mixes include flour, sugar, dry milk, leavening, and spices if they are in the recipe. These all keep well at room temperature and do not need to be refrigerated or frozen unless you intend to keep them several months or find it more convenient to store them that way.

I don't add nuts, margarine, or anything else that might get stale unless I plan to refrigerate or freeze the mix. It is always better to add those perishable ingredients at the last minute.

It's important to use standard measuring cups and spoons when you measure the ingredients for your mixes.

You can mix one extra batch when you are preparing a recipe or you can mix several batches at one time. If you want to do several batches at once, mix the ingredients thoroughly and then measure the total amount. Then divide by the number of batches you are making. Once you calculate individual amounts, bag each amount separately or put all of the mix in a large container ready to be measured along with the remaining ingredients and mixed when you need it. Label the mix with directions for preparation as well as the date you prepared it. For instance, the mix for Yellow Cake (see Index) would be as follows:

YELLOW CAKE

Ingredients	1 cake	4 cakes
Cake flour	2 cups	8 cups
Baking soda	½ teaspoon	2 teaspoons
Baking powder	1½ teaspoons	6 teaspoons (2 tablespoons)
Sugar	½ cup	2 cups
Dry buttermilk	3 tablespoons	12 tablespoons (¾ cup)
Total	2½ cups	10 cups

Note: This mix will need to be refrigerated because it contains dry buttermilk. It does not need to be refrigerated if nonfat dry milk is used.

Jan also thinks it's a good idea to use mixes when you go camping. She suggests putting the mix in a heavy plastic bag to which you can add the final ingredients after you get to the campsite, mixing everything right in the bag, which saves taking along bulky items and a mixing bowl.

Your own special mixes are also a thoughtful gift for special friends, especially if they also have diabetes. Decide which treat you want to send to them, put the ingredients in a pretty jar or other container, seal it well, tie the name and directions onto the container with a pretty ribbon, and give it to them.

You can prepare mixes for many different items. There is a recipe for Hot Cocoa Mix in this book (see Index). I also use mixes of my favorite spices. I mix a quantity of the spices, put them in a small container, and then use whatever amount I need when making the recipe. This is generally the total amount of spices in the recipe. The nutritive value of a spice mixture is negligible so you don't need to count them when you are analyzing a recipe unless it includes salt and you are on a low-salt diet. In this case you can omit the salt or use your favorite salt substitute. The most important step in preparing your spice mix is to blend it well. It also helps to use fresh spices and herbs. Here are some of my favorite spice mixes.

Minestrone Soup Seasoning Mix

Ideal for seasoning minestrone and other soups. Add 1–2 teaspoons to each quart of soup; then add more to taste as desired.

- **2 tablespoons salt**
- **2 teaspoons ground black pepper**
- **2 teaspoons sweet basil**
- **2 tablespoons oregano**
- **1 tablespoon thyme**
- **1 tablespoon garlic salt**

Italian Seasoning Mix

This mix is nice to have on hand for seasoning spaghetti sauce, lasagna, manicotti, and other Italian entrées. Add 1–2 teaspoons while browning meat or preparing sauce; then add more to taste as desired.

> 1 tablespoon ground oregano
> 1 tablespoon ground allspice
> ½ teaspoon ground cloves
> 1 tablespoon ground cumin
> 2 teaspoons paprika
> 2 teaspoons ground thyme
> 1 teaspoon ground basil
> Salt and pepper to taste

Mexican Seasoning Mix

This mix goes nicely in tacos, burritos, enchiladas, and other Mexican entrées. Start with 1–2 teaspoons and add more to taste.

> 3 tablespoons red chili powder
> 1 tablespoon salt
> 1 tablespoon garlic powder
> 2 tablespoons onion powder
> 1 tablespoon paprika
> 1 tablespoon ground cumin
> 1 tablespoon ground oregano
> 1 tablespoon sugar

Cake and Cookie Spice Mix

2 tablespoons ground cinnamon
1 tablespoon ground nutmeg
1 teaspoon ground cloves

If you want to start using your own favorite spice and herb mixtures, choose one of your favorite recipes, combine enough spices and/or herbs for several occasions, and mix well. Now you are prepared to save time and effort the next time you prepare the recipe.

STANDARD MEASURES

1½ teaspoons equal ½ tablespoon
3 teaspoons equal 1 tablespoon
4 tablespoons equal ¼ cup
5⅓ tablespoons equal ⅓ cup
8 tablespoons equal ½ cup
10⅔ tablespoons equal ⅔ cup
12 tablespoons equal ¾ cup
14 tablespoons equal ⅞ cup
16 tablespoons equal 1 cup
2 cups equal 1 pint
4 cups equal 1 quart
4 quarts equal 1 gallon

There are many mixes you can make depending upon your own needs and diet requirements. Many of the mixes you make will help simplify your meal preparation at a later date. I have several mixes I keep on hand because I know that I will be using them occasionally. There is one mix that I have been keeping on hand all of the time—my favorite oat bran mix which I can use several ways. Oat bran is an excellent addition to your diet and therefore I like to use it frequently.

Foods high in fiber, like oat bran, help slow the absorption of carbohydrate in the blood stream. This helps keep your blood glucose level more even during the day.

Oat Bran Mix

---

6 cups all-purpose flour
4 cups oat bran
1 cup nonfat dry milk
²/₃ cup packed brown sugar
¹/₃ cup baking powder
2 tablespoons wheat gluten (optional)
1 tablespoon baking soda
Dry sugar substitute equal to 1¹/₂ cups
    sugar
1 teaspoon salt

Put all ingredients in a mixer bowl and mix at low speed for 2 minutes or until thoroughly blended. Store in an airtight container until used. The mix does not need to be refrigerated or frozen unless you plan to keep it for several months. The mix yields 11 cups. Nutritive information is for 1 cup.

Nutritive Values Per Serving

CAL	CARBS (g)	PRO (g)	TOTAL FAT (g)	SAT. FAT (g)	CHOL (mg)	FIBER (g)	NA (mg)
45	9	2	trace	0	0	trace	157

Food exchanges per serving: ¹/₂ starch.
Low-sodium diets: Omit salt.
Sugar content per serving: .6 teaspoon.

Oat Bran Mix Muffins

---

2 large egg whites
1 cup water
2 tablespoons vegetable oil
1 teaspoon vanilla

2¹/₄ cups Oat Bran Mix
¹/₄ cup chopped nuts

Place egg whites, water, oil, and vanilla in mixer bowl and mix at low speed to blend. Add mix and nuts and mix at low speed only until blended. Fill 12 muffin cups that have been greased, sprayed with pan spray, or lined with paper liners about two-thirds full (level No. 16 dipper) and bake at 400°F for 18–20 minutes or until golden. Serve hot, if possible, using one muffin per serving.

Yields 12 muffins—12 servings

Nutritive Values Per Serving

CAL	CARBS (g)	PRO (g)	TOTAL FAT (g)	SAT. FAT (g)	CHOL (mg)	FIBER (g)	NA (mg)
130	20	5	4	0	0	1	340

Food exchanges per serving: 1¹/₂ starch.
Low-sodium diets: Omit salt.
Sugar content per serving: 1.2 teaspoons.

Oat Bran Mix Scones

1 cup Oat Bran Mix
¹/₂ teaspoon ground cinnamon
1 tablespoon packed brown sugar
2 tablespoons (¹/₄ stick) cold margarine
2 large egg whites
¹/₃ cup water at room temperature
2 tablespoons raisins

Place mix, cinnamon, brown sugar, and margarine in a bowl and cut the margarine into pea-size pieces as you would for pie crust. Add the egg whites, water, and raisins and mix lightly with a fork or large spoon. Shape into a 1¹/₄-inch-thick round in a pie tin that has been greased with margarine or sprayed with cooking spray. Bake in a preheated 400°F oven for 20 minutes or until golden brown. Cut into eight equal wedges and serve warm, if possible. Each wedge is one serving.

Yields 8 scones—8 servings

Nutritive Values Per Serving

CAL	CARBS (g)	PRO (g)	TOTAL FAT (g)	SAT. FAT (g)	CHOL (mg)	FIBER (g)	NA (mg)
100	16	3	3	0	0	trace	260

Food exchanges per serving: 1 starch.
Low-sodium diets: Omit salt.
Sugar content per serving: 1 teaspoon.

Oat Bran Mix Pancakes

1 cup Oat Bran Mix
1 large egg
½ cup water
1 tablespoon vegetable oil
Dry sugar substitute equal to 1 tablespoon
   sugar
1 teaspoon vanilla
¼ teaspoon salt

Place ingredients in a small bowl and mix until smooth.

Pour ¼ cup (level No. 16 dipper) batter onto a griddle that has been preheated to 375°F and sprayed with cooking spray. Cook about 3 minutes on one side or until bubbles form on the surface and the edges of the pancake are dry. Turn and cook 2–3 minutes on the other side or until nicely browned. Repeat with remaining batter. Serve hot using one pancake per serving. Yields six pancakes.

Note: If you want a larger pancake, use ½ cup batter for each pancake, which will double the exchange value to two starch and one fat per pancake.

Yields 6 pancakes—6 servings

Nutritive Values Per Serving

CAL	CARBS (g)	PRO (g)	TOTAL FAT (g)	SAT. FAT (g)	CHOL (mg)	FIBER (g)	NA (mg)
110	18	5	3	0	0	trace	410

Food exchanges per serving: 1 starch.
Low-sodium diets: Omit salt.
Sugar content per serving: 1 teaspoon.

Oat Bran Mix Pecan Spice Cookies

You can vary the spices in these cookies if you like. I sometimes use 1½ teaspoons Chinese 5-Spice powder instead of the cinnamon, nutmeg, and cloves.

> **1 cup Oat Bran Mix**
> **½ teaspoon baking soda**
> **1 teaspoon ground cinnamon**
> **¼ teaspoon ground nutmeg**
> **¼ teaspoon ground cloves**
> **⅓ cup packed brown sugar**
> **⅓ cup chopped pecans**
> **2 large egg whites**
> **6 tablespoons (¾ stick) softened margarine**
> **2 tablespoons water**

Place mix, soda, spices, brown sugar, and nuts in mixing bowl and mix at low speed to blend. Add egg whites, margarine, and water and mix at low speed to blend well. Drop by 1½ tablespoonfuls (level No. 40 dipper) onto cookie sheets that have been lined with aluminum foil or sprayed with cooking spray. Bake at 350°F for 10 minutes or until almost firm and lightly browned. Remove cookies to wire rack to cool to room temperature. Serve one cookie per serving. Yields 18 cookies.

Note: These cookies are gently rounded on top. If you want a flatter cookie, press each cookie lightly with the back of a spoon dipped in cold water before they are baked.

Yields 18 cookies—18 servings

Nutritive Values Per Serving

CAL	CARBS (g)	PRO (g)	TOTAL FAT (g)	SAT. FAT (g)	CHOL (mg)	FIBER (g)	NA (mg)
90	10	2	5	1	0	trace	180

Food exchanges per serving: 1 starch.
Low-sodium diets: May be used as written.
Sugar content per serving: 1.2 teaspoons.

20

Beverages

A good hot beverage or a well-chilled sugar-free soft drink can be a real lift when you are hot and tired—or cold and tired, too, for that matter. Beverages are such a part of our lives that we need to know what we can enjoy without going off our diet when we want something to drink.

It is also nice to have beverages you can serve for parties or when friends drop in. I make my own low-calorie cocoa mix that I think is extra special. A friend of mine who was counting her calories asked for some of it the other day, and she told me she liked it even better than the regular commercial kind.

When you go to a party, and it seems like food and socializing always go together, you can always walk around with a cup of black coffee or a glass of iced tea or sugar-free soft drink and have just as much fun as anyone else.

If you are home alone and hungry or thirsty and don't want to spend any more of your exchanges, you can have a twist of lemon in ice water (which is one of my favorites), or a cup of hot bouillon or tomato juice with a twist of lemon in it. When I was visiting Bud and Frances Gunsallus in Miami, I discovered that half of a lime from the tree in their backyard put a lot of life into a glass of ice water or sugar-free 7-Up.

In other words, use what is available in the line of sugarless beverages and enjoy the party—or get a real lift when you are tired and just need a pick-me-up.

Sparkling Punch

**2 .14- or .20-ounce packets of Wyler's
   unsweetened flavored soft drink mix or
   Kool-Aid unsweetened soft drink mix
   (2-quart size)**
1 quart water
**3 quarts chilled sugar-free 7-Up or sugar-
   free ginger ale**

Dissolve drink mix in water and refrigerate until needed. Place
in punch bowl along with a chunk of ice.

Add 7-Up or ginger ale to drink mix in bowl. Mix lightly and
serve a 4-ounce cup per serving.

I like to freeze some of the drink mix (which has been prepared with water according to directions on the package) in a
bowl or plastic container to be used instead of ice in the punch
bowl. This keeps the punch from being diluted as the ice melts.
To add a special touch, you can add a few grapes or strawberries
in with the mix you are freezing.

Yields 1 gallon—32 4-ounce cups

Nutritive Values Per Serving

CAL	CARBS (g)	PRO (g)	TOTAL FAT (g)	SAT. FAT (g)	CHOL (mg)	FIBER (g)	NA (mg)
1	0	0	0	0	0	0	25

Food exchanges per serving: None.
Low-sodium diets: May be used as written.
Sugar content per serving: None.

Hot Spiced Tea

This recipe is from Edith Robinson, a dietitian from Decatur, Georgia. Edith and I worked together at the Army Food Service Center in Chicago. She told me that she got the recipe from our commanding officer Colonel Cozad's wife, who served it one cold day when she and Colonel Cozad entertained the members of the department at their home.

> **12 cups water**
> **1 teaspoon whole cloves**
> **4 sticks cinnamon**
> **6 tea bags**
> **¼ cup lemon juice**
> **1 cup unsweetened pineapple juice**
> **1½ cups unsweetened orange juice**
> **Sugar substitute equal to ¾ cup sugar**

Combine water, cloves, and cinnamon and simmer, covered, for 5 minutes. Remove from heat. Add tea bags to hot liquid and steep for 5 minutes. Remove tea bags and spices.

Add juices to tea and mix lightly. Tea may be cooled to room temperature and refrigerated overnight at this stage, if desired. If tea is refrigerated, it should be reheated before it is served.

Add sugar substitute just before tea is served. Taste for flavor and add a little more lemon juice or sugar substitute, if desired. Serve one 4-ounce punch cup per serving.

Yields 15 cups—30 servings

Nutritive Values Per Serving

CAL	CARBS (g)	PRO (g)	TOTAL FAT (g)	SAT. FAT (g)	CHOL (mg)	FIBER (g)	NA (mg)
14	4	trace	trace	0	0	trace	22

Food exchanges per serving: ¼ fruit.
Low-sodium diets: May be used as written.
Sugar content per serving: None.

Hot Cocoa Mix

---

³/₄ cup cocoa
¹/₂ teaspoon salt
1 quart instant nonfat dry milk
Dry sugar substitute equal to 1–1¹/₂ cups
  sugar

Mix ingredients well and store in an airtight container in a moderately cool place. Use 2 tablespoons mix plus 6 ounces boiling water for one 6-ounce serving of cocoa.

Variations:
MEXICAN COCOA

Add 2–3 teaspoons ground cinnamon when mixing the total ingredients; or place a scant ¹/₈ teaspoon of cinnamon in a cup, 2 tablespoons of the mix, and 6 ounces boiling water for one serving.

MOCHA

Add ¹/₃ cup instant coffee when mixing the total ingredients; or place ¹/₂ teaspoon instant coffee in a cup, 2 tablespoons of the mix, and 6 ounces boiling water for one serving.

Yields mix for 32 6-ounce cups of cocoa

Nutritive Values Per Serving

CAL	CARBS (g)	PRO (g)	TOTAL FAT (g)	SAT. FAT (g)	CHOL (mg)	FIBER (g)	NA (mg)
39	6	3	trace	trace	2	.6	109

Food exchanges per serving: ¹/₂ skim milk (exchanges remain the same for the variations of the basic recipe).
Low-sodium diets: Omit salt.
Sugar content per serving: None.

Chocolate Milk Shake

This recipe from Patti Dillon, our Fayette County home econom- ics extension agent, is cool and refreshing and costs a lot less in calories and exchanges than you would expect.

> 1 cup skim milk
> 2 teaspoons cocoa
> 1 1-gram packet Equal (aspartame) sugar
> substitute
> 3 or 4 ice cubes

Place ingredients in blender or food processor and beat at high speed until frothy and thickened. Serve immediately. Total amount is one serving.

Yields 1 milk shake

Nutritive Values Per Serving

CAL	CARBS (g)	PRO (g)	TOTAL FAT (g)	SAT. FAT (g)	CHOL (mg)	FIBER (g)	NA (mg)
98	14	10	1	.6	5	1	128

Food exchanges per serving: 1 skim milk.
Low-sodium diets: May be used as written.
Sugar content per serving: None.

Chocolate Liqueur

I like to sprinkle a couple of tablespoons of this over a chocolate cake before I cut it and put the topping on it. It adds a certain something to the cake without increasing the food value very much. In fact, 3 tablespoons on one cake doesn't need to be counted since the amount per portion is so small. Gail Olson of Volga City, Iowa, gave me this recipe and the one following. They are both good over ice milk or served with an after-dinner drink.

2 cups vodka
1½ cups water
1½ cups Sugar Twin Brown Sugar
   Replacement
4 ounces chocolate extract
2 teaspoons vanilla
½ teaspoon peppermint extract (optional)

Combine ingredients and pour into a dark-colored glass bottle. Let stand for 2 weeks before it is used. Store as you would any liqueur. Consider 1 ounce (2 tablespoons) per serving when calculating nutritional values.

Yields 1 quart—32 1-ounce servings

Nutritive Values Per Serving

CAL	CARBS (g)	PRO (g)	TOTAL FAT (g)	SAT. FAT (g)	CHOL (mg)	FIBER (g)	NA (mg)
48	2	0	0	0	0	0	trace

Food exchanges per serving: ³/₄ other carbohydrate.
Low-sodium diets: May be used as written.
Sugar content per serving: None.

Orange Liqueur

Frances Nielsen taught me to appreciate the flavor of fruit and orange liqueur combined together, using about 1 tablespoon orange liqueur per serving of fruit. I had given that up because of the high carbohydrate content of liqueurs until Gail Olson of Volga City, Iowa, gave me this recipe. It is good over ice milk or served as an after-dinner drink, and it is marvelous with fruit.

2 cups water
Thin peel from 2 large oranges
2 teaspoons vanilla
1 teaspoon lemon flavoring
2 teaspoons orange flavoring

1 drop yellow food color
1 drop orange food color
2 cups vodka
Sugar substitute equal to ½ cup sugar

Combine water and orange peel and simmer, covered, over low heat for 5 minutes. Cool to room temperature.

Add remaining ingredients to simmered mixture. Pour into a glass or stainless steel container. Cover and keep in a dark place for 2 weeks. Strain and discard any solids. Pour into a dark glass bottle and store as you would any liqueur. Consider 1 ounce (2 tablespoons) per serving when calculating nutritional values.

Yields 1 quart—32 1-ounce servings

Nutritive Values Per Serving

CAL	CARBS (g)	PRO (g)	TOTAL FAT (g)	SAT. FAT (g)	CHOL (mg)	FIBER (g)	NA (mg)
38	1	trace	0	0	0	0	11

Food exchanges per serving: ⅔ other carbohydrate.
Low-sodium diets: May be used as written.
Sugar content per serving: None.

21

Canning and Freezing Foods

If you have been canning and freezing fruits and vegetables, don't stop now. This is a good time to take advantage of your expertise to save yourself some money. Canning for the low-cholesterol diabetic diet is no more complicated than any other kind of canning. You can can your fruits in a light or very light syrup as well as any commercial canner.

Sugar helps develop the flavor and color of canned fruits—so now that we can use small amounts of sugar in our diets (see Chapter 3), we can can fruits every bit as flavorful and tasty as any product on the market.

When we are canning fruits and vegetables for the low-cholesterol diabetic diet, we need only worry about the diabetic part of the diet. The only canned item I can think of that includes cholesterol is mincemeat that is made with suet. You can manage that by canning mincemeat without suet and adding some margarine to the mincemeat when you are ready to use it. (You can add ¼ cup sugar per quart of mincemeat, providing 1½ teaspoons of sugar per ½ cup, when you are canning it and then add sugar substitute to taste when you use it.)

We can buy or can fruits in unsweetened fruit juice. (Count the fruit juice when you use it as a fruit exchange according to the kind and amount you use.) Fruit can also be canned using very light syrup, light syrup, medium and heavy syrup. I'm sure you know we should use very light syrup and add sugar substitute if we like it sweeter. To make the syrup, heat water and sugar together until the sugar is dissolved, skimming off any foam that rises to the top of the liquid. Processing time for fruit is the same whether heavy or light syrup or fruit juice is used. Canning fruit in a very light syrup will add about 1 teaspoon of sugar per ½ cup serving, which is acceptable. One half cup fruit and juice canned in very light syrup is one fruit exchange. Here are the proportions for preparing the syrup.

Very light syrup for 9 pints or 4 quarts of fruit:
6½ cups water
¾ cup sugar

Organisms that cause food spoilage—molds, yeast, and bacteria—are present in the air, water, and soil. Enzymes that cause deterioration are always present in the fruit. Canning destroys the organisms that cause spoilage and inactivates the enzymes. Because fruits are high in acid they can be safely processed in a boiling-water canner or pressure cooker.

Choose fresh, firm, high-quality fruit. Wash all fruits thoroughly under running water or use several changes of water. Lift the food out of the water each time so dirt that has been washed off the fruit will not settle back on the fruit. Do not let fruits soak because they will lose flavor and nutritive value. Handle fruit gently to avoid bruising, and process fresh foods as soon as possible to avoid spoilage.

The amount of canned food from a given amount of fresh fruit will depend upon the quality, condition, variety, maturity, and size of the fruit, the size of the pieces packed, and whether the fruit is packed hot or raw. The amount of fresh fruit generally needed for 1 quart of canned fruit is as follows: 2 to 3 pounds apples, cherries, nectarines, peaches, or pears; 2 pounds apricots; 1 to 3 pounds berries; 2 pounds grapefruit or oranges; and 1 to 2 pounds plums.

Light-colored fruits, especially apples, apricots, peaches, and pears, darken when cut and exposed to air. This can be prevented by pretreating the fruit with an ascorbic acid solution. Keep the fruit in this solution until it is ready to be canned. The fruit should be drained well before it is placed in the jars. Ascorbic acid is available in several forms under various names. Look for it among the canning supplies in the grocery store or supermarket. (It also keeps fruit looking good when making fruit salads.)

Use only jars and lids made especially for canning. Mayonnaise jars and others that may look as if they could be used for canning should not be used because they are not made of the same quality glass, may break during processing, and are not made for use with the two-piece canning lids. These guidelines also apply when you are making jellies and jams. Throw away all those odd-shaped jars and get some meant for canning to avoid risk of breakage or spoilage.

Most people prefer to use the hot-pack method for canning fruit. To hot pack fruit, preheat fruit in a small amount of hot syrup, juice, or water. Pack into hot jars and cover with hot liquid. Wipe the rims of the jars, tighten the lids, and process according to instructions. Cold packing is also approved and may be used if desired. To cold pack fruit, pack the raw fruit in jars, add boiling hot syrup, juice, or water to cover the fruit, wipe the rims, tighten the lids, and process according to instructions. Always make sure you have covered the fruit with liquid because any fruit not covered will darken. In either case, process in a hot-water bath according to the time required for that particular fruit. Plan on ½ to 1½ cups liquid per quart.

The space between the fruit and liquid and the jar lid is called headspace. Generally speaking, you should allow ½ inch headspace for fruits and ¼ inch headspace for fruit juices and purées. It's a good idea to run a spatula down the side of the jar to remove any air bubbles.

To use a boiling-water canner, fill the canner halfway with water and preheat to 140°F for cold pack or 180°F for hot pack. Put sealed jars in the water, making sure the water can circulate freely around the jars. Add boiling water so that the water is 1 to 2 inches above the tops of the jars. Bring the water in the canner to a vigorous boil, adjust the heat to maintain a gentle boil, and cover. Keep the water boiling during the entire processing time (never reduce the specified boiling time), keeping the water at least 1 inch above the tops of the jars (keep the lid on the canner). Remove the jars from the canner and place them upright on folded towels or a rack. Allow them to cool away from drafts for 12 to 24 hours. Do not tighten the lids. To test the seals, press the center of the lids. If the lid is down and doesn't move, the jar is sealed. Remove the screw bands carefully after the jars are cool. Wash the jars, if necessary, dry, label, and store them in a cool, dark place. If any of the jars haven't sealed, put them in the refrigerator and use them within a few days. Fruit can be placed in another jar and reprocessed but the flavor is never as good after the second processing. Canned fruit is safe as long as the jar remains sealed. Never use fruits that show mold or if the jar leaks liquid.

To use a pressure canner, partially fill the canner with 2 to 3 inches of water. Place a jar rack in the canner, put the jars on the rack, fasten the lid, and turn the heat on high. After the steam exhausts for 10 minutes, add weighted gauge or close the petcock. Allow the canner to reach the designated pressure. Start timing when the designated pressure is reached. Regulate heat to maintain a uniform pressure. Process for the recommended time. (Do not reduce the processing time.) When the processing time is ended, remove the pressure cooker from the heat. Let the canner cool at room temperature until the canner is fully depressurized, which will probably take from 30 to 60 minutes depending upon the type of canner. Do not try to reduce the time of cooling by setting the canner in cold water or by running cold water over the canner. Never attempt to hasten the pressure reduction by lifting the weight or opening the vent. When the pressure is reduced, carefully open the petcock or remove the weighted gauge. Wait 2 minutes and then slowly release and remove the canner lid. After the jars are removed from the canner, set them upright on a rack or folded cloth away from drafts. Do not tighten the screw bands. Allow jars to cool for 12 to 24 hours and then check to be sure that all of the jars are sealed correctly. If they aren't sealed correctly, refrigerate them and use the fruit within a few days. The fruit can be canned again but it is not as good the second time. To test the seal, press the center of the lid. If the lid is down and doesn't move, the jar is sealed. It is best to keep your canned fruit in a cool, dark place. Canned fruit is safe as long as the jar is sealed, but never use canned fruit that is leaking or that shows any sign of mold.

I want to stress to you that canning food safely at home is not difficult, but it does require you to follow specific directions exactly. Always use tested recipes and directions from a reliable source. Ignoring the recommended procedures can result in loss of your canned goods and sickness for your family. However, you have a lot to gain if you do some canning and I urge you to try it. The rewards can be great.

The following charts will show you processing times for various foods at different altitudes.

Recommended Processing Time for Fruit in a Boiling-Water Canner

Type of Fruit	Pack	Jar Size	Minutes of Processing at Altitudes (ft.)			
			0–1,000	1,001–3,000	3,001–6,000	Over 6,000
Apples	Hot	Pints or quarts	20	25	30	35
Apple juice	Hot	Pints or quarts	5*	10	10	15
		Half gallons	10	15	15	20
Applesauce	Hot	Pints	15	20	20	25
		Quarts	20	25	30	35
Berries	Hot	Pints or quarts	15	20	20	25
	Raw	Pints	15	20	20	25
		Quarts	20	25	30	35
Cherries	Hot	Pints	15	20	20	25
		Quarts	20	25	30	35
	Raw	Pints or quarts	25	30	35	40
Fruit cocktail	Raw	Half or full pints	20	25	30	35
Fruit purées	Hot	Pints or quarts	15	20	20	25
Grapefruit and orange sections	Raw	Pints or quarts	10	15	15	20
Grape juice	Hot	Pints or quarts	5*	10	10	15
		Half gallons	10	15	15	20

Peaches, apricots, or nectarines	Hot	Pints	20	25	30	35
		Quarts	25	30	35	40
	Raw	Pints	25	30	35	40
		Quarts	30	35	40	45
Pears	Hot	Pints	20	25	30	35
		Quarts	25	30	35	40
Plums	Hot or raw	Pints	20	25	30	35
		Quarts	25	30	35	40

*Foods processed under 10 minutes must be canned in sterile jars. Washing the jars is not sufficient. They should be washed well with hot soapy water, rinsed, and then immersed in boiling water for 11 minutes.

Processing Time for Some Acid Foods in a Dial-Gauge Pressure Canner

Type of Fruit	Pack	Jar Size	Process Time (Min.)	Canner Pressure (PSI) at Altitudes (ft.)			
				0–2,000 6 lb.	2,001–4,000 7 lb.	4,001–6,000 8 lb.	6,001–8,000 9 lb.
Applesauce	Hot	Pints	8	6	7	8	9
		Quarts	10	6	7	8	9
Apples, sliced	Hot	Pints or quarts	8	6	7	8	9
Berries, whole	Hot	Pints or quarts	8	6	7	8	9
	Raw	Pints	8	6	7	8	9
		Quarts	10	6	7	8	9
Cherries, sour or sweet	Hot	Pints	8	6	7	8	9
		Quarts	10	6	7	8	9
	Raw	Pints or quarts	10	6	7	8	9
Fruit purées	Hot	Pints or quarts	8	6	7	8	9
Grapefruit and orange sections	Hot	Pints or quarts	8	6	7	8	9
	Raw	Pints or quarts	10	6	7	8	9
Nectarines, apricots, or peaches	Hot or raw	Pints or quarts	10	6	7	8	9
Pears	Hot	Pints or quarts	10	6	7	8	9
Plums	Hot or raw	Pints or quarts	10	6	7	8	9
Rhubarb	Hot	Pints or quarts	8	6	7	8	9

Processing Time for Some Acid Foods in a Weighted-Gauge Pressure Cooker

Type of Fruit	Pack	Jar Size	Process Time (Min.)	Canner Pressure (PSI) at Altitudes (ft.)	
				0– 1,000	Above 1,000
				5 lb.	10 lb.
Applesauce	Hot	Pints	8	5	10
	Hot	Quarts	10	5	10
Apples, sliced	Hot	Pints or quarts	8	5	10
Berries, whole	Hot	Pints or quarts	8	5	10
	Raw	Pints	8	5	10
		Quarts	10	5	10
Cherries, sour or sweet	Hot	Pints	8	5	10
		Quarts	10	5	10
	Raw	Pints or quarts	10	5	10
Fruit purées	Hot	Pints or quarts	8	5	10
Grapefruit and orange sections	Hot	Pints or quarts	8	5	10
	Raw	Pints	8	5	10
		Quarts	10	5	10
Nectarines, peaches, or apricots	Hot or raw	Pints or quarts	10	5	10
Pears	Hot	Pints or quarts	10	5	10
Plums	Hot or raw	Pints or quarts	10	5	10
Rhubarb	Raw	Pints or quarts	8	5	10

There is little difference, nutritionally, between vegetables canned at home and vegetables purchased already canned. Several large packers are now offering low-sodium canned foods so it is no longer as difficult to follow a low-sodium diet using canned vegetables. If you want to can low-sodium vegetables at home, prepare and process them according to directions, without adding any salt. They will keep as well as vegetables canned with salt.

It is important that you use the latest information when you are canning vegetables since research has shown that it is better to process foods for longer periods of time than we used to think was necessary. Vegetables, except for tomatoes, should always be canned in a pressure canner. Information on that process is available from the makers of pressure canners, your county extension agent, the library, the makers of canning jars, and numerous other publications.

The only food that needs salt when it is being prepared for canning is pickles. The pickles don't need salt for preservation but for drawing the liquid out of the vegetables to be pickled so it can be replaced by the vinegar-sugar solution that makes them crisp and flavorful. There are some recipes for making pickles without salt but they must be kept refrigerated or frozen and cannot be canned.

You can make pickles without sugar, if you like. In fact, there are some brands of pickles now available that are sugar-free, and they are very good. Dill pickles are made without sugar and are readily available, but I prefer a sweet pickle. Now that we can have some sugar in our diets, I worked on making sweet pickles and developed a couple of recipes I like well enough to include them at the end of this chapter.

Freezing fruits and vegetables is often faster and easier than canning. We generally think of fruits frozen with sugar but they can also be frozen without sugar. I like them IQF (individually quick frozen). In order to do that, clean the fruits, blot them dry with a paper towel, and spread them on a cookie sheet lined with aluminum foil or wax paper. Put them in the freezer, uncovered, until they are frozen and then put them in a freezer bag, label them, and return them to the freezer until you need them. Strawberries, blueberries, gooseberries, currants, and rhubarb all respond well to being individually frozen. Of course all of these fruits except cranberries should be washed and drained before they are frozen.

I also like to cook cranberries, rhubarb, and applesauce without sugar, freeze them in containers and then add sugar substitute when I'm ready to serve them. I love those frozen fruits during the winter when fresh fruit is not always all that good and available.

Squeeze as much air as possible out of the freezer bags before storage. Leave ½-inch headspace for expansion in rigid containers. Fruit should be stored at 0°F or colder and used within 8 to 12 months for best quality. Partially defrosted fruits taste best to me although they should generally be defrosted for use in salad or dessert. Fruit can be defrosted in the container in the refrigerator although it can also be defrosted by submerging the container in water. Once again, consult the authorities if you have questions about proper procedures.

Mrs. Riley's Pickles

This recipe is based on that old standby, 14-day pickles. We call them Mrs. Riley's Pickles because my cousin Virginia Ballantine's grandmother, Mrs. Riley, used to make them every year.

Make only enough for one year because they are wonderful the first year—sweet, spicy, and crisp—but they lose some of their quality the second year.

> 2½ quarts vinegar
> 2 cups sugar
> 2 tablespoons celery seed
> 1 ounce stick cinnamon
> 10 drops green or red vegetable coloring (optional)
> 2 gallons washed and sliced medium-size firm cucumbers with the ends removed
> 1 gallon boiling water
> 2 cups pickling salt
> 1 gallon boiling water (day 7)
> 1 tablespoon alum
> 1 gallon boiling water (day 9)
> 1 gallon boiling water (day 10)
> Sugar substitute equal to 1½ cups sugar

Heat together vinegar, sugar, celery seed, cinnamon, and vegetable coloring. Cool to room temperature and return to the vinegar container. Cover tightly and let stand until needed. (I like to use some coloring because it enhances the color of the pickles and makes them look more like the commercial sweet pickle slices. I sometimes make a red batch for gifts and to use on relish trays on special occasions.)

Place cucumbers in empty glass gallon jars, stainless-steel pots, or crocks. Dissolve pickling salt in 1 gallon boiling water and then pour over cucumbers. Let stand, covered loosely, for 1 week. Remove any mold on top of the cucumbers at the end of 7 days.

On the seventh day, drain cucumbers well. Pour 1 gallon boiling water over them and let them stand, covered loosely, for 2 days.

On the ninth day, drain cucumbers well. Dissolve the alum in 1 gallon boiling water and pour over cucumbers.

On the tenth day, drain cucumbers well and cover with 1 gallon boiling water. On the eleventh day, drain cucumbers well and pack into 7 quart or 14 pint sterilized jars.

Strain the reserved vinegar mixture. Throw away the spices and heat the vinegar. Add sugar substitute and pour over the sliced cucumbers in the jars. (Do not use Equal [aspartame] since it is not stable to heat.) Cover and seal the jars and process in a boiling-water canner for the time recommended in the accompanying chart. Serve 2 tablespoons per serving.

Yields 7 quarts or 14 pints

Nutritive Values Per Serving

CAL	CARBS (g)	PRO (g)	TOTAL FAT (g)	SAT. FAT (g)	CHOL (mg)	FIBER (g)	NA (mg)
10	3	trace	0	0	0	trace	292

Food exchanges per serving: 2 tablespoons are free, ¼ cup is 1 vegetable.
Low-sodium diets: This recipe is not suitable.
Sugar content per serving: .4 teaspoon.

Recommended Processing Time in a Boiling-Water Canner
Minutes of Processing at Altitudes (ft.)

Pack	Jar Size	0–1,000	1,001–6,000	Above 6,000
Raw	Pints	5	10	15
	Quarts	10	15	20

Zucchini Pickles

There are so many zucchini around that I thought I'd try to make some pickles from them. I used the recipe that I always use for bread-and-butter pickles and it really worked well. Everyone liked them very much.

>1 gallon thinly sliced 6- to 8-inch-long
>   zucchini
>4 cups sliced white onions
>½ cup salt
>2 quarts cracked ice
>5 cups cider vinegar
>3 cups water
>1½ teaspoons turmeric
>1 teaspoon celery seed
>1 tablespoon mustard seed
>Sugar substitute to taste

Combine zucchini, onions, salt, and ice in a large bowl and mix well. Cover with a plate with a weight on top of it so that all of the zucchini slices are covered with the salted ice water formed as the ice melts. Let them stand for 3 hours and then drain them well. Place in a large saucepan.

Thoroughly mix vinegar, water, turmeric, celery seed, and mustard seed and add to zucchini. Bring almost to a boil but do not let mixture boil, stirring frequently with a wooden spoon. Pack the hot pickles in pint jars.

Add sugar substitute to taste to the hot liquid. I use about ¼ cup of liquid sugar substitute, but you may prefer them a little sweeter or even a little less sweet. (Do not use Equal [aspartame] to sweeten the pickles because it is not stable to heat and the pickles are processed in a hot water bath.) Pour the hot liquid over the pickles to about ½ inch from the top. Cover and seal. Process in a boiling-water canner for the time indicated in the accompanying chart. Serve 2 tablespoons pickles per serving.

Yields 5 pints—80 servings

Nutritive Values Per Serving

CAL	CARBS (g)	PRO (g)	TOTAL FAT (g)	SAT. FAT (g)	CHOL (mg)	FIBER (g)	NA (mg)
10	2	trace	trace	0	0	trace	84

Food exchanges per serving: 2 tablespoons are free, ¼ cup is 1 vegetable.
Low-sodium diets: This recipe is not suitable.
Sugar content per serving: None.

Recommended Processing Time in a Boiling-Water Canner
Minutes of Processing at
Altitudes (ft.)

Pack	Jar Size	0–1,000	1,001–6,000	Above 6,000
Raw	Pints or			
	quarts	10	15	20

Frozen Sliced Sweet Dill Pickles

1 pound 3-inch unwaxed cucumbers
2 cups packed, sliced yellow onions
4 teaspoons salt
2 tablespoons water
¼ cup sugar
1 tablespoon Weight Watchers Low Calorie Sweetener
½ cup white vinegar
¼ cup garlic wine vinegar
1 tablespoon dry dill weed

Wash cucumbers and slice them about ⅛ inch thick. Place cucumbers, onions, salt, and water in a 2-quart glass or stainless-steel bowl (don't use aluminum) and let stand for 2 hours at room temperature or overnight in the refrigerator. Drain cucumbers and onions, but do not rinse.

Combine sugar, sugar substitute, vinegars, and dill weed. Stir until sugar is dissolved and then add vegetables. The liquid should cover vegetables. Cover and refrigerate 2 hours.

Pack pickles lightly in jars or plastic containers, leaving 1 inch at top for expansion. Seal tightly and freeze. The pickles may be kept in the freezer for 6 months. Use within 3 or 4 days after defrosting. Two days of freezing is enough if you want to use them right away. Use ¼ cup per serving.

1 quart—16 servings

Nutritive Values Per Serving

CAL	CARBS (g)	PRO (g)	TOTAL FAT (g)	SAT. FAT (g)	CHOL (mg)	FIBER (g)	NA (mg)
29	7	trace	0	0	0	trace	167

Food exchanges per serving: 1 vegetable.
Low-sodium diets: Rinse pickles after they are drained before vinegar is added.
Sugar content per serving: .8 teaspoon.

Glossary

There are some words and phrases used in a discussion of diabetes that are important for you to understand when discussing your diabetes and its treatment with health professionals.

The *Exchange Lists* for meal planning contain an excellent glossary so I decided to include the information in that publication here. I hope being familiar with these terms will help you to cope with your diabetes and its treatment.

Alcohol—An ingredient in a variety of beverages, including beer, wine, liqueurs, cordials, and mixed straight drinks. Pure alcohol itself yields about 7 calories per gram.

Calories—A unit used in expressing the heat or energy value of food. Calories come from carbohydrate, protein, fat, and alcohol.

Carbohydrate—One of the three major energy sources in foods. The most common carbohydrates are sugars and starches. Carbohydrates yield about 4 calories per gram. Carbohydrates are found primarily in foods from the milk, vegetable, fruit, and starch exchange lists.

Certified Diabetes Educator (CDE)—Health educators who specialize in diabetes and have passed the Certification Examination for Diabetes Educators are certified by the American Association of Diabetes Educators. These educators stay up to date on diabetes care and can help you with your diabetes management.

Cholesterol—A fat-like substance normally found in blood. A high level of cholesterol in the blood has been shown to be a major risk factor for developing heart disease. Dietary cholesterol is found in all animal products, but is especially high in egg yolks and organ meats. Eating foods high in dietary cholesterol and saturated fat tends to raise the level of blood cholesterol. Foods of plant origin such as fruits, vegetables, grains, and dried beans and peas contain no cholesterol. Cholesterol is found in foods from the milk, meat, and fat exchange lists.

Dietitian—A registered dietitian (RD) is recognized by the medical profession as the primary provider of nutritional care, education, and counseling. The initials RD after a dietitian's name ensure that he or she has met the standards of the American Dietetic Association. Look for those credentials when you seek advice on nutrition.

Exchanges—Foods grouped together on a list according to similarities in food. Measured amounts of foods within the group may be exchanged or traded in planning meals.

Fat—One of the three major energy sources in food. A concentrated source of calories—about 9 calories per gram. Fat is found in foods from the fat and meat lists. Some kinds of milk also have fat; some foods from the starch list also contain fat.

Saturated fat—Type of fat that tends to raise blood cholesterol levels. It comes primarily from animals and is usually hard at room temperature. Examples of saturated fat are butter, lard, meat fat, solid shortening, palm oil, and coconut oil.

Polyunsaturated fat—Type of fat that is usually liquid at room temperature and is found in vegetable oils. Safflower, sunflower, corn, and soybean oils contain the highest amount of polyunsaturated fats. Polyunsaturated fats such as corn oil can help lower high blood cholesterol levels when they are part of a healthful diet.

Monounsaturated fat—Type of fat that is liquid at room temperature and is found in vegetable oils, such as canola and olive oils. Monounsaturated fats can help lower high blood cholesterol levels when they are part of a lower-fat diet.

Fiber—An indigestible part of certain foods. Fiber is important in the diet as roughage or bulk. Fiber is found in foods from the starch, vegetable, and fruit exchange lists.

Glucose—A simple sugar, the main source of energy in the body. Insulin helps utilize glucose for energy, so if you lack insulin, glucose remains in the bloodstream and you will have a high glucose count.

Glycosylated hemoglobin test—A test that shows your average blood sugar levels during the past 8 to 10 weeks. This test is done in the doctor's office or a laboratory.

Gram—A unit of mass and weight in the metric system. An ounce is about 30 grams.

Hyperglycemia—High glucose levels. Symptoms include fatigue, excessive thirst, and frequent urination. Mild to moderate hyperglycemia over a period of time may be the cause of many diabetic complications.

Hypoglycemia—Low blood sugar levels. Symptoms may include dizziness, irritability, and loss of consciousness. It may come on slowly or quickly and can be very serious if it is not treated.

Insulin—A hormone produced by the pancreas that helps the body use glucose for energy. Insulin, which is also manufactured commercially, is injected into the body to replace the insulin no longer manufactured by your pancreas.

Meal plan—A guide showing the number of food exchanges to use in each meal and snack to control distribution of carbohydrates, proteins, fats, and calories throughout the day.

Mineral—Substance essential in small amounts to build and repair body tissue and/or control functions of the body. Calcium, iron, magnesium, phosphorus, potassium, sodium, and zinc are minerals.

Nephropathy—A condition in which the kidneys can't filter wastes out of the bloodstream into the urine. Kidney failure may result from this complication.

Neuropathy—A complication of diabetes in which the nerves are damaged.

Nutrient—Substance in food necessary for life. Carbohydrates, proteins, fats, minerals, vitamins, and water are nutrients.

Oral agent—A medication that helps control blood glucose in some people with Type 2 diabetes.

Protein—One of the three major nutrients in food. Protein provides about 4 calories per gram. Protein is found in foods from the milk and meat exchange lists. Smaller amounts of protein are found in foods from the vegetable and starch lists.

Renal threshold—The glucose level at which excess glucose in the blood starts spilling out into the urine.

Retinopathy—A complication of diabetes in which blood vessels in the eye are damaged. This can result in blindness if it isn't treated, but it can be effectively slowed or stopped with laser beam treatment if it is discovered before permanent damage is done.

Sodium—A mineral needed to maintain life, found mainly as a component of salt. Many individuals need to cut down the amount of sodium (and salt) they eat to help control high blood pressure.

Starch—One of the two major types of carbohydrate foods. Foods consisting mainly of starch come from the starch list.

Sugars—One of the two main types of carbohydrate. Foods including naturally present sugars are those from the milk, vegetable, and fruit lists. Added sugars include common table sugar and the sugar alcohols (sorbitol, mannitol, etc.).

Triglycerides—Fats normally present in the blood that are made from food. Gaining too much weight or consuming too much fat, alcohol, or carbohydrate may increase the blood triglycerides.

Vitamins—Substances found in food, which are needed in small amounts to assist in body processes and functions. These include vitamins A, D, E, the B-complex, C, and K.

Index